Maximising Triathlon Health and Performance: The State of the Art

Maximising Triathlon Health and Performance: The State of the Art

Guest Editors

Veronica Vleck
Maria Francesca Piacentini

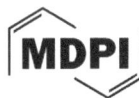

Basel • Beijing • Wuhan • Barcelona • Belgrade • Novi Sad • Cluj • Manchester

Guest Editors

Veronica Vleck
CIPER Faculdade de
Motricidade Humana
University of Lisbon
Lisbon
Portugal

Maria Francesca Piacentini
Department of Movement
Human and Health Sciences
University of Rome "Foro Italico"
Rome
Italy

Editorial Office
MDPI AG
Grosspeteranlage 5
4052 Basel, Switzerland

This is a reprint of the Special Issue, published open access by the journal *Sports* (ISSN 2075-4663), freely accessible at: https://www.mdpi.com/journal/sports/special_issues/Maximising_Triathlon_Health.

For citation purposes, cite each article independently as indicated on the article page online and as indicated below:

Lastname, A.A.; Lastname, B.B. Article Title. *Journal Name* **Year**, *Volume Number*, Page Range.

ISBN 978-3-7258-3591-1 (Hbk)
ISBN 978-3-7258-3592-8 (PDF)
https://doi.org/10.3390/books978-3-7258-3592-8

Cover image courtesy of Nigel Farrow

© 2025 by the authors. Articles in this book are Open Access and distributed under the Creative Commons Attribution (CC BY) license. The book as a whole is distributed by MDPI under the terms and conditions of the Creative Commons Attribution-NonCommercial-NoDerivs (CC BY-NC-ND) license (https://creativecommons.org/licenses/by-nc-nd/4.0/).

Contents

About the Editors vii

Veronica Vleck and Maria Francesca Piacentini
Maximising Triathlon Health and Performance: The State of the Art
Reprinted from: *Sports* **2025**, *13*, 66, https://doi.org/10.3390/sports13030066 1

David Procida, Jocelyn Mara, Lachlan Mitchell and Naroa Etxebarria
How Do Age-Group Triathlon Coaches Manage Training Load? A Pilot Study
Reprinted from: *Sports* **2024**, *12*, 261, https://doi.org/10.3390/sports12090261 12

Héctor Arévalo-Chico, Sergio Sellés-Pérez and Roberto Cejuela
Applying a Holistic Injury Prevention Approach to Elite Triathletes
Reprinted from: *Sports* **2024**, *12*, 225, https://doi.org/10.3390/sports12080225 22

Veronica Vleck, Luís Miguel Massuça, Rodrigo de Moraes, João Henrique Falk Neto, Claudio Quagliarotti and Maria Francesca Piacentini
Work, Training and Life Stress in ITU World Olympic Distance Age-Group Championship Triathletes
Reprinted from: *Sports* **2023**, *11*, 233, https://doi.org/10.3390/sports11120233 39

Alba Cuba-Dorado, Veronica Vleck, Tania Álvarez-Yates and Oscar Garcia-Garcia
Gender Effect on the Relationship between Talent Identification Tests and Later World Triathlon Series Performance
Reprinted from: *Sports* **2021**, *9*, 164, https://doi.org/10.3390/sports9120164 70

João Henrique Falk Neto, Eric C. Parent, Veronica Vleck and Michael D. Kennedy
The Training Characteristics of Recreational-Level Triathletes: Influence on Fatigue and Health
Reprinted from: *Sports* **2021**, *9*, 94, https://doi.org/10.3390/sports9070094 81

Atsushi Aoyagi, Keisuke Ishikura and Yoshiharu Nabekura
Exercise Intensity during Olympic-Distance Triathlon in Well-Trained Age-Group Athletes: An Observational Study
Reprinted from: *Sports* **2021**, *9*, 18, https://doi.org/10.3390/sports9020018 96

Sebastian Seifarth, Pavel Dietz, Alexander C. Disch, Martin Engelhardt and Stefan Zwingenberger
The Prevalence of Legal Performance-Enhancing Substance Use and Potential Cognitive and or Physical Doping in German Recreational Triathletes, Assessed via the Randomised Response Technique
Reprinted from: *Sports* **2019**, *7*, 241, https://doi.org/10.3390/sports7120241 113

Candace S. Brown
Motivation Regulation among Black Women Triathletes
Reprinted from: *Sports* **2019**, *7*, 208, https://doi.org/10.3390/sports7090208 124

Jørgen Melau, Maria Mathiassen, Trine Stensrud, Mike Tipton and Jonny Hisdal
Core Temperature in Triathletes during Swimming with Wetsuit in 10 °C Cold Water
Reprinted from: *Sports* **2019**, *7*, 130, https://doi.org/10.3390/sports7060130 140

Casper Grim, Ruth Kramer, Martin Engelhardt, Swen Malte John, Thilo Hotfiel and Matthias Wilhelm Hoppe
Effectiveness of Manual Therapy, Customised Foot Orthoses and Combined Therapy in the Management of Plantar Fasciitis—A RCT
Reprinted from: *Sports* **2019**, *7*, 128, https://doi.org/10.3390/sports7060128 149

Guillermo Olcina, Miguel Ángel Perez-Sousa, Juan Antonio Escobar-Alvarez and Rafael Timón
Effects of Cycling on Subsequent Running Performance, Stride Length, and Muscle Oxygen Saturation in Triathletes
Reprinted from: *Sports* **2019**, *7*, 115, https://doi.org/10.3390/sports7050115 . . . . **161**

Joel A. Walsh
The Rise of Elite Short-Course Triathlon Re-Emphasises the Necessity to Transition Efficiently from Cycling to Running
Reprinted from: *Sports* **2019**, *7*, 99, https://doi.org/10.3390/sports7050099 . . . . **171**

Pauline Neidel, Petra Wolfram, Thilo Hotfiel, Martin Engelhardt, Rainer Koch, Geoffrey Lee and Stefan Zwingenberger
Cross-Sectional Investigation of Stress Fractures in German Elite Triathletes
Reprinted from: *Sports* **2019**, *7*, 88, https://doi.org/10.3390/sports7040088 . . . . **189**

Maria Francesca Piacentini, Luca A Bianchini, Carlo Minganti, Marco Sias, Andrea Di Castro and Veronica Vleck
Is the Bike Segment of Modern Olympic Triathlon More a Transition towards Running in Males than It Is in Females?
Reprinted from: *Sports* **2019**, *7*, 76, https://doi.org/10.3390/sports7040076 . . . . **199**

Joao Henrique Falk Neto, Martin Faulhaber and Michael D. Kennedy
The Characteristics of Endurance Events with a Variable Pacing Profile—Time to Embrace the Concept of "Intermittent Endurance Events"?
Reprinted from: *Sports* **2024**, *12*, 164, https://doi.org/10.3390/sports12060164 . . . . **208**

Thilo Hotfiel, Isabel Mayer, Moritz Huettel, Matthias Wilhelm Hoppe, Martin Engelhardt, Christoph Lutter, et al.
Accelerating Recovery from Exercise-Induced Muscle Injuries in Triathletes: Considerations for Olympic Distance Races
Reprinted from: *Sports* **2019**, *7*, 143, https://doi.org/10.3390/sports7060143 . . . . **230**

Naroa Etxebarria, Iñigo Mujika and David Bruce Pyne
Training and Competition Readiness in Triathlon
Reprinted from: *Sports* **2019**, *7*, 101, https://doi.org/10.3390/sports7050101 . . . . **247**

Jørgen Melau, Martin Bonnevie-Svendsen, Maria Mathiassen, Janne Mykland Hilde, Lars Oma and Jonny Hisdal
Late-Presenting Swimming-Induced Pulmonary Edema: A Case Report Series from the Norseman Xtreme Triathlon
Reprinted from: *Sports* **2019**, *7*, 137, https://doi.org/10.3390/sports7060137 . . . . **262**

About the Editors

Veronica Vleck

Veronica Vleck, in addition to holding a Ph.D. in triathlon training and injury, has over 30 years of sports science support and/or coaching experience with multiple levels of triathletes, from novices to Olympic medallists. She is a previous long-term chair of the Medical and Research Committee of the European Triathlon Union, and a former Laboratory Director of the National Sports Medicine Institute of the UK. Dr Vleck has authored almost 100 peer-reviewed academic papers/book chapters on triathlon, including upon invitation from both the IOC and from World Triathlon.

Maria Francesca Piacentini

Maria Francesca Piacentini is a Professor at the University of Rome "Foro Italico". She holds a Ph.D. in human physiology from the Vrije Universiteit Brussel (B) and a Master's degree from the University of California Berkeley (USA). Her main area of research is endurance and ultra endurance sports with a specific focus on monitoring training in the prevention of overtraining or non-functional overreaching, pacing strategies, and central fatigue. Professor Piacentini collaborates with the Vrije Universiteit Brussels with whom she developed an online monitoring system to prevent overtraining in athletes. She is chair of the scientific committee of the European College of Sports Science and has collaborated with various National Federations. Furthermore, Prof. Piacentini has authored more than 100 peer-reviewed publications.

Editorial

Maximising Triathlon Health and Performance: The State of the Art

Veronica Vleck [1,*] and Maria Francesca Piacentini [2]

[1] CIPER, Faculdade de Motricidade Humana, Universidade de Lisboa, Cruz Quebrada, 1499-002 Lisbon, Portugal
[2] Department of Movement, Human and Health Sciences, University of Rome 'Foro Italico', 00135 Rome, Italy; mariafrancesca.piacentini@uniroma4.it
* Correspondence: research.vleck@gmail.com

It is with great pleasure that Professor Piacentini and I present this closing Editorial for the Special Issue of Sports on "Maximising Triathlon Health and Performance: The State of the Art". Thirty-four papers—of which 52% were accepted for publication—were submitted to this Special Issue. At the time of writing in December 2024, the 18 published papers had already been viewed over 106,000 times. Vleck et al.'s publication (Paper (P)3), entitled "Work, Training and Life Stress in ITU World Olympic Distance Age-Group Championship Triathletes", has been shortlisted for the Sports Paper of the Year 2023 award. Our featured authors (listed below) include many world-renowned experts in the field. Many other subject experts, including the coach of an Olympic medallist, devoted significant time and expertise to this project as reviewers. Notably, several of the submissions (e.g., P16, Hotfiel et al., 2019) resulted from collaborations between researchers and National Federation staff. We are privileged that our contributors chose to publish their research findings, including that of a randomised control trial (P10, Grim et al., 2019), with us. We are happy to have also featured first author papers from several (then) Ph.D. students- the incoming generation of triathlon subject experts. We extend our congratulations to those authors who have since been awarded their doctorates: Dr Claudio Quagliarotti (ITA) [1], Dr Alba Cuba-Dorado (ESP) [2], Dr Joel Walsh (AUS) [3], and Dr Jørgen Melau (NOR) [4]. Dr Thibaut Ledanois (FR) [5], Dr Stuart Evans (AUS) [6], and Dr Christian Weich (GER) [7] also recently obtained their triathlon-related doctorates. João Henrique Falk Neto (CAN), who proved himself an outstanding compère of the Edmonton 2020/2021 ITU Science and Triathlon conference; Héctor Arévalo-Chico (ESP), who both conducted research with and recently accompanied members of the Spanish team to the Paris Olympic Games; and Atsushi Aoyagi (JPN), whose papers we also feature in our Special Issue—are all close to submitting their Ph.D.'s [8–10]. We sincerely thank Atsushi Aoyagi for kindly accepting Dr Vleck's invitation to include his paper on the exercise intensity at which age group triathletes race in Olympic distance triathlons in this Special Issue. In common with many of the other papers in the Special Issue, Aoyagi et al.'s paper is surely destined to become regarded as a classic in the field.

The number- 10- and the submission dates, which are reasonably close to each other, of all the aforementioned doctoral theses is a testament to how scientific research related to our sport has evolved. The first triathlon paper was published just forty years ago. To our knowledge, the first doctorates on triathlons (both of which included National Squad athletes in their subject groups) were awarded to Professor Grégoire Millet (in 1999) [11], followed by myself [12]. Professor Millet was a former French National Olympic distance triathlon champion and a French National Triathlon Squad coach. In 2000, he was British

Received: 24 December 2024
Accepted: 6 January 2025
Published: 21 February 2025

Citation: Vleck, V.; Piacentini, M.F. Maximising Triathlon Health and Performance: The State of the Art. Sports 2025, 13, 66. https://doi.org/10.3390/sports13030066

Copyright: © 2025 by the authors. Licensee MDPI, Basel, Switzerland. This article is an open access article distributed under the terms and conditions of the Creative Commons Attribution (CC BY) license (https://creativecommons.org/licenses/by/4.0/).

Triathlon's Performance Director for triathlon's first Olympic Games. As such, he was an exemplar of what is an increasingly distinguishing feature of those who are involved in triathlon research. The fact that so many of our peers are actively researching *and* coaching *and/or* training for/racing triathlon (and sometimes all three at the same time), as Grégoire himself pointed out, is likely to facilitate the successful dissemination of our research findings. Almost all of the individuals whose work is featured in this Special Issue possess these same characteristics. Importantly, we were privileged to have published contributions from several researchers with a fourth, immensely valuable feature. As doctors, paramedics, physiotherapists, and/or surgeons, they have active field-, medical tent-, and/or hospital-based experience of protecting the health and safety of athletes. Dr Jørgen Melau—a paramedic and the safety director of the Norseman Xtreme triathlon, who is now the holder of a Ph.D. on physiological changes induced by cold water swimming [4]—personifies these outstanding individuals. Importantly, our authors also include those who have been (Engelhardt, Vleck) longstanding representatives on the committees or boards of either their respective continental governing bodies or World Triathlon. Thus, all of our contributors were uniquely placed to bring this collation of papers, with its stated aim of acting as a spur to the instigation and expansion of collaborative research projects that have the potential to improve applied practice in the sport, to fruition.

In 2007, Millet and I, together with David Bentley, published an invited commentary [13] on the extent to which a reciprocal relationship existed between the development of the sport of triathlon and the nature of the scientific investigation that was directly related to both it and to endurance sport in general. This Editorial provides us with a timely opportunity to revisit the questions that we first posed in the *International Journal of Sports Physiology and Performance* (IJSPP) 17 years ago. They fall under three main headings. Has science influenced the knowledge and practices in a given sport? Is sports science part of the development of the sport? Is sports science an important parameter for the emergence of new practices (i.e., training or testing methods and technological development) or coach education, and vice versa?

In Table 1, we provide selected examples of the above issues being addressed in the literature as a whole. We do the same for the three areas for which this Special Issue invited submissions, namely:

(a) Triathlon health in training and/or competition (health evaluation, event medical care, open water swimming, and heat acclimation) (Papers 7, 9, 13, 16, and 18).

(b) Training and risk factors for maladaptation (as evidenced by injury, illness, and non-functional overreaching and/or performance stagnation), including how it may change with athlete age, ability level, and event distance specialisation (Papers 3 and 5).

(c) Optimising training and race preparation- at the cutting edge (preparation for the Olympic Games, what can scientists tell coaches, what can coaches tell scientists, what do athletes want, and how technology can change the game, e.g., as regards research into both the aetiology and the prediction of maladaptation) (Papers 1, 2, 4, 6, 8, 10–12, 14–15, and 17).

Table 1. Comments on the extent of reciprocity between the development of triathlons and that of triathlon-related research.

Question	Comment	Selected Examples	
		The Literature	This Special Issue
1a. Has science influenced the knowledge and practices in a given sport?	Yes, regarding event medical care. The OWS rules for both open-water swimming and triathlon swimming were amended in 2013 in light of research that was unfortunately precipitated by the death of Fran Crippen in a 10 km event in the UAE (see Miller and Wendt, 2012 [14]). At the time of Crippen's death, only lower and not upper water temperature limits for OWS existed. Saycell et al. later conducted research to provide a scientific rationale for lower water temperature and wetsuit rules for elite and sub-elite triathletes. They recommended a minimum water temperature of 12 °C for racing in wetsuits and of 16 °C without wetsuits. The ITU rules for racing were changed accordingly (January 2017).	Bradford et al., 2015 [15]; Saycell et al., 2018 [16].	Too early to say, but several papers have implications for applied practice, e.g., (both 2019 studies by Melau et al.) P9. Core Temperature in Triathletes during Swimming with Wetsuit in 10 °C Cold Water; and P18. Late-Presenting Swimming-Induced Pulmonary Edema: A Case Report Series from the Norseman Xtreme Triathlon; P16. Hotfiel et al., 2019. Accelerating Recovery from Exercise-Induced Muscle Injuries in Triathletes: Considerations for Olympic Distance Races; and P17. Extebarria, Mujika & Pyne, 2019. Training and Competition Readiness in Triathlon.
	Harris et al. [17] showed that the SCD rate for triathlons is higher in the swim section than it is in the cycling and running sections. It is not yet clear why. IM swimming has introduced staggered swim starts. We are not aware of any studies having yet compared the death/medical incident rates before and after this rule change—presumably there are not enough data yet available to carry out such an analysis. See https://triathlon.org/medical/ppe for details on the recommendations and regulations of WT as regards periodic health evaluation.	Di Masi et al. (2022) [18]; Harris et al., (2017) [17]; Windsor, Newman & Shephard (2020) [19].	
1b. Can it?	Yes, regarding event medical care (see the comments in the main text regarding the GTSD), but considerably more research is warranted. Several published papers to date have important implications for event medical care. Rimmer and Coniglione [20] and Felletti et al. [21] show that it may be possible, once enough quality data are collected and analysed, to both optimise the medical staff/athlete support ratios, and tailor the specificity of staff medical training, to different locations around the race course as a function of event distance, event format, athlete ability, and environmental conditions. Event medical guidelines, e.g., those of WT, include recommended staff/athlete staffing ratios, but given the paucity of research into this subject, it is difficult to determine on what basis these ratios have been set and to what extent they are valid and/or could be improved. This point applies to several other aspects of current race-related medical guidelines. For example, "the current World Triathlon heat policy that is used for Para athlete events is based on recommendations for non-disabled persons. Future studies should explore whether a specific heat policy for Para triathletes is needed, tailored in a similar manner to the exertional heat stroke policy for Para athletes" [22]. There is still no academic consensus statement on the definition and reporting of injuries and illness in triathlons.	Rimmer & Coniglione, 2012 [20]; Felletti et al., 2022 [21]; Nilssen et al., 2023, 2024 [23,24]; Johnson et al., 2023 [25]; Cho et al., 2024 [26].	

Table 1. *Cont.*

Question	Comment	Selected Examples	
		The Literature	This Special Issue
1c. Is the sport benefiting from science?	Yes. We are aware of several doctoral theses (e.g., Malcata, 2014 [27]; Ledanois, 2023 [5]) that focused on a particular country's preparation for the Olympic Games.		Again, it is still too early to say, but several papers have implications for applied practice, e.g., P4. Alba Cuba et al., 2017 regarding talent ID, whose findings are themselves largely explained by P14. Piacentini et al., 2019's analysis of WTS events.
1d. Is science benefiting from the sport?	Yes e.g., hyponatremia research. Triathlon studies on thermoregulation and fluid balance were instrumental in the formulation of international recommendations on preparation for endurance sports (e.g., the ACSM position stand on exercise and fluid replacement, [28]), plus work into the decline of performance with ageing. Dasa et al., 2024 [29] "questions the validity of the current metabolic limits" and "suggests a new perspective on what is physiologically achievable in world-class athletes". However, surprising gaps exist in the literature as regards several issues that have wider implications outside the sport (e.g., the effect of triathlon participation on cardiac function, the injury and long-term health implications of multi-disciplinary cross-training across the lifespan).	Convertino et al., 1996 [28]; Noakes et al., 1985 [30]; Speedy et al., 1987 [31].	P15. Falk Neto et al., 2024. The Characteristics of Endurance Events with a Variable Pacing Profile—Time to Embrace the Concept of "Intermittent Endurance Events"?
1e. Is science influenced or stimulated by a given sport?	Yes. See the above.		
1f. Are investigations of specific interest for athletes, coaches, medical staff and administrators who are involved in that sport?	Athletes	Jeukendrup, Jentjens & Mosely, 2012 [32].	P2. Arevalo Chico et al., 2024; P17. Extebarria, Mujika & Pyne, 2019.
	Coaches	Van Schuylenburgh, Eynde & Hespel, 2004 [33]; Jacko et al., 2024 [34]; Christensen, 2025 [35].	P2. Arévalo-Chico et al., 2024; P3. Vleck et al., 2023; P14. Piacentini et al., 2019.
	Medical staff	Gailey and Hartsch, 2009 [36]; Chalmers et al., 2021 [37]; Armstrong et al., 2024 [38].	P10. Grim et al., 2019 (plantar fasciitis therapy, RCT); P18. Melau et al., 2019.
	Administrators	Wicker et al., 2012 [39]; Downs et al., 2020 [40]; Heilman et al., 2024 [41]; Bevins, 2024 [42].	P7. Seifarth et al., 2019; P8. Brown, 2019.
2a. Is sports science part of the development of the sport?	Yes, e.g., MTAR research.	Ledanois et al., 2023 [43].	Bike run transition research, e.g., P11. Olcina et al., 2019; P12. Walsh, 2019.

Table 1. *Cont.*

Question	Comment	Selected Examples — The Literature	Selected Examples — This Special Issue
2b. Are the scientific topics modified by the change in rules or development stages in the sport?	Yes, see the above and Millet, Bentley & Vleck, 2007 [13] for detailed charts.		P15. Falk Neto et al., 2024.
2c. With the emergence of a sport, did it renew interest or influence the scientific investigation by providing new topics, "new borders"?	Yes regarding hyponatremia-related research. The newish Arena Games triathlon may provide a useful model for future talent identification (see Stapley et al., 2024 [44]).	See 1d.	P15. Falk Neto et al., 2024.
3a. What is the relationship between scientists, athletes, coaches, and administrators?	It exists on mostly individual bases. At a world level, it could be made more coherent and better structured. The formation of both WT coaching course accreditation and the Global Triathlon Safety Task Force (see https://education.triathlon.org/mod/page/view.php?id=10899) were very promising developments.	Nilssen et al., 2023; 2024; Johnson et al., 2023, Cho et al., 2024 (GTSD analyses of 30 years of IM data) [23–26].	P16. Hotfiel et al., 2019 is one of the multiple examples in this Special Issue of this relationship working beautifully.
3b. Are the continental or international governing bodies supporting scientific projects or congresses?	A triathlon chapter was included in Caine, Harmer, and Schiff's *IOC Encyclopaedia of Sports Medicine Series* book on "Epidemiology of Injury in Olympic Sports".	Vleck (2010) [45].	
	The *"Triathlon Medicine"* book was supported by WT.	Migliorini (Ed.), 2010 [46].	
	GTSD (see the main text). See also https://education.triathlon.org/mod/page/view.php?id=10899.		
	Several ITU Science of Triathlon World Congresses have taken place (Alicante 2011, Macolin 2013, Paris 2015, Edmonton 2020/2021).		
	OWS temperature limits research was funded by FINA, the IOC Medical Commission and the ITU. Saycell et al. (2018) [16] was funded by the Joint Medical Committee of the IOC, FINA, and ITU.	Bradford et al., 2015; Saycell et al., 2018 [15,16].	
3c. Are the scientists involved directly with elite or national teams or with developing junior or youth athletes?	Yes. Multiple Ph.D. theses undertaken thus far were in collaboration with National Federations and/or National Squad athletes (e.g., those of Ledanois (FR) [5], Cuba-Dorado (ESP) [2], Vleck (GBR) [12], Millet (FR) [11], Malcata (NZ) [27], Extebarria (GBR) [47] and Comotto (ITA) [48]); and several published scientists (e.g., Bottoni, Cejuela, Millet, Piacentini, and Vleck) work(ed) with National Squads.	Cuba-Dorado, 2017 [2]; Ledanois, 2023 [5].	P2. Arévalo-Chico et al., 2024; P13. Neidel et al., 2019; P14. Piacentini et al., 2019; P17. Extebarria, Mujika & Pyne, 2019; P4. Alba Cuba et al., 2021.

Table 1. *Cont.*

Question	Comment	Selected Examples	
		The Literature	This Special Issue
3d. Is sports science an important parameter for the emergence of new practices (training or testing methods, technological development) or coach education?	Yes, but its transfer into applied practice could perhaps be improved (see Quagliarotti et al., 2024 [49]; Wells et al., 2024 [50]) as could the amount of research that is undertaken on, e.g., paralympic triathletes and minority groups. See also Vleck, 2018 [51]. The "Health Triathlon Coaching program" of FFTri and the French Ministry of Sport (see Coste et al., 2020 [52] for an overview) is an inspiring example of a training program that enables triathlon coaches to work with individuals who have stable chronic diseases and in so doing, take advantage of the potential advantages of swim, cycle and run/walk training for general health.	Weich et al., 2022 [53].	P1. Procida et al. 2024; P3. Vleck et al., 2024; P8. Brown, 2019.
3e. Is a given sport only a vehicle for general scientific investigation, or are there some sport-science research initiatives specific to it?	Sports-specific initiatives exist, e.g., wetsuit research, bike-run transition research, and pacing research (including, most recently, those related to the MTAR).	Ledanois et al., 2023 [43].	P12. Walsh, 2019.

Key: ACSM, American Society of Sports Medicine; ESP, Spain; FINA, Fédération Internationale de Natation; FFTri, Fédération Française de Triathlon; FR, France; ID, identification; IM, Ironman distance triathlon; ITA, Italy; ITU, International Triathlon Union (now WT, World Triathlon); GBR, Great Britain; GTSD, Global Triathlon Safety Database; IOC, International Olympic Committee; MTAR, triathlon Mixed Team Athlete Relay; NZ, New Zealand; OD, Olympic Distance triathlon; OWS, open water swimming; P, paper (see the numbered list of contributors and papers); Qu, Question; re, regarding; RCT, randomised control trial; SCD, sudden cardiac death; UAE, United Arab Emirates; WTS, World Triathlon Series.

Essentially, our reply to the above key questions about whether reciprocity exists between the sport and research related to it is "yes, to some extent, but more work is needed". We highlight the fact that the event guidelines for open-water swimming have been revised on the basis of research that was commissioned and funded by this sport's governing body, amongst others. Research that has the potential to directly improve event medical care (e.g., P10, Melau et al., 2019. Late-Presenting Swimming-Induced Pulmonary Edema: A Case Report Series From The Norseman Xtreme Triathlon) is continuously being published. Surprisingly, however (and especially given the opportunities that amateur triathlon's unique age-group system provides for research into the effects of multi-disciplinary exercise training in ageing populations), few comprehensive studies of either triathlon training or of its long-term effects exist. The latter point is relevant to medical issues (e.g., the incidence of skin cancer; see [40]). It also applies to research into how triathlon participation might offset the effects of ageing and (given that it is a multi-disciplinary sport) might affect those at the other end of the age spectrum, e.g., motor skill development of younger athletes (of less than 8 years of age) [54,55]. There also appears to have been little investigation to date on the extent to which triathlon participation can either positively [56]) or negatively [57] impact mental health, and/or non-communicable disease [51]. It would prove useful if how triathletes actually train were better researched- both for those who take part in the sport and, probably, for sports science in general. We further recommend that more research be carried out into the extent to which current coaching accreditation courses and coaches themselves are both up to date with and implement findings from the triathlon literature. We applaud the sterling work of Professor Romuald Lepers on the decline of performance with age in masters athletes [58–61]. Lepers' work to make the practical implications of his findings available to the wider exercising public (Lepers, 2021 [62]) sets an excellent example for us all.

We are privileged that this Special Issue was met with such an enthusiastic, collaborative response from the triathlon community worldwide. We are confident that the papers contained within it should also prove relevant to its component sports, and we extend our grateful thanks to everyone who was involved and continues to support research in our sport. We note that the analysis that I conducted in 2007 for the IJSPP commentary [13] was based on the 278 articles with triathlon or triathlete in the title that were published in PubMed between the first published paper in 1984 and the end of 2006. After four decades of research https://lida.sport-iat.de/dtu-triathlon/ (LIDA)- the database of scientific literature related to triathlon that is based on a collaboration between the Deutschen Triathlon Union (DTU) and the Institute of Applied Training Science Leipzig (IAT), now numbers over 1440 triathlon articles and over 19,000 triathlon related items. This database is freely available. In closing this Editorial, we therefore extend a special thank you to Birgit Franz, who was working on the aforementioned database when I started my triathlon-related Ph.D. over thirty years ago, and still works on it, for her significant contribution to the sport.

Finally, we wish to both acknowledge the work of Professor (Doug) Hiller, M.D., and make a related announcement. Professor Hiller was one of the first three members of the medical committee of the International Triathlon Union (ITU, now World Triathlon) in 1989. He (together with Pamela S. Douglas M.D. and Professor Mary L. O'Toole) was one of the initial leading trio of researchers to publish on triathlon and was involved with drafting the first set of medical guidelines for what would eventually become USA Triathlon. He was inducted into the Hall of Fame of the ITU in August 2019 for his lifetime contributions to this evolving Olympic sport.

The triathlon chapter in the 2010 IOC book on epidemiology of injury and illness in Olympic sports [45] concluded with these words: "It is strongly urged that a collaborative research team of race organizers, technical officials, coaches, athletes, medical support staff, and researchers working at both the grass-roots and the top end of the sport be established, for an adequate database of injury data to be compiled and used to drive continuous improvement in triathlon training and competition practice, as well as education of athletes, coaches, and both technical and medical staff". Professor Hiller and Professor Christopher Connolly of Washington State University have now set up such a global triathlon safety database (GTSD, www.globaltrisafety.org). The GTSD is both a medical data repository and provides secure data management and analysis for triathlon organizations worldwide. To date, it is supported by the World Triathlon, Ironman Triathlon, and USA Triathlon. In addition to the LIDA database and the recently established Triathlon Research Initiative (www.triathlonresearchinitiative.com), it is likely to prove to be a critically valuable resource for the sport.

We strongly encourage all of our colleagues in the sport to make use of the GTSD and, in so doing, improve the translation of research findings into improvement in applied practice because

"Nothing is more important than the health and safety of the athlete."

(Hiller, undated quote).

Sincerely,

Veronica Vleck, Ph.D.

Professor Maria Francesca Piacentini, Ph.D.

Author Contributions: Original draft preparation, V.V.; review, M.F.P. All authors have read and agreed to the published version of the manuscript.

Funding: CIPER—Centro Interdisciplinar para o Estudo da Performance Humana (unit 447) acknowledges the support of the "Fundação para a Ciência e Tecnologia", as expressed by Grant UIDB/00447/2020.

Acknowledgments: We thank Christopher Connolly, Stuart Evans, João Henrique Falk Neto, William Douglas Hiller, Romauld Lepers, Dennis Sandig, and Jørgen Melau for their comments on the penultimate draft of this manuscript.

Conflicts of Interest: The authors declare no conflicts of interest.

List of Contributors and Papers

1. Procida, D.; Mara, J.; Mitchell, L.; Etxebarria, N. How Do Age-Group Triathlon Coaches Manage Training Load? A Pilot Study. *Sports* **2024**, *12*, 261. https://doi.org/10.3390/sports12090261.
2. Arévalo-Chico, H.; Sellés-Pérez, S.; Cejuela, R. Applying a Holistic Injury Prevention Approach to Elite Triathletes. *Sports* **2024**, *12*, 225. https://doi.org/10.3390/sports12080225.
3. Vleck, V.; Massuça, L.M.; de Moraes, R.; Falk Neto, J.H.; Quagliarotti, C.; Piacentini, M.F. Work, Training and Life Stress in ITU World Olympic Distance Age-Group Championship Triathletes. *Sports* **2023**, *11*, 233. https://doi.org/10.3390/sports11120233.
4. Cuba-Dorado, A.; Vleck, V.; Álvarez-Yates, T.; Garcia-Garcia, O. Gender Effect on The Relationship between Talent Identification Tests and Later World Triathlon Series Performance. *Sports* **2021**, *9*, 164. https://doi.org/10.3390/sports9120164.
5. Falk Neto, J.H.; Parent, E.C.; Vleck, V.; Kennedy, M.D. The Training Characteristics of Recreational-Level Triathletes: Influence on Fatigue and Health. *Sports* **2021**, *9*, 94. https://doi.org/10.3390/sports9070094.
6. Aoyagi, A.; Ishikura, K.; Nabekura, Y. Exercise Intensity During Olympic-Distance Triathlon in Well-Trained Age-Group Athletes: An Observational Study. *Sports* **2021**, *9*, 18. https://doi.org/10.3390/sports9020018.
7. Seifarth, S.; Dietz, P.; Disch, A.C.; Engelhardt, M.; Zwingenberger, S. The Prevalence Of Legal Performance-Enhancing Substance Use and Potential Cognitive and Or Physical Doping in German Recreational Triathletes, Assessed Via The Randomised Response Technique. *Sports* **2019**, *7*, 241. https://doi.org/10.3390/sports7120241.
8. Brown, C.S. Motivation Regulation among Black Women Triathletes. *Sports* **2019**, *7*, 208. https://doi.org/10.3390/sports7090208.
9. Melau, J.; Mathiassen, M.; Stensrud, T.; Tipton, M.; Hisdal, J. Core Temperature in Triathletes during Swimming with Wetsuit in 10 °C Cold Water. *Sports* **2019**, *7*, 130. https://doi.org/10.3390/sports7060130.
10. Grim, C.; Kramer, R.; Engelhardt, M.; John, S.M.; Hotfiel, T.; Hoppe, M.W. Effectiveness of Manual Therapy, Customised Foot Orthoses and Combined Therapy in the Management of Plantar Fasciitis—A RCT. *Sports* **2019**, *7*, 128. https://doi.org/10.3390/sports7060128.
11. Olcina, G.; Perez-Sousa, M.Á.; Escobar-Alvarez, J.A.; Timón, R. Effects of Cycling on Subsequent Running Performance, Stride Length, and Muscle Oxygen Saturation in Triathletes. *Sports* **2019**, *7*, 115. https://doi.org/10.3390/sports7050115.
12. Walsh, J.A. The Rise of Elite Short-Course Triathlon Re-Emphasises the Necessity to Transition Efficiently from Cycling to Running. *Sports* **2019**, *7*, 99. https://doi.org/10.3390/sports7050099.
13. Neidel, P.; Wolfram, P.; Hotfiel, T.; Engelhardt, M.; Koch, R.; Lee, G.; Zwingenberger, S. Cross-Sectional Investigation of Stress Fractures in German Elite Triathletes. *Sports* **2019**, *7*, 88. https://doi.org/10.3390/sports7040088.
14. Piacentini, M.F.; Bianchini, L.A.; Minganti, C.; Sias, M.; Di Castro, A.; Vleck, V. Is the Bike Segment of Modern Olympic Triathlon More a Transition towards Running in Males than It Is in Females? *Sports* **2019**, *7*, 76. https://doi.org/10.3390/sports7040076.
15. Falk Neto, J.H.; Faulhaber, M.; Kennedy, M.D. The Characteristics of Endurance Events with a Variable Pacing Profile—Time to Embrace the Concept of "Intermittent Endurance Events"? *Sports* **2024**, *12*, 164. https://doi.org/10.3390/sports12060164.

16. Hotfiel, T.; Mayer, I.; Huettel, M.; Hoppe, M.W.; Engelhardt, M.; Lutter, C.; Pöttgen, K.; Heiss, R.; Kastner, T.; Grim, C. Accelerating Recovery from Exercise-Induced Muscle Injuries in Triathletes: Considerations for Olympic Distance Races. *Sports* **2019**, *7*, 143. https://doi.org/10.3390/sports7060143.
17. Etxebarria, N.; Mujika, I.; Pyne, D.B. Training and Competition Readiness in Triathlon. *Sports* **2019**, *7*, 101. https://doi.org/10.3390/sports7050101.
18. Melau, J.; Bonnevie-Svendsen, M.; Mathiassen, M.; Mykland Hilde, J.; Oma, L.; Hisdal, J. Late-Presenting Swimming-Induced Pulmonary Edema: A Case Report Series from the Norseman Xtreme Triathlon. *Sports* **2019**, *7*, 137. https://doi.org/10.3390/sports7060137.

References

1. Quagliarotti, C. Valutazione ed Ottimizzazione della Performance nel Triathlon [Evaluation and Optimization of Triathlon Performance]. Ph.D. Thesis, University of Rome "Foro Italico", Rome, Italy, 2023. Available online: https://www.uniroma4.it/wp-content/uploads/2023/10/Abstract-PhD-35-Thesis-Quagliarotti-Claudio.pdf (accessed on 17 December 2024).
2. Cuba-Dorado, A. La Detección y Selección de Talentos en Triatlón—Análisis y Propuesta [Talent detection and selection in triathlon—Analysis and proposal]. Ph.D. Thesis, University of Vigo, Pontevedra, Spain, 2017. Available online: https://www.investigo.biblioteca.uvigo.es/xmlui/handle/11093/809 (accessed on 29 November 2024).
3. Walsh, J.A. Neuromotor Control of Eccentric Cycling. Ph.D Thesis, University of Wollongong, Wollongong, Australia, 2023. Available online: https://hdl.handle.net/10779/uow.27666867.v1 (accessed on 29 November 2024).
4. Melau, J. Physiological Changes Following Swimming in Cold Water in Triathlon and Military Operations: Temperature Physiology and Cold Water Swimming with Wetsuit or Drysuit. Ph.D. Thesis, Oslo Medical Hospital, Oslo, Norway, 2022. Available online: https://www.duo.uio.no/handle/10852/94205 (accessed on 17 December 2024).
5. Ledanois, T. Les Stratégies et L'environnement dans la Performance Sportive de Haut-Niveau en Triathlon [The Strategies and Environment in High Performance Triathlon]. Ph.D. thesis, Université Paris Cité, Paris, France, 2023. Available online: https://theses.fr/2023UNIP7101 (accessed on 19 December 2024).
6. Evans, S. A Sensor-Based Approaching to Understanding Trunk Motion in Cycling and Running in Sprint Distance Triathlon: A Triaxial Tool for the Triathlete. Ph.D. Thesis, Charles Darwin University, Casuarina, Australia, 2022.
7. Weich, C. The Attractor Method and its Application in Running, Bicycling and Nordic Skiing. Ph.D. Thesis, University of Konstanz, Konstanz, Germany, 2021. Available online: https://www.researchgate.net/publication/350544258_The_Attractor_Method_and_its_application_in_running_bicycling_and_Nordic_skiing (accessed on 12 December 2024).
8. Falk Neto, J.H. (University of Alberta, Edmonton, AB T6G 2R3, Canada). The Physiological Consequences of Repeated Sprints in the Anaerobic Power Zone (Provisional title). Personal communication. Ph.D. Thesis to be submitted in early 2025.
9. Arévalo-Chico, H. (University of Alicante, 03690 Alicante, Spain). Actualización en los Factores de Rendimiento y el Entrenamiento en Triatlón. [Updates on performance factors and training in triathlon] (Provisional Title). Personal communication. Ph.D. Thesis to be submitted in early 2025.
10. Atsushi, A. (University of Tsukuba, Tsukuba 305-8577, Japan). A Study of the Physiological Determinants of Running Performance in Triathletes (Provisional title). Personal communication. Ph.D. Thesis to be submitted in early 2025.
11. Millet, G.P. Facteurs Déterminants de la Performance et Spécificité de l'Entraînement [Determinant Factors of the Performance and Specificity of Training]. Ph.D. Thesis, University of Montpellier, Montpellier, France, 1999.
12. Vleck, V.E. Ph.D. Thesis, Staffordshire University, Staffordshire, UK; Published as Vleck, V.; *Triathlete Training and Injury Analysis: An Investigation in British National Squad and Age-Group Triathletes*; VDM Verlag Dr Müller GmbH & Co. K.G.: Saarbrucken, Germany, 2010; ISBN 978-3-639-21205-1.
13. Millet, G.P.; Bentley, D.J.; Vleck, V.E. The Relationships Between Science and Sport: Application In Triathlon. *Int. J. Sports Physiol. Perf.* **2007**, *2*, 315–322. [CrossRef] [PubMed]
14. Miller, J.J.; Wendt, J.T. The Lack of Risk Communication at an Elite Sports Event: A Case Study of the FINA 10 K Marathon Swimming World Cup. *Int. J. Sport Commun.* **2012**, *5*, 265–278. [CrossRef]
15. Bradford, C.D.; Lucas, S.J.; Gerrard, D.F.; Cotter, J.D. Swimming in Warm Water is Ineffective in Heat Acclimation and is Non-Ergogenic for Swimmers. *Scand. J. Med. Sci. Sports* **2015**, *25*, 277–286. [CrossRef] [PubMed]
16. Saycell, J.; Lomax, M.; Massey, H.; Tipton, M. Scientific Rationale for Changing Lower Water Temperature Limits for Triathlon Racing to 12 °C With Wetsuits and 16 °C Without Wetsuits. *Br. J. Sports Med.* **2018**, *52*, 702–708. [CrossRef] [PubMed]
17. Harris, K.M.; Creswell, L.L.; Haas, T.S.; Thomas, T.; Tung, M.; Isaacson, E.; Garberich, R.F.; Maron, B.J. Death and Cardiac Arrest in U.S. Triathlon Participants, 1985 to 2016: A case series. *Ann. Intern. Med.* **2017**, *167*, 529–536. [CrossRef]
18. Di Masi, F.; Costa e Silva, G.; Mello, D.; Szpilman, D.; Tipton, M. Deaths in Open Water Races. *Int. J. Exerc. Sci.* **2022**, *15*, 1295–1305. [PubMed]

19. Windsor, J.S.; Newman, J.; Sheppard, M. Cardiovascular Disease and Triathlon-Related Deaths in the United Kingdom. *Wilderness Env. Med* **2020**, *31*, 31–37. [CrossRef]
20. Rimmer, T.; Coniglione, T. A Temporal Model for Nonelite Triathlon Race Injuries. *Clin. J. Sport Med.* **2012**, *22*, 249–253. [CrossRef] [PubMed]
21. Feletti, F.; Saini, G.; Naldi, S.; Casadio, C.; Mellini, L.; Feliciani, G.; Zamprogno, E. Injuries in Medium to Long-Distance Triathlon: A Retrospective Analysis of Medical Conditions Treated in Three Editions of the Ironman Competition. *J. Sports Sci. Med.* **2022**, *21*, 58–67. [CrossRef]
22. Borg, D.N.; Gibson, A.D.; Bach, A.J.E.; Beckman, E.M.; Tweedy, S.M.; Stewart, I.B. The Influence of Water and Air Temperature on Elite Wheelchair Triathlon Performance. *Temperature* **2024**, *11*, 363–372. [CrossRef]
23. Nilssen, P.K.; Connolly, C.P.; Johnson, K.B.; Cho, S.P.; Cohoe, B.H.; Miller, T.K.; Laird, R.H.; Sallis, R.E.; Hiller, W.D. Medical Encounters and Treatment Outcomes in Ironman-Distance Triathlon. *Med. Sci. Sports Exerc.* **2023**, *55*, 1968–1976. [CrossRef] [PubMed]
24. Nilssen, P.K.; Johnson, K.B.; Hiller, W.D.B.; Miller, T.K.; Connolly, C.P. Exercise-Associated Muscle Cramps in Ironman-Distance Triathletes over 3 Decades. *Clin. J. Sport Med.* **2024**, *Online ahead of print*.
25. Johnson, K.B.; Connolly, C.P.; Cho, S.P.; Miller, T.K.; Robert, E.; Sallis, R.E.; Hiller, W.D.B. Clinical Presentation of Exercise-Associated Hyponatremia in Male and Female IRONMAN® Triathletes over Three Decades. *Scand. J. Med. Sci. Sports* **2023**, *33*, 1841–1849. [CrossRef] [PubMed]
26. Cho, S.P.; Connolly, C.P.; Hiller, D.B.; Miller, T.K. Reoccurrence of Adverse Medical Incidents in Repeat Ultraendurance Triathlon Competitors. *J. Sports Med. Phys. Fitness* **2024**, *64*, 1340–1347. [CrossRef]
27. Malcata, R.M. Modelling Progression of Competitive Sport Performance. Ph.D. Thesis, Auckland University of Technology, Auckland, New Zealand, 2014. Available online: https://hdl.handle.net/10292/7442 (accessed on 11 December 2024).
28. Convertino, V.A.; Armstrong, L.E.; Coyle, E.F.; Mack, G.W.; Sawka, M.N.; Senay, L.C., Jr.; Sherman, W.M. ACSM Position Stand: Exercise and Fluid Replacement. *Med. Sci. Sports Exerc.* **1996**, *28*, 1–7. [CrossRef]
29. Dasa, M.S.; Bu, O.A.; Sandbakk, Ø.; Rønnestad, B.R.; Plasqui, G.; Gundersen, H.; Kristoffersen, M. Training Volume and Total Energy Expenditure of an Olympic and Ironman World Champion: Approaching the Upper Limits of Human Capabilities. *J. Appl. Physiol.* **2024**, *137*, 1535–1540. [CrossRef]
30. Noakes, T.D.; Goodwin, N.; Rayner, B.L.; Branken, T.; Taylor, R.K.N. Water Intoxication: A Possible Complication during Endurance Exercise. *Med. Sci. Sports Exerc.* **1985**, *17*, 370–375. [CrossRef]
31. Speedy, D.B.; Faris, J.G.; Hamlin, M.; Gallagher, P.G.; Campbell, R.G. Hyponatremia and Weight Changes in an Ultradistance Triathlon. *Clin. J. Sport Med.* **1997**, *7*, 180–184. [CrossRef]
32. Jeukendrup, A.E.; Jentjens, R.L.P.G.; Moseley, L. Nutritional Considerations in Triathlon. *Sports Med.* **2005**, *35*, 163–181. [CrossRef] [PubMed]
33. Van Schuylenbergh, R.; Eynde, B.V.; Hespel, P. Prediction of Sprint Triathlon Performance from Laboratory Tests. *Eur. J. Appl. Physiol.* **2004**, *91*, 94–99. [CrossRef]
34. Jacko, T.; Bartsch, J.; von Diecken, C.; Ueberschär, O. Validity of Current Smartwatches for Triathlon Training: How Accurate are Heart Rate, Distance, And Swimming Readings? *Sensors* **2024**, *24*, 4675. [CrossRef]
35. Christensen, P.M. Aerobic Energy Turnover and Exercise Economy Profile during Race Simulation in a World-Record-Breaking Male Full-Distance Triathlete. *Int. J. Sports Physiol. Perform.* **2025**, *20*, 161–167. [CrossRef] [PubMed]
36. Gailey, R.; Harsch, P. Introduction to Triathlon for the Lower Limb Amputee Triathlete. *Prosthet. Orthot. Int.* **2009**, *33*, 242–255. [CrossRef] [PubMed]
37. Chalmers, S.; Shaw, G.; Mujika, I.; Jay, O. Thermal Strain during Open-Water Swimming Competition in Warm Water Environments. *Front. Physiol.* **2021**, *12*, 785399. [CrossRef] [PubMed]
38. Armstrong, L.E.; Johnson, E.C.; Adams, W.M.; Jardine, J.F. Hyperthermia and Exertional Heatstroke during Running, Cycling, Open Water Swimming, and Triathlon Events. *Open Access J. Sports Med.* **2024**, *15*, 111–127. [CrossRef]
39. Wicker, P.; Hallmann, K.; Prinz, J.; Weimar, D. Who Takes Part In Triathlon Events? A Application Of Lifestyle Segmentation to Triathlon Participants. *Int. J. Sport. Mark.* **2012**, *12*, 1–24. [CrossRef]
40. Downs, N.J.; Axelsen, T.; Parisi, A.V.; Schouten, P.W.; Dexter, B.R. Measured UV exposures of Ironman, Sprint and Olympic-distance Triathlon Competitors. *Atmosphere* **2020**, *11*, 440. [CrossRef]
41. Heilman, N.J.; Martin, D.; Huggins, R.A.; Stearns, R.L.; Casa, D.J. FACSM. Ironman Triathlon-Related Fatalities from 2017–2022: A Case Series: 792. *Med. Sci. Sports Exerc.* **2024**, *56*, 279. [CrossRef]
42. Bevins, R.L. Paratriathlon Race Performance in Elite Ambulatory Athletes with Physical Impairments. *Am. J. Phys. Med. Rehabil.* **2024**, *Online ahead of print*. [CrossRef]
43. Ledanois, T.; Hamri, I.; De Larochelambert, Q.; Libicz, S.; Toussaint, J.F.; Sedeaud, A. Cutoff Value for Predicting Success in Triathlon Mixed Team Relay. *Front. Sports Act. Living* **2023**, *5*, 1096272. [CrossRef] [PubMed]

44. Stapley, P.J.; Lepers, R.; Heming, T.; Gremeaux, V. The Arena or E-Games Triathlon as a Unique Real World and Virtual Mixed-Model Endurance Sports Event. *Front. Sports Act. Living* **2024**, *6*, 1444385. [CrossRef]
45. Vleck, V.E. Triathlon injury. In *Epidemiology of Injury in Olympic Sports*; International Olympic Committee 'Encyclopaedia of Sports Medicine' Series; Blackwell Publications: Hoboken, NJ, USA, 2010; pp. 294–320.
46. Migliorini, S. (Ed.) *Triathlon Medicine*; Springer: Cham, Switzerland, 2019.
47. Extebbaria, N. Physiology and Performance of Cycling and Running during Olympic Distance Triathlon. Ph.D. Thesis, Loughborough University, Loughborough, UK, 2013. Available online: https://hdl.handle.net/2134/12530 (accessed on 29 November 2024).
48. Comotto, S. Analisi Della Prestazione nel Triathlon. Dai Kids agli Atleti Junior [Triathlon Performance Analysis. From Kids to Junior Athletes]. Ph.D. Thesis, University of Rome Foro Italico, Rome, Italy, 2012.
49. Quagliarotti, C.; Villanova, S.; Marciano, A.; López-Belmonte, Ó.; Caporali, C.; Bottoni, A.; Lepers, R.; Piacentini, M.F. Warm-up in Triathlon: Do Triathletes Follow the Scientific Guidelines? *Int. J. Sports Physiol. Perform.* **2024**, *19*, 1473–1479. [CrossRef]
50. Wells, L.A.; Bruce, L.; Hoffmann, S.M.; Kremer, P.; Dwyer, D.B. Differences Between Australian Triathlon Coaching Practices and Evidence-Based Training Load Management Recommendations. *Int. J. Sports Sci. Coach.* **2024**, *20*(1), 17479541241305677. [CrossRef]
51. Vleck, V. The Changing Relationship between Multidisciplinary (Triathlon) Exercise and Health Across the Lifespan. Movimento Humano, cultura e saúde: Situação atual e abordagem educacional (Human movement, culture and health). In *Research on Human Kinetics—Multidisciplinary Perspectives*; Lisbon University Press: Lisbon, Portugal, 2018. Available online: https://www.researchgate.net/publication/337085493_The_changing_relationship_between_multidisciplinary_triathlon_exercise_and_health_across_the_lifespan_In_Research_on_Human_Kinetics-_multidisciplinary_perspectives_Eds_Alves_F_Rosado_O_Pereira_LM_Arau (accessed on 29 November 2024).
52. Coste, O.; Lieux, R.; Gremeaux-Bader, V.; Dupont, A.-C.; Marble, C. Health Coaching Triathlon: A Model of Involvement in a Sports Federation. *Dtsch Z Sportmed.* **2020**, *71*, 258–262. [CrossRef]
53. Weich, C.; Barth, V.; Killer, N.; Vleck, V.; Erich, J.; Treiber, T. Discovering the Sluggishness of Triathlon Running—Using the Attractor Method to Quantify the Impact of the Bike-Run Transition. *Front. Sports Act. Living* **2022**, *4*, 1065741. [CrossRef]
54. Bergeron, M.F.; Mountjoy, M.; Armstrong, N.; Chia, M.; Côté, J.; Emery, C.A.; Faigenbaum, A.; Hall, G.; Kriemler, S.; Léglise, M.; et al. International Olympic Committee Consensus Statement on Youth Athletic Development. *Br. J. Sports Med.* **2015**, *49*, 843–851. [CrossRef] [PubMed]
55. Bergeron, M.F. The Youth Triathlete. In *Triathlon Medicine*; Migliorini, S., Ed.; Springer: Cham, Switzerland, 2020.
56. Parsons-Smith, R.L.; Barkase, S.; Lovell, G.P.; Vleck, V.; Terry, P.C. Mood profiles of amateur triathletes: Implications for mental health and performance. *Front. Psychol.* **2022**, *13*, 925992. [CrossRef] [PubMed]
57. Muros, J.J.; Ávila-Alche, Á.; Knox, E.; Zabala, M. Likelihood of Suffering from an Eating Disorder in a Sample of Spanish Cyclists and Triathletes. *J. Eat. Disord.* **2020**, *8*, 70. [CrossRef] [PubMed]
58. Lepers, R.; Sultana, F.; Bernard, T.; Hausswirth, C.; Brisswalter, J. Age-Related Changes in Triathlon Performances. *Int. J. Sports Med.* **2010**, *31*, 251–256. [CrossRef]
59. Lepers, R.; Knechtle, B.; Stapley, P.J. Trends in Triathlon Performance: Effects of Sex and Age. *Sports Med.* **2013**, *43*, 851–863. [CrossRef]
60. Lepers, R.; Stapley, P.J. Master Athletes are Extending the Limits of Human Endurance. *Front. Physiol* **2016**, *12*, 613. [CrossRef]
61. Valenzuela, P.L.; Maffiuletti, N.A.; Joyner, M.J.; Lucia, A.; Lepers, R. Lifelong Endurance Exercise as a Countermeasure Against Age-Related Decline: Physiological Overview and Insights from Masters Athletes. *Sports Med.* **2020**, *50*, 703–716. [CrossRef]
62. Lepers, R. *Athlète Master—S'entraîner et Performer à 40,50 Ans et Plus [The Masters Athlete—Training and Performing at Age 40, 50 and Over]*; Editions Outdoor: Lyon, France, 2021; ISBN 249032909X.

Disclaimer/Publisher's Note: The statements, opinions and data contained in all publications are solely those of the individual author(s) and contributor(s) and not of MDPI and/or the editor(s). MDPI and/or the editor(s) disclaim responsibility for any injury to people or property resulting from any ideas, methods, instructions or products referred to in the content.

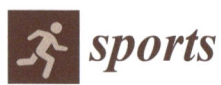 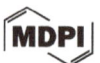

Article

How Do Age-Group Triathlon Coaches Manage Training Load? A Pilot Study

David Procida [1], Jocelyn Mara [1], Lachlan Mitchell [2] and Naroa Etxebarria [1,*]

[1] Discipline of Sport and Exercise Science, University of Canberra Research Institute of Sport and Exercise, Canberra 2617, Australia; david@procida.com.au (D.P.); jocelyn.mara@canberra.edu.au (J.M.)
[2] Victorian Institute of Sport, Melbourne 3206, Australia; lachlan.mitchell@vis.org.au
* Correspondence: naroa.etxebarria@canberra.edu.au

Abstract: Multidisciplinary sports like triathlons require combining training for three different sports, and it is unclear how triathlon coaches manage this. During a 10-week period, we provided four age-group triathlon coaches with summary reports of the training completed by their athletes (n = 10) in the previous week. Coaches were then asked if the information provided to them was used to inform training prescription for the following week. The information provided to coaches included relative acute training load (rATL) and training stress scores (TSSs). Weekly fluctuations in rATL of >10% (spikes) were 83% (swim), 74% (bike) and 87% (run). Coaches adapted training loads for the upcoming week in 25% of all rATLs reported, and only 5% (swim), 33% (bike) and 9% (run) of the adjusted loads avoided spikes. Consequently, there were 22 single-discipline acute training load spikes vs. 14 spikes when combining all three disciplines. Only 1.5% of training was lost to injury, mostly after a large running-based training load spike (>30%). Coaches largely overlooked the information provided in the report when prescribing exercise for the following week, and when adjusted, it failed to bring weekly load variability <10%.

Keywords: multidisciplinary sports; swimming; running; cycling; training management; load quantification; coach behavior

Citation: Procida, D.; Mara, J.; Mitchell, L.; Etxebarria, N. How Do Age-Group Triathlon Coaches Manage Training Load? A Pilot Study. *Sports* **2024**, *12*, 261. https://doi.org/10.3390/sports12090261

Academic Editors: Veronica Vleck, Jared Coburn and Maria Francesca Piacentini

Received: 21 April 2024
Revised: 22 July 2024
Accepted: 10 September 2024
Published: 20 September 2024

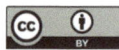

Copyright: © 2024 by the authors. Licensee MDPI, Basel, Switzerland. This article is an open access article distributed under the terms and conditions of the Creative Commons Attribution (CC BY) license (https://creativecommons.org/licenses/by/4.0/).

1. Introduction

Multidisciplinary sports such as triathlon require intentional planning of weekly training sessions for three different sports [1,2]. To be adequately prepared for endurance events of this nature, the volume of training is significant [3]; hence, monitoring and reviewing training loads is crucial to enhance training adaptations and consequent performance [4–6]. Enhancing training adaptations requires combining adequate types, intensity levels, and volumes of training stimuli interspersed with effective recovery periods [7]. However, prescribed external (objective) training loads might differ from the loads athletes complete [8]; hence, coaches should consider completed workloads by athletes instead of relying on original exercise prescription when planning future training loads.

Suboptimal training preparation may result in compromised performance outcomes for athletes, but perhaps in age-group triathletes, injury prevention comes before performance optimization. Triathlon studies have characterized training undertaken by age-group triathletes [9,10]. Inappropriate training loads may result in injury, illness, or non-functional over-reaching [11–13], with injury reported to affect between 29 and 91% of adult triathletes at some stage during training and competition [14]. Injury results in a loss of training consistency, which has a negative impact on individual athletic success [15]. Although no single marker of an athlete's response to training load consistently predicts maladaptation or injury [16], avoiding abrupt increases or decreases in training load seems to be key to avoid them [17,18]. This is why there are numerous ways to monitor load in endurance sports, such as Training Impulse (TRIMP) [19], training stress scores (TSSs) [20], and relative acute training load (rATL) [21] as well as acute/chronic workload ratio (ACWR) [22].

Most training-load-related outcome measures require context around them and have their limitations in explaining training load; hence, they should be interpreted carefully. Given that age-group or amateur triathletes would comprise a very high portion of registered triathletes world-wide (compared to professional or elite athletes), their training load management and enhancement warrant further research.

In order to identify exercise programming aspects that might negatively affect triathletes, it is crucial to capture training-related data consistently and accurately. The increase in readily available wearable technologies in combination with the growth of online-based athlete monitoring systems make capturing training data a reasonably easy venture. However, despite the ability to capture exercise training metrics such as running distance, intensity of exercise, power output in cycling, etc., it is unclear how this information may be used by coaches to amend or enhance future training prescription, hence the urgency to expand on the understanding and education of coach knowledge and practices on coach behavior in relation to training load management.

It is unclear how triathlon training data are used to inform future exercise prescription in an attempt to align with fundamental principles of training metrics relating to the volume, intensity, frequency, and type of exercise. However, evidence from other sports suggests that sudden increases in training load can increase the likelihood of injury. Such sports include team sports [21,23], as well as individual endurance sports including swimming [24] and running [25]. Coach behavior regarding weekly training load fluctuations would provide insights into how age-group triathlon coaches manage athlete training loads in triathlon, both for each individual discipline and also the combined overall weekly load distribution. Therefore, the primary aim of this study was to investigate if the exercise training load prescribed by triathlon coaches is informed by or adjusted according to the training load undertaken in the previous week(s) or not, in order to avoid substantial fluctuations in training load.

2. Materials and Methods

2.1. Design

This exploratory observational study focused on a 10-week training data collection period (competition season, May–September) where the training loads of a cohort of age-group athletes were monitored. Coaches were provided with weekly summary reports with the completed loads by athletes in the previous week and were asked whether they used the information provided on training load monitoring metrics to inform the training plan for the following week. All athletes performed standardized time trial-based field testing in all three disciplines (swim, bike and run) prior to commencing the study to determine their basal individual threshold intensities. These data were required to calculate individualized training loads derived from the various relative training intensities.

This study was approved by the Committee for Ethics in Human Research at the University of Canberra (project ID 2030) and all participants provided their written informed consent prior to participating in the study.

2.2. Participants

In total, 10 (n = 10) age-group triathletes (females, n = 6; males, n = 4) and 4 (n = 4) male nationally accredited age-group coaches were recruited via a post on social media to participate in this study. The triathletes were 38 ± 6 years old (mean ± SD) and the coaches were 46 ± 8 years old. The coaches had 3.0 ± 1.6 years of experience in coaching age-group triathletes with 13 ± 6 h of weekly commitment. Three coaches had a triathlon development coach accreditation (Level II out of III, AusTriathlon, Milton, QLD, Australia). One coach had an equivalent accreditation as a running coach but coached all three disciplines of triathlon. All coaches would be considered non-elite development coaches. Coaches had 11 ± 6 years of personal triathlon competition experience at the age-group level. All coaches used TrainingPeaks™ (Boulder, CO, USA) as their athlete monitoring system and had 2.3 ± 1.2 years of experience using this system. Coaches coached their athletes face-to-face and also remotely. All participating triathletes were coached by one of the participant coaches. The triathletes had 1 to 4 years of triathlon training experience at age-group competition level. Athletes had completed a wide range of race distances, predominantly Sprint and Olympic distance, and one of them had completed a Half-Ironman. Triathletes had to be healthy when the field-based testing took place and have been training for triathlon races for at least 12 months.

2.3. Data Collection

All the athletes used Garmin GPS-enabled smart devices to record training data across the swim, bike, and run. All sessions recorded training time, distance, and pace/speed. For the bike and run sessions, heart rate was recorded using Garmin chest strap-based technology. All data were uploaded to the online athlete monitoring system TrainingPeaks™. The participant coaches were required to use the online platform TrainingPeaks™ as their athlete monitoring system [11], which conveniently provides the training load data required for this study. All athletes performed time trial-based field testing in all three disciplines (swim, bike, and run) prior to commencing the study to determine their basal individual threshold intensities. The field testing consisted of a 1000 m time trial (TT) for swimming, a 30 min TT for the bike (flat open road), and a 30 min TT for the run. These time trials were common field-based tests undertaken by the athletes during a season to monitor progress. Since we were interested in looking at chronic training load and acute training load, we only needed the threshold so that we could determine the intensity factor for each session. The intensity factor and the session duration were then used to calculate the training stress score, which was used for the CTL and ATL. These data were required to calculate individualized training loads derived from the various relative training intensities.

Coaches were provided with several familiarization sessions with the lead researcher (DP) prior to the commencement of the study. The lead researcher provided the coaches with mentoring about all the data collection and outcome measures involved in the study. Coaches completed a questionnaire at the start of the study which included information on the coaches' background (experience, weekly commitments to coaching, coaching delivery modes), certifications and education relating to coaching, and athletic history. The athletes completed their questionnaire at the start of the study and included information on training and competition experience and a brief injury history summary.

All athlete training data were gathered via the athlete's smart training devices and the associated sensor and uploaded to TrainingPeaks™ via the athlete's smartphone application. At the end of each week, the lead researcher accessed the following information: total number of sessions (and per discipline), training session duration, intensity of training, training stress score (TSS), chronic training load, and acute training load for each discipline. The lead researcher then provided the coaches with a summary feedback report for each individual athlete on a Sunday. The next day on the Monday, coaches released the training program for the following week. The summary feedback provided by the research team to the coaches included (i) the weekly average intensity factor (*mean percentage of threshold intensity for a given session*, e.g., *a session completed at 65% of threshold intensity would have an IF of 0.65*); (ii) the training stress score ($IF^2 \times Volume\ (hours) \times 100$), [26] representing the total training load for the week; (iii) the number of sessions planned by the coach; (iv) the number of sessions completed by the athlete; (v) chronic training load: exponentially weighted moving average of the training stress score over the previous 42 days; (vi) acute training load: (vii) exponentially weighted moving average of the training stress score over the previous 7 days; (viii) relative acute training load (rATL): difference in acute training load between the current week and the previous week (%), used to calculate weekly variability in training load; and (ix) acute/chronic workload ratio (ACWR). Although the role of ACWR as a risk injury predictor is contested [27], it was used as a complementary measure to monitor training load overtime.

Given the 42-day period used to calculate chronic load (for each discipline as well as for all three disciplines combined), the threshold testing was performed 42 days prior to the collection of any training load data for the study. During this period, athletes continued training as per usual. The results of both training load metrics for the previous week were color-coded green if they were within the pre-defined range (<10% in rATL, ACWR between 0.8 and 1.5 [28], and compliance between 80 and 110%). When the difference fell outside of these ranges, the metrics were color-coded red. We defined a >10% change in week-to-week training load fluctuations in rATL to be enough to consider it a spike.

Training compliance was monitored as the percentage of prescribed sessions completed by the athlete in the previous week. Finally, the coaches were asked to provide a binary response to the question "Did you use the rATL/ACWR feedback metric to alter training load in the subsequent week?" This information was used to determine whether the coaches considered the training load metrics from the previous week when prescribing their athletes' training loads for the following week. In instances where the coach indicated that the feedback metrics were not used to adjust the training load, the coaches were asked to provide a reason for it (open text).

2.4. Data Analysis

Data analysis was conducted using R version 4.01 in RStudio (version 1.3.959, RStudio Inc., Boston, MA, USA). Descriptive statistics are reported as mean ± SD, unless otherwise stated. In addition, training load and training load prescription were highly individualized and achieved large inter-athlete variation. Therefore, we provided 'per athlete' and 'per coach' descriptive statistics to present individual athlete data. In instances where the coach indicated that the feedback metrics were not used to adjust the training load, the coaches were asked to provide a reason as a short response. These responses were summarized into codes, which were then used to determine themes using thematic analysis [29] to understand coach behavior regarding training load management.

3. Results
3.1. Training Load

A total of 770 training sessions were prescribed by the coaches over 10 weeks, and 640 training sessions (663 h of training) were completed by the participant athletes. Out of all the training sessions, only three athletes missed training sessions due to injury or illness, twelve sessions due to injury and fourteen sessions due to illness. Ten of the sessions lost to injury relate to the same athlete and after a rATL of >30% (running-related).

There were no missing data or non-responses from the coaches. Cycle training consistency was highest with 88 ± 36% of sessions being completed, followed by run training (84 ± 29%) and swim training (81 ± 35%). Overall training compliance was 84 ± 25%. A summary of the overall training volume, intensity, and total stress scores for the training sessions during the 10-week period is shown in Table 1.

Table 1. Training load data over the 10-week data collection period (mean ± SD).

Discipline	TSS	IF (%)	Volume (h)
Swim	128 ± 118	85 ± 37	1.3 ± 1.0
Bike	215 ± 161	70 ± 25	3.6 ± 2.6
Run	168 ± 91	83 ± 22	2.2 ± 1.2
Overall	507 ± 245	86 ± 15	6.6 ± 3.1

IF = intensity factor (mean percentage of threshold intensity for a given session, e.g., a session completed at 65% of threshold intensity would have an IF of 0.65); TSS = training stress score (IF^2 × volume (hours)) × 100).

For the purpose of this study, rATL and ACWR metrics were only used as signposts to guide the training load completed by the athletes (as opposed to predictive outcomes). The weekly training load fluctuations for the 90 person-weeks, each with 3 separate rATLs (1 per discipline), were recorded, with a total of 270 week-to-week fluctuations in rATLs recorded, showing that 71% of them were >10% (Figure 1). Weekly variations in rATL of >10% were 83% for swimming, 74% for cycling, and 87% for running. Moreover, there was a substantial number of weekly fluctuations in rATL of >30% in training load (52% for swimming, 53% for cycling, and 51% for running). There were 32% of weekly fluctuations in rATL >30% for overall training load. All rATLs for each individual athlete for the 10-week data collection period for each discipline (swim, bike, and run) are shown in Figure 2. Coaches considered 23%, 27%, and 24% of the swim, bike, and run (respectively) of all rATL summary feedback reports provided to them (Table 2).

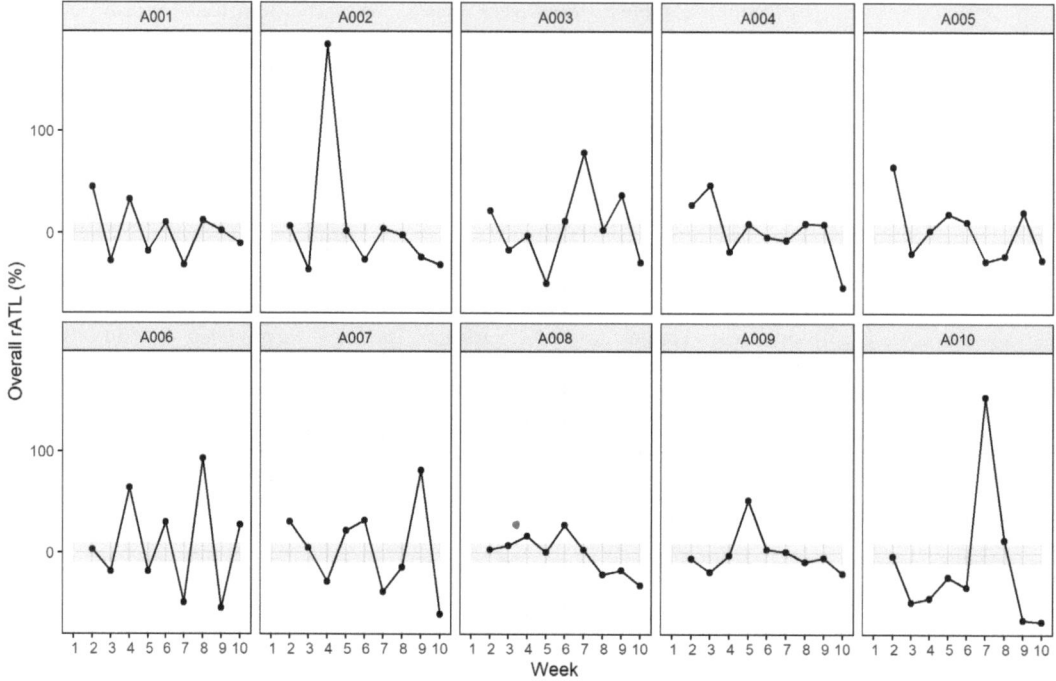

Figure 1. Overall rATL per athlete. A00× indicates the athlete identification number. Gray shaded bands represent ±10% relative acute training load (rATL) range. Symbols indicate whether the coach for each athlete modified the training load based on the rATL feedback metric provided: '•' = feedback was used.

Table 2. Number of weeks and athletes each coach was responsible for and the corresponding number of weeks where coaches considered the relative acute training load (rATL) to adapt their training load prescribed to the athletes for the following week; 100% of rATLs considered were calculated as follows: # of athletes X # of weeks × 3 (disciplines). Key: # = number.

			rATL Considered by Coaches (# of Weeks)			
Coaches	# of Athletes	# of Athletes × 10 (# of Weeks)	Swim	Bike	Run	% of rATL Considered
C1	2	20	0	0	1	2
C2	3	30	20	23	21	58
C3	1	10	1	1	0	7
C4	4	40	0	0	0	0
Total	10	100	21	24	22	22

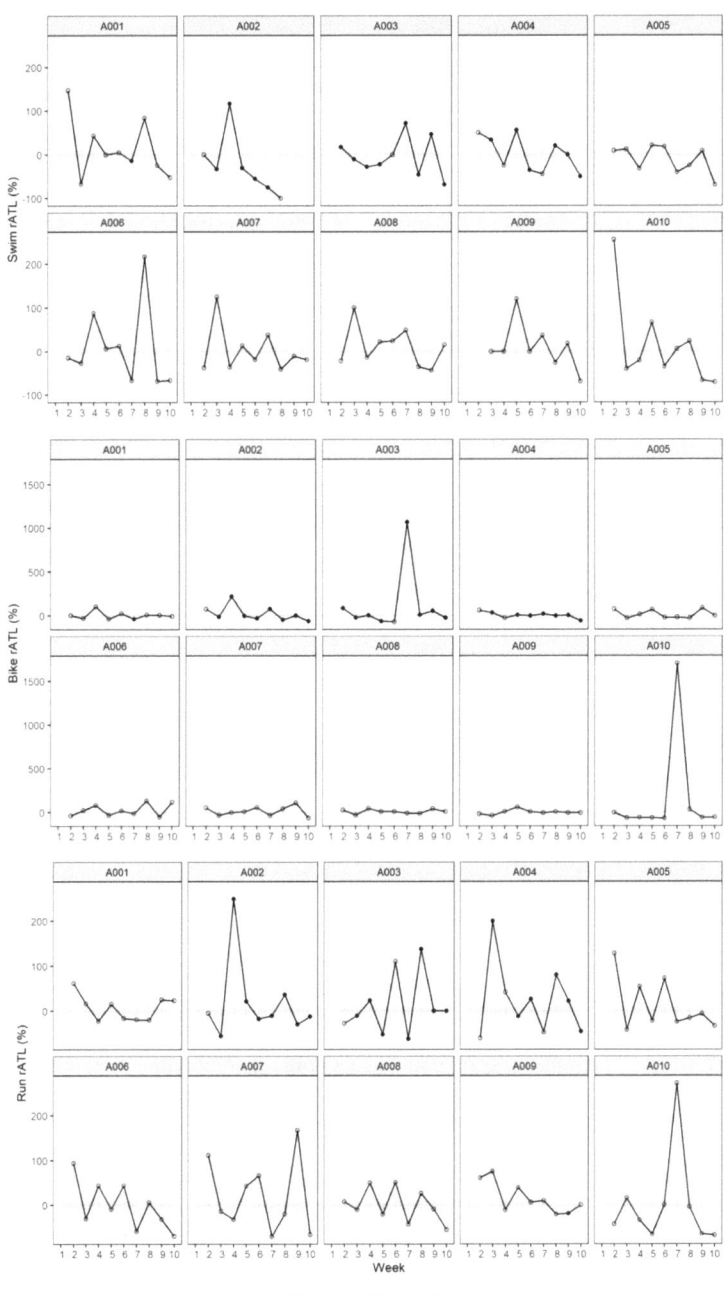

Figure 2. Swim, bike, and run rATL per athlete. A00× indicates the athlete identification number. Gray shaded bands represent ±10% relative acute training load (rATL) range. Symbols indicate whether the coach for each athlete modified the training load based on the rATL feedback metric provided: '○' = feedback was not used, '●' = feedback was used.

3.2. Weekly Reports

From the summary feedback reports where rATL was considered, only 5%, 33%, and 9% of swim, bike, and run rATLs fell within the ±10% variability range the following week. Only 48% (swim), 67% (bike), and 57% (run) of the ACWRs fell between the recommended 0.8 and 1.5, and coaches considered 20% (swim), 23% (bike), and 21% (run) of the ACWR information provided. From the summary feedback reports where ACWR was considered, only 33%, 50%, and 59% of swim, bike, and run rATLs fell within the recommended 0.8 and 1.5. The majority (95%) of the weekly reports considered came from the same coach, who had a higher education degree (i.e., Sport and Recreation with a Coaching Major) and was the most experienced (>5 years). Only 5% of the reports were considered by the others with less experience (1–3 years).

3.3. Coach Behavior

The main reason, in 66% of cases, for coaches to not consider the summary report was because they wanted to avoid changing the training they had already planned. The second reason for not considering the summary report was related to environmental constraint (18%), where the training environment impacted the ability of the athlete to train. Illness/injury and work/life constraints combined explained 13% of the cases to not consider the feedback report. Coaches gave the athlete the freedom to decide on training load for that week in 3% of cases.

4. Discussion

This exploratory study reports a high incidence of large (10–30%) and ad hoc weekly training load fluctuations in the training prescription of amateur (age-group) triathletes. When faced with the use of an externally provided summary of training metrics (that coaches already have access to) with added interpretation, coaches in most cases did not consider the information provided and relied instead on pre-existing planning for future load prescription. It is unclear whether capturing and processing other information on the weekly reports would have been more valuable for the coaches. High weekly training variation did not result in a high incidence of injuries. It is unclear how effective this training prescription approach would be when the priority is to enhance training adaptations.

There were larger fluctuations in weekly training load metrics when training load was observed separately for each discipline than when the training load of the three disciplines was combined. This outcome underpins the importance of studying each individual discipline separately as well as considering the combined load. The weight-bearing nature of running probably contributed to how most of the injuries in this study were linked to weekly running load fluctuations of >30%, in agreement with previous research [25]. Running results in higher musculoskeletal load compared to the non-weight-bearing exercise like swimming and cycling, and most injuries in triathlon result from it [30]. Running-related training load would be the priority for triathlon coaches to monitor and alter, if needed, in order to minimize injuries. Endurance sports exercise prescription is dominated by remote coaching practices and digital technology [31]. Training management systems such as TrainingPeaks™ allow coaches to amend sessions remotely with ease. Coaches might need to be responsive to adjustments required in training loads at short notice, especially with running, to ensure a progressive and incremental model for training and avoid abrupt spikes.

The weekly training volume undertaken by the triathletes in this study is similar to that described in the literature for recreational triathletes [9]. Athletes and coaches understandably push close to the limits of tolerance of the given athlete to promote performance gains without compromising good health and the risk of injury. Suboptimal training stimuli may preserve good health but might not produce the best performance, while a more aggressive approach with training load might jeopardize the athlete's health.

Consistency in training has been shown to be a key factor in athletic success [15], where training load is progressive and incremental, fundamentally, despite many different ways to periodize endurance training. Despite the low illness/injury incidence registered over the relatively short 10-week period, with over half of the weekly load fluctuations being >30% across all three single disciplines, it is unclear if the training process is adequate for enhancing adaptations [16]. A combination of failure to consider recently completed workloads by athletes to inform training prescription for the coming week, and athlete compliance factors (i.e., adherence to the prescribed exercise intensity during training sessions), likely contributed to large fluctuations in training load. These two factors are key when athletes and coaches work remotely, and should be the focus when athletes and coaches discuss strategies for training and competition.

Most coaches favored the already-planned workload for the upcoming week without checking the work completed by the athletes in the previous week. Perhaps this decision making is related to the metrics provided to them in the weekly summary reports, or perhaps it is because of coaches expecting/assuming athletes to complete exactly the load prescribed. It could also be that coaches in this study did not have a problem with substantial week-to-week load variations, and they perceive this to not have any negative consequences. These findings in themselves are very interesting, provided that there is limited evidence on the concept of how the exercise prescribed by coaches and the exercise completed by athletes align. Little is understood about how coaches go about exercise prescription and whether the completed exercise by the athletes reflects the exercise prescribed by the coach.

We acknowledge that this exploratory study has a limited number of coach and athlete observations, and provided that there are very limited data on how triathlon coaches use training data to inform future prescription, this study provides some preliminary insights and would encourage future research to include more coaches and athletes in their study designs. Although the present study is limited by a low number of observations, it raises some important and fundamental questions that future research should aim to address, for example, identifying the factors that influence coaches' training load management decisions in multi-sport environments. The discrepancy or alignment between training load prescription by coaches and training load completion by athletes, not only in terms of sessions completed or not but also in relation to the intensity of the work undertaken (vs. prescribed), is a topic that requires investigating. This knowledge will assist in evaluating the importance of acting on work undertaken instead of relying on work that was planned to inform future exercise prescription.

The practical implications for age-group triathlon coaches include the following:

- Rapid changes (increases) in weekly training load derived from individual disciplines (swimming, cycling, running) might be masked when observed as the overall training load combining all disciplines (swim, cycle and run) compared with the training load of isolated disciplines.
- Running-related workloads are to be monitored more carefully, as the injuries experienced by athletes in this study occurred mostly after a large increase (>30%) in running load.
- Identifying a system to increase responsiveness to adjust future workloads based on previous work undertaken might be advantageous in avoiding large weekly fluctuations that might negatively affect some athletes.

5. Conclusions

This study provides preliminary insights into how variable training prescription by coaches and corresponding training load completed by athletes is in age-group triathlons. Coaches were more likely to adhere to pre-determined training loads rather than modifying them based on completed training load feedback metrics, even at the expense of exposing athletes to high training load differentials from one week to the next. The incidence of injuries was mostly related to large weekly fluctuations in running training load, but not all athletes were affected by it, suggesting there is substantial inter-individual variability. Moreover, even when the feedback provided was considered, this did not always avoid a spike in training load (both single-discipline and combined training loads) the following week. This pilot study indicates that the outcome measures chosen in this study might not have been useful for coaches, that coaches might not always seek to avoid large weekly training load fluctuations, and/or that coaches might prescribe training loads that athletes might not adhere to or follow accurately.

Author Contributions: D.P. and N.E. conceived and designed the research project. D.P. conducted the data collection and drafted the manuscript. D.P., J.M., L.M. and N.E. contributed to the data analysis and editing of the manuscript. All authors have read and agreed to the published version of the manuscript.

Funding: Authors declare no competing financial or non-financial interests and no external funding contributed to the completion of the study.

Institutional Review Board Statement: The study was approved by the University of Canberra Human Research Ethics Committee and conforms to the Code of Ethics of the World Medical Association (Declaration of Helsinki), project ID 2030 approved in June 2019.

Informed Consent Statement: All participants provided their written informed consent prior to participating in the study.

Data Availability Statement: The data are not publicly available due to privacy and ethical restrictions.

Acknowledgments: The authors would like to acknowledge all the participants, both athletes and coaches, who participated in this study and volunteered their time.

Conflicts of Interest: The authors declare no conflicts of interest.

References

1. Millet, G.P.; Vleck, V.E.; Bentley, D.J. Physiological requirements in triathlon. *J. Hum. Sport. Exerc.* **2011**, *6*, 184–204. [CrossRef]
2. Mujika, I. Olympic preparation of a world-class female triathlete. *Int. J. Sport. Physiol. Perform.* **2014**, *9*, 727–731. [CrossRef] [PubMed]
3. Vleck, V.; Millet, G.P.; Alves, F.B. The impact of triathlon training and racing on athletes' general health. *Sport. Med.* **2014**, *44*, 1659–1692. [CrossRef]
4. Etxebarria, N.; Mujika, I.; Pyne, D.B. Training and competition readiness in triathlon. *Sports* **2019**, *7*, 101. [CrossRef] [PubMed]
5. Mujika, I. Quantification of Training and Competition Loads in Endurance Sports: Methods and Applications. *Int. J. Sport. Physiol. Perform.* **2017**, *12*, S29–S217. [CrossRef]
6. Seiler, S. What is best practice for training intensity and duration distribution in endurance athletes? *Int. J. Sport. Physiol. Perform.* **2010**, *5*, 276–291. [CrossRef]
7. Jakovlev, N. *Sportbiochemie*; Barth: Leipzig, Germany, 1977.
8. Foster, C.; Florhaug, J.A.; Franklin, J.; Gottschall, L.; Hrovatin, L.A.; Parker, S.; Doleshal, P.; Dodge, C. A new approach to monitoring exercise training. *J. Strength. Cond. Res.* **2001**, *15*, 109–115.
9. Falk Neto, J.H.; Parent, E.C.; Vleck, V.; Kennedy, M.D. The Training Characteristics of Recreational-Level Triathletes: Influence on Fatigue and Health. *Sports* **2021**, *9*, 94. [CrossRef]
10. Vleck, V.; Massuca, L.M.; de Moraes, R.; Falk Neto, J.H.; Quagliarotti, C.; Piacentini, M.F. Work, Training and Life Stress in ITU World Olympic Distance Age-Group Championship Triathletes. *Sports* **2023**, *11*, 233. [CrossRef]
11. Halson, S.L. Monitoring training load to understand fatigue in athletes. *Sport. Med.* **2014**, *44* (Suppl. S2), S139–S147. [CrossRef]
12. Foster, C. Monitoring training in athletes with reference to overtraining syndrome. *Med. Sci. Sport. Exerc.* **1998**, *30*, 1164–1168. [CrossRef] [PubMed]
13. Burns, J.; Keenan, A.M.; Redmond, A.C. Factors associated with triathlon-related overuse injuries. *J. Orthop. Sport. Phys. Ther.* **2003**, *33*, 177–184. [CrossRef] [PubMed]
14. Vleck, V.; Millet, G.P.; Alves, F.B. Triathlon Injury—An update. *Schweiz. Z. Med. Traumatol.* **2013**, *61*, 10–16.
15. Drew, M.K.; Raysmith, B.P.; Charlton, P.C. Injuries impair the chance of successful performance by sportspeople: A systematic review. *Br. J. Sport. Med.* **2017**, *51*, 1209–1214. [CrossRef]
16. Borresen, J.; Lambert, M.I. The quantification of training load, the training response and the effect on performance. *Sport. Med.* **2009**, *39*, 779–795. [CrossRef]
17. Jones, C.M.; Griffiths, P.C.; Mellalieu, S.D. Training load and fatigue marker associations with injury and illness: A systematic review of longitudinal studies. *Sport. Med.* **2017**, *47*, 943–974. [CrossRef] [PubMed]
18. Meeuwisse, W. Assessing causation in sport injury: A multifactorial model. *Clin. J. Sport. Med.* **1994**, *4*, 166–170. [CrossRef]
19. Banister, E.W.; Morton, R.H.; Fitz-Clarke, J. Dose/response effects of exercise modeled from training: Physical and biochemical measures. *Ann. Physiol. Anthropol.* **1992**, *11*, 345–356. [CrossRef] [PubMed]

20. Allen, H.; Coggan, A. *Training and Racing with a Power Meter*, 2nd ed.; Velopress: Boulder, CO, USA, 2010.
21. Hulin, B.T.; Gabbett, T.J.; Blanch, P.; Chapman, P.; Bailey, D.; Orchard, J.W. Spikes in acute workload are associated with increased injury risk in elite cricket fast bowlers. *Br. J. Sport. Med.* **2014**, *48*, 708–712. [CrossRef]
22. Hulin, B.T.; Gabbett, T.J.; Caputi, P.; Lawson, D.W.; Sampson, J.A. Low chronic workload and the acute:chronic workload ratio are more predictive of injury than between-match recovery time: A two-season prospective cohort study in elite rugby league players. *Br. J. Sport. Med.* **2016**, *50*, 1008–1012. [CrossRef]
23. Gabbett, T.J.; Hulin, B.T.; Blanch, P.; Whiteley, R. High training workloads alone do not cause sports injuries: How you get there is the real issue. *Br. J. Sport. Med.* **2016**, *50*, 444–445. [CrossRef] [PubMed]
24. Hellard, P.; Avalos, M.; Guimaraes, F.; Toussaint, J.F.; Pyne, D.B. Training-related risk of common illnesses in elite swimmers over a 4-yr period. *Med. Sci. Sport. Exerc.* **2015**, *47*, 698–707. [CrossRef] [PubMed]
25. Nielsen, R.O.; Parner, E.T.; Nohr, E.A.; Sorensen, H.; Lind, M.; Rasmussen, S. Excessive progression in weekly running distance and risk of running-related injuries: An association which varies according to type of injury. *J. Orthop. Sport. Phys. Ther.* **2014**, *44*, 739–747. [CrossRef]
26. Coggan, A. Normalized Power, Intensity Factor and Training Stress Score. 2020. Available online: https://www.trainingpeaks.com/learn/articles/normalized-power-intensity-factor-training-stress/ (accessed on 12 March 2020).
27. Impellizzeri, F.M.; Tenan, M.S.; Kempton, T.; Novak, A.; Coutts, A.J. Acute:Chronic Workload Ratio: Conceptual Issues and Fundamental Pitfalls. *Int. J. Sport. Physiol. Perform.* **2020**, *15*, 907–913. [CrossRef]
28. Gabbett, T.J. The training-injury prevention paradox: Should athletes be training smarter and harder? *Br. J. Sport. Med.* **2016**, *50*, 273–280. [CrossRef]
29. Braun, V.; Clarke, V. What can "thematic analysis" offer health and wellbeing researchers? *Int. J. Qual. Stud. Health Well-Being* **2014**, *9*, 26152. [CrossRef] [PubMed]
30. Zwingenberger, S.; Valladares, R.D.; Walther, A.; Beck, H.; Stiehler, M.; Kirschner, S.; Engelhardt, M.; Kasten, P. An epidemiological investigation of training and injury patterns in triathletes. *J. Sport. Sci.* **2014**, *32*, 583–590. [CrossRef]
31. Kirkland, A.; Cowley, J. An exploration of context and learning in endurance sports coaching. *Front. Sport. Act. Living* **2023**, *5*, 1147475. [CrossRef]

Disclaimer/Publisher's Note: The statements, opinions and data contained in all publications are solely those of the individual author(s) and contributor(s) and not of MDPI and/or the editor(s). MDPI and/or the editor(s) disclaim responsibility for any injury to people or property resulting from any ideas, methods, instructions or products referred to in the content.

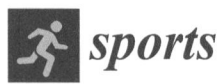

Article

Applying a Holistic Injury Prevention Approach to Elite Triathletes

Héctor Arévalo-Chico, Sergio Sellés-Pérez * and Roberto Cejuela

Physical Education and Sports, Faculty of Education, University of Alicante, 03690 San Vicente del Raspeig, Spain; hector.arevalochico@ua.es (H.A.-C.); roberto.cejuela@ua.es (R.C.)
* Correspondence: sergio.selles@gcloud.ua.es; Tel.: +34-649-22-32-70

Abstract: (1) Background: Studies on injury prevention programs are lacking for triathletes. The aim of the present study was to describe the results of a holistic (injury) training prevention program (HITP), based on training load control and strength training, in elite triathletes. (2) Methods: The study was conducted over 2021–2023 and involved 18 males and 10 females from the same training group. The HITP itself included various methods of fatigue monitoring, strength training focused on the prevention of overuse injuries (OIs), cycling skills training, and recovery strategies. The total number and type of injuries that were sustained, subsequent training/competition absence time, and injury incidence were determined. (3) Results: Twenty-four injuries were recorded over all three seasons, i.e., 0.65 injuries per 1000 h of training and competition exposure. Fourteen injuries were traumatic injuries (TIs) and ten were OIs. Of the OIs, four were of minimal severity, two were mild, three were moderate, and one was severe (accounting for 1–3, 4–7, 8–28, and >28 days of training absenteeism, respectively). A total of 46.4% of the participants did not present any type of injury and 71,4% did not incur any OIs. Average absenteeism was 17.3 days per injury. (4) Conclusions: The HITP design and implementation resulted in low OI and severe injury incidence. Due to their unpredictable nature, the number of TIs was not reduced. The TIs were suffered more frequently by men. Women are more likely to suffer from OIs, so it is particularly important to prevent OIs in women.

Keywords: multifactorial injury prevention; endurance training; strength training; triathlon

Citation: Arévalo-Chico, H.;
Sellés-Pérez, S.; Cejuela, R. Applying a Holistic Injury Prevention Approach to Elite Triathletes. *Sports* **2024**, *12*, 225. https://doi.org/10.3390/sports12080225

Academic Editors: Veronica Vleck, Maria Francesca Piacentini and François Billaut

Received: 19 June 2024
Revised: 13 August 2024
Accepted: 15 August 2024
Published: 19 August 2024

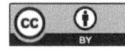

Copyright: © 2024 by the authors. Licensee MDPI, Basel, Switzerland. This article is an open access article distributed under the terms and conditions of the Creative Commons Attribution (CC BY) license (https://creativecommons.org/licenses/by/4.0/).

1. Introduction

Triathlon is an Olympic sport in which swimming, cycling, and running are timed consecutively. The most common distance in the short-distance triathlon is the so-called Olympic distance (i.e., 1.5 km swimming, 40 km cycling, and 10 km running) [1].

Triathletes are subjected to high training loads when preparing for competition because of the multidisciplinary nature of the sport. A professional triathlete racing in the elite category may average weekly training volumes of 15–27 h over the course of a full season [2,3]. Triathlon may present lower sport-related injury (SI) incidence than several other risk or contact sports [4], but high training loads can result in frequent overuse injuries (OIs) or traumatic injuries (TIs) [5–7]. Previous studies have indicated that injury prevalence during the competition phase ranges from 2% to 15% [8]. Vleck et al. [9] showed that the most common types of SIs among high-level triathletes are OIs (with 72% reporting at least one) followed by TIs (with 43% of athletes reporting at least one). Moreover, the most frequent anatomical location of injuries is in the lower limbs [7,10]. This is due to the high impact of the run, the exercise mode in which most injuries occur [7].

SIs are a major concern for coaches [11]; not only do they affect the athlete's health, but, because they impede training, they can also lead to poorer performance.

This is why SI prevention should be regarded as a key component of an effective training plan. However, to the best of our knowledge, no studies have hitherto presented any specific injury prevention programs for triathletes [5–8,12,13]. The nature of SIs in triathlon is multifactorial and complex, prompting a holistic prevention approach [14,15]. In such prevention programs, knowledge of risk factors must be translated into real training contexts [15]. The fundamental aspects of a holistic injury training prevention program (HITP) would include systematic strength training; indeed, a recent systematic review and meta-analysis demonstrated that a 10% strength training volume increase reduces SI risk by over four percentage points [16]. Nonetheless, triathletes often overlook strength training, owing to misconceptions about the use of concurrent training as well as because of practical considerations [17]. The adequate monitoring of training load is a second important aspect of a successful HITP. Proper management of both internal loads (e.g., rating of perceived exertion (RPE), heart rate) and external loads (e.g., training duration and intensity) helps balance performance enhancement and injury risk. Research shows that sudden changes in training load and excessive or insufficient training can significantly increase injury rates [15,18]. Therefore, systematic monitoring and adjustment of training loads are essential for optimizing performance and reducing the risk of injury [19]. Other techniques such as deep tissue massage and myofascial release not only enhance muscle recovery but also improve flexibility and circulation, thereby reducing injury risk. Consistent application of massage therapy has been shown to prevent common sports injuries by maintaining muscle integrity and optimizing an athlete's overall functional capacity [20]. Suarez et al. [21] provide a good illustration of an HITP involving these topics. They developed a program for professional football players that embraced strength training interventions, physiotherapy, load control, and constant technical staff feedback. The aforementioned HITP had important results in practice. It reduced the total number of SIs that were sustained by the athletes by more than half over the seasons during which it was implemented.

The issue of injury has been a recurring subject in the field of sports science over the last decade. A number of descriptive and experimental studies have addressed both the causes of injury, and rehabilitation and prevention protocols [22–24]. However, much of such literature has focused on more popular sports, such as football or basketball [25,26]. In the domain of endurance sports, some triathlon-related studies have been published on swimming [27], cycling [28], and running [29]. They found that the implementation of injury prevention protocols (including strength, stretching, and physiotherapy) reduced OI risk. Nevertheless, to our knowledge, no studies with high-performance athletes, detailing the characteristics of the HITP and its effects on injury incidence, have been conducted in the sport of triathlon. A comprehensive description of such a triathlon-specific program that thoroughly describes all the strategies used would likely help coaches and athletes to improve their training plans. This could consequently lead to a reduction in their risk and/or severity of sports injury.

Thus, the aim of the present study was to provide an in-depth account of an HITP proposal that was implemented in high-level triathletes over a 3-year period, together with its effects.

2. Materials and Methods
2.1. Participants

A total of 28 athletes participated in the study, of whom 18 were men and 10 were women. Based on McKay's framework for sport science research [30], of the male triathletes, 4 were categorized as tier 5 (world-class level) athletes, 6 as tier 4 (elite/international level) athletes, and 13 as tier 3 (highly trained national level) athletes. That is, 10 males were international-level and 13 were national-level triathletes. Of the female triathletes, 4 were tier 4 and 6 were tier 3. Overall, the study participants included 4 triathletes with at least one podium finish in the World Triathlon Series, 5 with at least one podium finish in the World Triathlon Cup, 9 with a top 10 finish in the World Triathlon Cup, and 9 national champions. The triathletes were of 7 different nationalities. The athletes belonged to the same triathlon team, followed the same training methodology, and were led by the same coaches (i.e., AT, HA, RC, and SS). The data presented in this work correspond to athletes who were part of the training group for at least one year over the 2021, 2022, and 2023 seasons.

As regards the male triathletes, their mean and standard deviation (SD) for age, height, and weight were 22.1 (4.2) years, 179.3 (8.7) cm, and 68.2 (5.3) kg, respectively. For the women, average age, height, and weight were 20.7 (4.6) years, 169.3 (7.5) cm, and 58.2 (4.1) kg, respectively. All the study participants had over 5 years of experience in triathlon training and competition. They underwent a medical check-up at the start of each season to confirm their physical readiness for intense exercise. The study participants also gave written informed consent in advance for their data to be used in the study. The study procedures were approved by the Ethics Committee (Expedient UA 2022-09-29_1) of the University of Alicante and followed the data collection guidelines of the Declaration of Helsinki.

2.2. Study Design

The present study was a longitudinal prospective descriptive study. The data were collected over the course of three entire calendar years, in the years 2021, 2022, and 2023.

The triathletes performed an HITP that was itself divided into 5 different sections (i.e., strength training, training load control, session development control, bike skills training, and physiotherapy treatment), all of which were worked on continuously throughout the season. All the interventions were coordinated with each other. Effective communication between the staff and medical team was strongly focused on throughout, with the athletes' health being regarded as the priority.

2.3. Injuries and Exposure

Only SIs that were attributed to triathlon training or competition were recorded. SI diagnosis and treatment were performed by the medical team. In more severe SI cases, the clinical diagnosis was verified via magnetic resonance imaging. A record book was used to take note of SI type, its anatomical location, and the (subsequent) duration of sports-related inactivity.

In line with previous studies [5,7,31], SIs causing absence from participation in at least one training session of any discipline were considered as recordable. Depending on the underlying injury mechanism, the SIs were categorized either as TIs (e.g., due to a bike crash) or as OIs (e.g., stress fracture). The SIs were categorized by anatomical location, as either lower body or upper body injuries. Injury recovery was considered complete when the participant was able to return to training in all three triathlon disciplines. SI severity was determined by the duration of the interval between the date on which the injury occurred and the triathlete's return to full training. Injury severity was categorized as follows: minimal (1–3 days of missed active participation), mild (4–7 days missed), moderate (8–28 days missed), or severe (over 28 missed days) [21].

Injury rate (IR) was determined as the number of total injuries that were recorded per 1000 h of training and competition. To calculate training and competition volume, all the study participants recorded their triathlon training and competition sessions using their training recording devices. The specific training analysis instrument that was used for monitoring endurance sports was the COROS Training Hub software (COROS Wearables Inc., Irvine, CA, USA).

2.4. Intervention

The HITP was implemented in the same way for all the study participants throughout each of the three seasons for which the study ran. Priority was given to some of the topics of the HITP depending on the season period, as illustrated in Table 1.

Table 1. Order of priority per section of the holistic training prevention program during the season.

		Strength Training	Training Load Control	Session Control	Physiotherapy Treatment	Bike Skills
Traditional periodization	General preparatory Period	****	***	****	**	***
	Specific Preparatory Period	***	****	****	****	****
	Competition Period	**	**	***	***	***
Block periodization	Accumulation Block	***	***	***	*	**
	Transformation Block	**	****	***	***	***
	Realization Block	*	**	**	**	**

* = Degree of importance of the topic from 1 to 4 stars, with a 4-star rating being the most important.

2.4.1. Strength Training

The strength training planning was structured based on the athlete's schedule of competitions and training sessions (Figure 1). Each season was planned according to each athlete's individual competition calendar. Due to the characteristics of the athlete's competitive calendar, a first training block of traditional-style periodization, followed by a second phase of block periodization (ATR style), was implemented [32]. The first, traditional periodization block of the season was the longer of the two blocks. The traditional periodization model can be useful for athletes who do not have an excessive number of competitions during this period. The athletes can benefit from a multi-task training program by developing several capacities and abilities at the same time, while the accumulated fatigue and any negative training transfer effects that can occur between such capacities are taken into account [32]. The second block was significantly shorter. In view of the residual training effect of the first block, it was decided to employ an ATR model for this second block of the season. Given the increased number of scheduled competitions within the aforesaid period, it was necessary for the athletes to work on different skills over a shorter period of time. The ATR model was deemed the most suitable model under such conditions [32]. The introduction of several methods of strength training was proposed because studies have shown that endurance athletes improve their strength levels and economy more with strength training programs that contain several methods (e.g., plyometric and maximum strength training) as opposed to a single method [33].

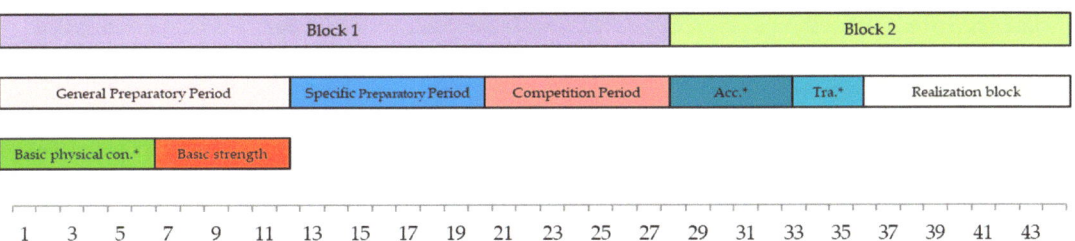

Figure 1. Timeline of the strength plan. * Acc = accumulation; Tra = transformation; Con = conditioning.

A submaximal load–velocity profiling test [34] was realized to estimate the one repetition maximum (1RM) of each triathlete, and then to set his/her individual loads on the basis of this, for each of the basic strength exercises that were utilized by the program.

- Block I (traditional-style periodization):

This period lasted 28 ± 3 weeks and included the entire general preparatory period (of 12 ± 2 weeks), the specific preparatory period (of 8 ± 1 weeks), and the competitive period (8 ± 2 weeks). During the general preparatory period, a first, basic physical conditioning phase, which involved 4 weekly sessions, unfolded for 6 weeks. The sessions focused on developing endurance strength using low loads (40–60% RM), with a 1 min rest period between sets. They involved two different types of (1) unilateral exercises; (2) complementary mobility hip and scapula exercises; and (3) complementary strengthening exercises of the core, Achilles tendon, tibial muscles, peroneal muscles, as well as of intrinsic foot and gluteus muscles. Figure 2 shows an example of hip mobility exercises. In this phase, isometric strength "Iso-Hold" hip-type exercises were also performed in 2–3 sets of 2–3 repetitions, lasting from 10 to 30 s on each side [35]. This training was conducted at the beginning of the season to generate a general muscular physical conditioning in the athlete, to avoid muscular decompensation, and to work on the stabilizing musculature. This should allow for the accumulation of more training load, as well as for strength training with higher loads [32,36].

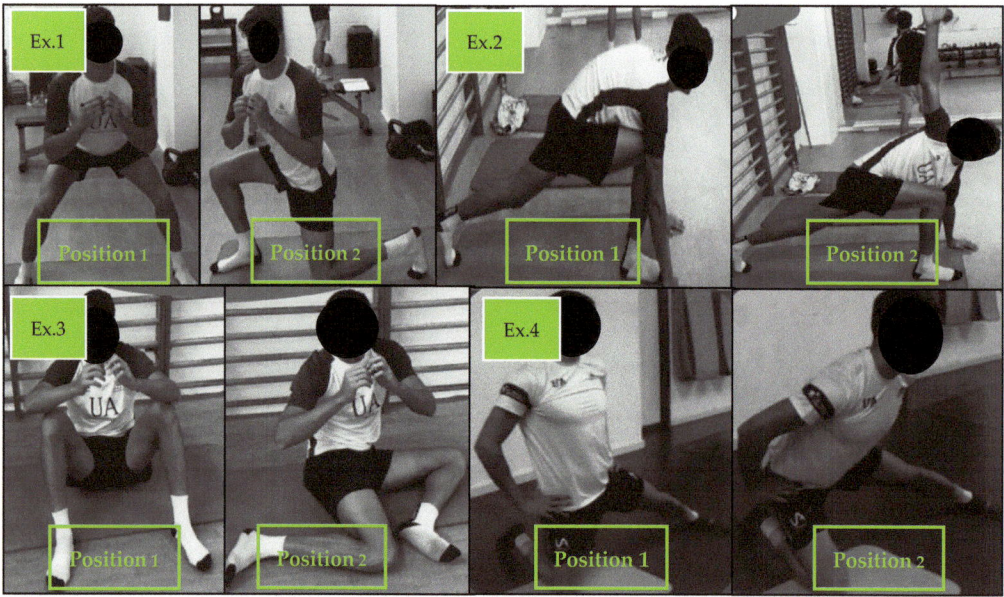

Figure 2. Examples of different exercises for hip mobility training.

The second phase of the general preparatory period was the basic strength development phase, which lasted 6 ± 1 weeks. In this phase, 3 sessions were performed per week. The workload that was performed was between 65 and 75% of 1RM, in 3–4 sets of 5–8 repetitions and with a 3′ rest between sets, i.e., of medium–low-level effort. This design was implemented so as to produce maximum strength improvement while avoiding the development of excessive fatigue that could then affect the athletes' main endurance training sessions. In this way, we avoid the excessive accumulation of metabolites and muscle damage, as well as the generation of hypertrophy, which is unnecessary for endurance sports [33,37,38]. The exercises that were performed were a total of 5 multi-joint exercises, divided into upper body (pull-ups and bench press) and lower body (deadlift, hip thrust, squat, and Bulgarian squat) exercises. In each session, 2 lower body exercises were alternated with one upper body exercise. There were no exercise repetitions in consecutive workouts. A reduced range of exercises was chosen so as to ensure technique mastery and to optimize the use of training time [39]. Once they had mastered the exercise technique, the triathletes were encouraged to move the load as quickly as possible, so as to generate adaptations at the neural level. This high-velocity movement training has been shown to improve high-velocity athletic performance, particularly among well-trained athletes [40]. During this phase, the athletes continued to perform the same "hip Iso-hold" work and introduced "Iso-push" exercises in 2–3 sets of 2–3 repetitions of 3 s on each side with 1 min rests between sets. Figure 3 shows examples of the "Iso-hold" and the "Iso-push" exercises.

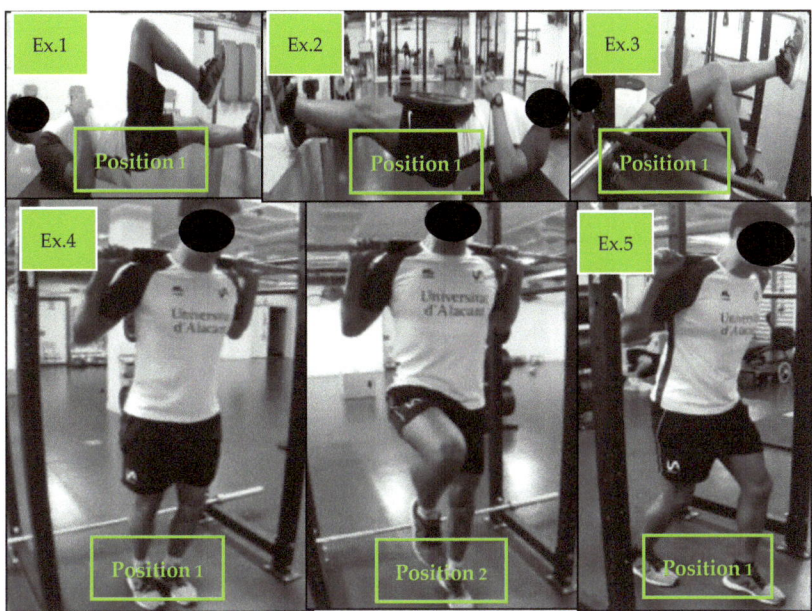

Figure 3. Examples of different exercises for iso-hold and iso-push hip training.

During the specific preparatory period, training frequency was 2 sessions per week. The exercises that were performed were identical to those that had been implemented within the previous training phase. The load was 60–70% of the athlete's 1RM, in 2–3 sets of 4–6 repetitions each. In this phase, "contrast training" was included; following the upper body strength series, medicine ball throwing exercises were performed (4–6 repetitions), and after the lower body exercises, hurdle jumps or box jumps were carried out (4–6 repetitions). Figures 4 and 5, respectively, show examples of the upper body contrast exercises and lower body contrast exercises that were utilized. Over this period, the "Iso hold" work was halted, and the "Iso-push" work was maintained, with the load for the latter being increased to 3–4 sets of 3–4 repetitions of 3" on each side. The contrast method has been shown to generate positive effects on both absolute strength gain and running economy [35].

In the competitive period, strength training frequency was reduced to 1 session per week. The same basic strength development sessions were performed along with contrasts. The number of sets was reduced to 1–2, while the number of repetitions and loads was maintained as before. "Iso-pushes" exercises were only performed as contrast training.

- Block II (ATR periodization)

This period lasted 16 ± 2 weeks and comprised a first accumulation period (of 5 ± 1 weeks' duration), a (3-week) transformation period, and a realization period (lasting 8 weeks). During the accumulation period, the training protocol that corresponded to the basic strength development phase of the general preparatory period was repeated. In the transformation period, the protocol of the specific preparatory period was repeated. In the performance period, the competitive period protocol of block I was repeated.

Throughout the season, complementary strength work was maintained on at least 3 days per week. Hip and ankle mobility exercises were carried out to warm up before running training sessions. Scapular mobility exercises were also performed before any swimming training sessions. The same periodization was implemented for the female triathletes as for the males, apart from the fact that that they performed one more upper body exercise in all the basic strength development sessions.

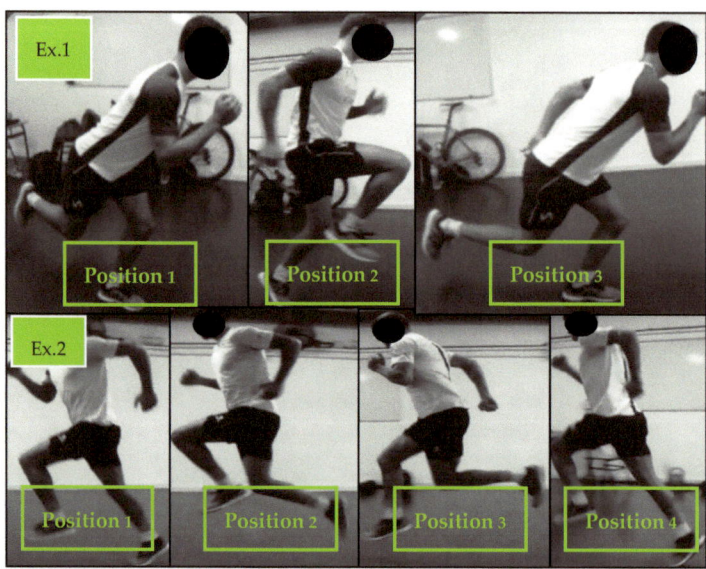

Figure 4. Examples of different exercises for lower body contrast training.

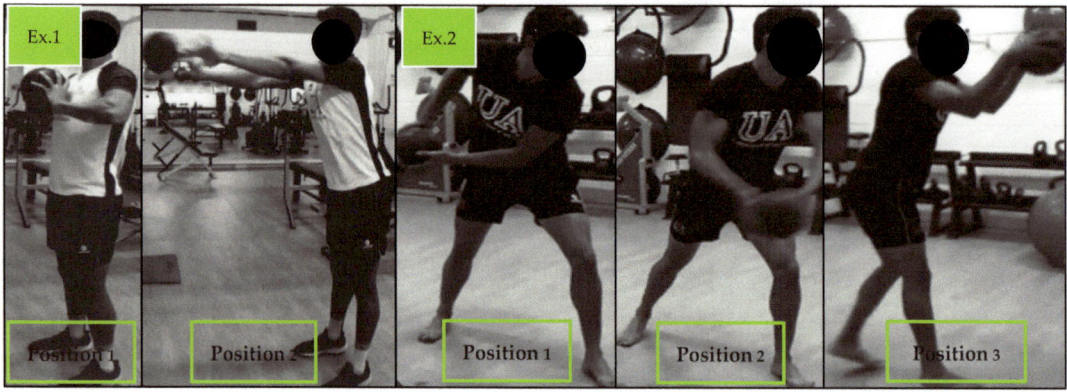

Figure 5. Examples of different upper body throw exercises for contrast training.

The objective, in so doing, was to increase work volume and to thus minimize the strength differences that existed between the upper and the lower limbs (this being accentuated in women [41]. The females were also given a larger volume of supplemental training than were the males, in order to minimize the occurrence of overuse injuries [24].

2.4.2. Training Load Control

To calculate and control the training load, the Objective Load Equivalent (ECO) methodology was employed. To summarize, based on laboratory performance tests with cardiorespiratory and lactate analysis, 8 intensity zones were defined for swim, cycling, and run. These zones were correlated with an individual RPE scale ranging from 1 to 10 [42]. Training load was determined by multiplying the duration (in minutes) of training time that was spent in each training zone (1–8) by a score value that ranged from 1 to 50 (and was based on that training zone), and then by applying specific weighting factors for running, swimming, and cycling. Subjective Load Equivalents (ECS) were also assessed, allowing athletes to subjectively quantify session difficulty on a scale of 0 to 5. The ECOs were calculated using the All in Your Mind Training 143 system®. Subjective data such as hours of sleep and ECS were recorded by the athletes in online training logs.

Special attention was paid to maintaining a balance in training loads, by alternating development sessions and recovery sessions. Generally, in an average training week, Tuesdays, Wednesdays, Thursdays, Saturdays, and Sundays were dedicated to developing different abilities depending on the time of the season, while Mondays and Fridays were active recovery days. The training load was reduced on recovery days, so as to avoid the development of states of excessive fatigue that could themselves lead to injury [42].

As a rule, the weekly training load was increased by 10–15% compared to the previous week in the development microcycles, and decreased by 20–25% in the recovery microcycles of the program. An undulating periodization model was used during the competition period. The training load was reduced compared to previous periods, maintaining intensity but lowering volume [42].

The athletes and the coaches were in continuous communication with each other throughout the season. If an athlete recorded excessive ECS values or transmitted subjective feelings of excessive fatigue, the training load was reduced to avoid states of non-functional overreaching that could lead to injuries.

2.4.3. Session Development Control

To monitor their adherence to session intensity and goals, the athletes were asked to remember and respect the intensity zones and their associated speed/power, heart ranges, and RPE. Low-intensity workouts (zones 1 and 2) were mostly guided by heart rate and RPE, while speed and power were used to regulate sessions of moderate to high exercise intensity (zones 3–8).

At least one coach (i.e., AT, HA, RC, or SS) was present to monitor the session in all training sessions. Additionally, the participants recorded their training sessions using training devices. The COROS Training Hub software (COROS Wearables Inc., Irvine, CA, USA) facilitated the control and monitoring of the athletes' training by their support team.

2.4.4. Cycling Skills Training

During the general preparatory period, the emphasis was on the refinement of fundamental skills that are essential for overall cycling proficiency and safety. A weekly, technique-only training session was conducted. This technical session was designed to enhance various cycling skills, including riding in a group, cornering, the ability to do U-turns, mounting and dismounting the bike, and other bike handling skills.

In the specific preparatory period, the athletes' bike skills were further improved via the use of brick (bike and run) sessions, once a week. The brick sessions took place on a closed circuit and involved 3 curves per kilometer. These sessions were carried out in groups, and close to or at exercise intensities resembling that of competitions, so as to replicate actual competition conditions as closely as possible. By simulating race-like conditions and incorporating targeted skill development, athletes were primed to optimize their performance and confidence in competitive events. It is also possible to conduct some group cycling training at high speeds, practicing skills such as draft relays. These exercises replicate the movements that occur within competitive cycling groups. Within the peloton, positions are alternated to achieve higher speeds more efficiently.

2.4.5. Physiotherapy

The athletes worked with the physiotherapist throughout the season and this collaboration played a key role in the HITP program of each triathlete. As a rule, one physiotherapy session took place per week. Some athletes had two sessions per week during peak season and these sessions were carried out on their recovery days. Myofascial induction techniques were performed to readjust the connective tissue mechanical properties and to facilitate drainage and recovery. In the case of injury having occurred, the medical team carried out the diagnosis. They designed the specific injury treatment and readaptation plan that was to be implemented for the injury in question jointly with the physiotherapist.

2.5. Data Analysis

A descriptive analysis was conducted using the means and standard deviation of the variables that were recorded within the study. Injury rate was calculated as the number of injuries per 1000 h of triathlon training and competition. The analyses were performed using a Microsoft Office Excel 2016 spreadsheet.

The nonparametric Mann–Whitney U test was performed to detect the statistical differences between the variables for men and women. Spearmans' bivariate correlation coefficient was used to determine the existence of any inter-relationships between the occurrence of injuries and the time of exposure and the years of experience performing HITP. The statistical software Statistical Package for Social Sciences (SPSS) version 22.0 (SPSS Inc., Chicago, IL, USA) was used to analyze the data. For all analyses, significance was accepted at $p < 0.05$.

3. Results

A total of 28 triathletes (10 females, 18 males) were prospectively followed across the three consecutive years of the study (Figure 6). The number of participating male athletes was 11, 12, and 14 for 2021, 2022, and 2023, respectively. A total of six, five, and seven female athletes took part in 2021, 2022, and 2023, respectively. Seven male and three female athletes were present throughout all 3 consecutive years of the program.

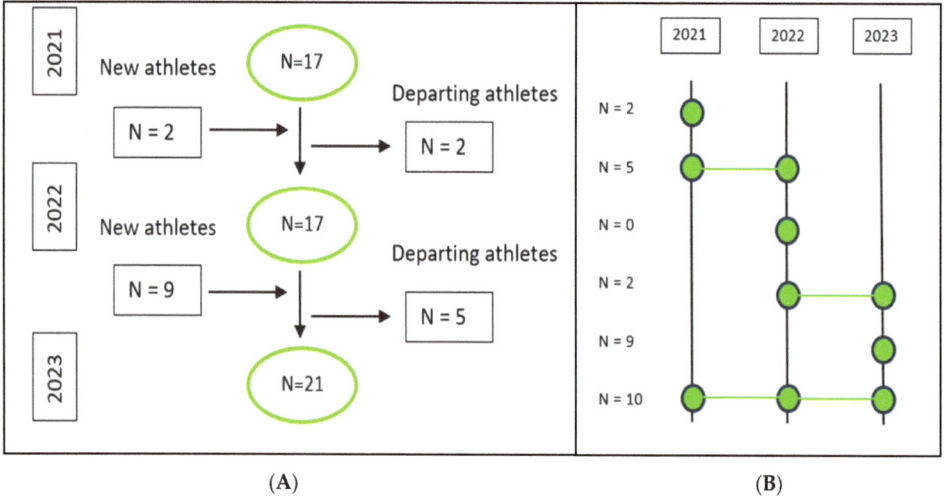

Figure 6. (**A**) The number of new and departing athletes each season. (**B**) The number of athletes in the training group across each season.

Mean and standard deviation (SD) participant exposure per calendar year was 660 (122) hours. The men's exposure was slightly higher (671 (33) hours) than that of the women (649 (89) hours), but not significantly so. Table 2 presents the corresponding injury data of the athletes. During the recording period, 24 SIs occurred overall, across all 28 study participants. Ten injuries (41.6% of the total SIs) were OIs and fourteen (58.3% of the total SIs) were TIs. The number of TIs that were incurred was significantly higher among the men than among the women (i.e., twelve TIs for the men vs. two for the women). Of the 28 athletes that participated in the study (i.e., regardless of the number of years that they participated in the program), the overall percentages of athletes affected by injury were 53.6% for any kind of injury, 28.6% for OI, and 35.7% for TI. In the males, the percentage of athletes affected by injury was 55.6% for any kind of injury, 27.7% for OI, and 44.4% for TI. The corresponding values for the male participants recorded 30% for any kind of injury, 30% for OI, and 20% for TI. A statistically significant difference between the sexes was found in the percentage of athletes who suffered a TI. Among the ten athletes who took part in all three years of the study, the highest percentage of athletes being affected by injuries was noted in 2021 (i.e., 50%). In 2022, this value decreased to 30%. The lowest percentage of athletes being affected by injuries was noted in 2023, at 20%.

Table 2. Injury data and comparison between male and female triathletes.

	Overall (n = 28)	Male (n = 18)	Female (n = 10)
Training and Competition Exposure per season			
Total (mean hours (SD))	660 (122)	671 (33)	649 (89)
Injuries during the three seasons			
Total (n)	24	18	6
Overuse (n)	10	6	4
Traumatic (n)	14	12 *	2 *
Absenteeism (mean days (SD))	17.3 (54.2)	22.6 (55.6) *	5.83 (8.7) *
Overall % of athletes affected by injury			
Among all participants (n = 28)	53.6	55.6	30
In first year of following the HITP (n = 28)	35.7	38.9	30
In second year of following the HITP (n = 17)	31.6	30.8	33.3
In third year of following the HITP (n = 10)	20	28.6	0
by OI, among all participants (n = 28)	28.6	27.7	30
by TI, among all participants (n = 28)	35.7	44.4 *	20 *
Overall Injury Severity, 2021–2023			
Minimal (n)	10	6	4
Mild (n)	6	4	1
Moderate (n)	6	6 *	1 *
Severe (n)	2	2	0
Overuse Injury Severity 2021–2023			
Minimal (n)	4	1	3
Mild (n)	2	1	0
Moderate (n)	3	3	1
Severe (n)	1	1	0
Traumatic Injury Severity, 2021–2023			
Minimal (n)	6	5	1
Mild (n)	4	3	1
Moderate (n)	3	3	0
Severe (n)	1	1	0
Injury rate/1000 h of training and competition			
Overall	0.65	0.68	0.61
Overuse	0.27	0.23	0.41
Traumatic	0.38	0.46 *	0.2 *
Anatomical location of injury			
Upper body (n)	2	2	0
Lower body (n)	22	16	6

* = sex group statistically significant difference. ($p < 0.05$); OI = overuse injury, TI = traumatic injury.

When, even if the athletes in question did not take part in all three years of the study, the number of years of experience of the HITP program was considered, the highest percentage of athletes affected by injuries was recorded during the first year of performing the HITP (e.g., 35.7%, n = 28). In the second year, this value decreased to 31.6% (n = 17). The lowest percentage of athletes affected by injuries was recorded in the third year of performing the program, with 20% affected (n = 10).

In terms of injury severity, significant differences were found between the sexes for the number of moderate-severity injuries that were sustained, with the men recording six and the women one. For the injuries that did occur, average and standard deviation (SD) absenteeism was 17.3 (54.2) days. Statistically significant differences were found between the men's absenteeism and women's absenteeism as a result of injury. This was 22.6 (55.6) days and 5.83 (8.7) days for men and women, respectively ($p < 0.05$). The registered IR during the recording period, which did not differ with sex, was 0.65 injuries per 1000 h overall. This equated to 0.68 injuries per 1000 h of training and competition exposure for the men and 0.61 injuries per 1000 h of training and competition exposure for the women. IR due to trauma was higher in men than it was in women (at 0.46 vs. 0.2 injuries per 1000 h of training and competition exposure, respectively). The IR for overuse injury was higher in women (at 0.41 injuries per 1000 h of exposure) than it was in men (at 0.23 injuries per 1000 h of training and competition exposure) but the difference was not statistically significant.

A small but statistically significant negative correlation was noted between the number of years that participants had been involved in the HITP program and the number of injuries they experienced during the year ($\varrho = -0.395$; $p < 0.05$). No such statistically significant correlations were found for TI ($\varrho = -0.034$; $p > 0.05$). No statistically significant correlations were found between exposure time in training and competition and the number of OIs ($\varrho = -0.22$; $p > 0.05$) or TI ($\varrho = 0.14$; $p > 0.05$) that were sustained by the athletes.

4. Discussion

The study objectives were to present an HITP proposal together with the results of its implementation over a 3-year period, in high-level triathletes. The main findings were that the implementation of an HITP resulted in low injury incidence (and particularly overuse injury incidence). Among the ten athletes who participated in all three years of the study, the percentage of athletes who were affected by injury decreased over the course of the three consecutive years. We also noted a small, but statistically significant, negative correlation between the individual athletes' years of experience of participation in the HITP and the number of overuse injuries that were suffered during the season by the study participants. Nevertheless, the most frequent kinds of injury that occurred were traumatic injuries. Men showed significant differences in the number of traumatic injuries that were incurred over the course of the study compared to women. Women presented a larger number of overuse injuries compared to males, but the difference was not statistically significant. Most of the injuries that occurred were of mild or minimal severity.

Over 2021–2023, i.e., the three years that the present study lasted, 53.6% of the participants (regardless of the years they participated in the program) suffered at least one sporting injury. These values are lower compared to the limited information that is available on this topic from previous prospective studies of elite triathletes. Vleck et al. [15], in a seven-month longitudinal prospective study of 71 members of the 1996 Great Britain National and Scottish National Triathlon Squads, noted a total of 80.4% of athletes that were affected by injury (regardless of severity). Crunkhorn et al. [43], in their four-year, prospective study of 50 Australian national elite squad triathletes, reported 92% of the athletes to have been injured over 2018–2021. It is important to note that this study, unlike the present one, also noted non-time loss injuries. In the Crunkhorn et al. [43] study, 67.3% of the injuries resulted in a period of time loss. We note, however, that differences in methodologies complicate the comparison between studies [7].

As regards the ten triathletes who participated in all three years of the HITP program, the highest percentage of those who were affected by injuries occurred in 2021 (e.g., 50%). This percentage dropped to 30% in 2022, and then to its lowest value in 2023, with 20% of athletes affected. Based on the years of experience in the program, it can be observed that during the first year performing the HITP, 35.7% of the overall cohort of 28 athletes suffered at least one injury. This percentage decreased in the next year for the 17 athletes who continued in the program for a second year (i.e., 31.6%). Among the 10 athletes that performed the program for three consecutive years, in the third and last year, this value was 20%. It can be observed that by implementing an HITP, the percentage of athletes who suffered an injury seems to decrease each year. HITP experience may enhance the injury prevention capacity of the program. This may be due to the adaptations that are generated year after year. It may also be due to the increased ability of athletes to perform the program successfully.

A higher number of lower body SIs were also recorded in the present study, which is consistent with most literature results [10,44] and is probably due to the impact generated by the run.

The injury incidence rate in this study was 0.65 injuries per 1000 h of training and competition exposure. This value is also lower than that of previous studies on elite triathletes, which reported values of between 17.5 and 58.1 per 1000 h of training exposure in seven consecutive months [15]. However, this comparison may not be completely correct because of the different data registration periods of the two studies. Unlike the present study (which collected data throughout the year), Vleck et al.'s [15] investigation was carried out between the months of February and August, when traditionally there is more training load and competitions. This may have increased the injury risk. In running, injury incidence has been reported to vary between 2.5 injuries per 1000 h of training and competition exposure (in a study of long-distance track and field athletes) and a maximum value of 33.0 injuries per 1000 h of training and competition exposure (in a study of amateur runners [29]). In the present study, no correlation was found between the training exposure time of the athletes and the amount of sporting injuries that were incurred by the triathletes. This may show the possible effectiveness of the HITP in terms of injury prevention.

In terms of injury absenteeism, an average of 17.3 days spent without being able to train in at least one discipline was reported in the present study. Vleck et al. [10], in a retrospective study, reported an average absenteeism of 29.3 days off running training for national squad athletes who were racing non-drafting competition. However, Vleck et al. [15], in their prospective seven-month study on elite triathletes, found an average length of time that injury lasted between 12.8 days and 5.6 days, depending on the area affected by the injury. On the other hand, Crunkhorn et al. [43] noted an injury burden calculated across the 4-year surveillance period of 68.39 days of time loss per 365 days. Again, the differences in the study design complicate the comparison between studies.

Regarding the origin of the SI, we can observe that in the present study, the percentage of athletes who were affected by injury (at 28.6% and 35.7% for OI and TI, respectively), the IR (at 0.27 and 0.38 injuries per 1000 h of training and competition exposure for OI and TI, respectively), and the amount of injuries (at 14 OI and 10 TI, respectively) were higher when the injuries were traumatic than when they were classified as being due to overuse. These injury data together with the negative relationship found between the years of experience of performing the HITP and the number of OIs that were sustained may indicate that the HITP program that was presented in this study can be an effective one, especially as regards OI. Although we cannot be sure that the effectiveness of HITP is due to strength training alone, it has been frequently shown that strength work can prevent OI occurrence [45]. Complementary strength training that focuses on higher-SI-risk joints also contributes to injury prevention [36]. The structure created for strength training can also benefit triathletes' performance. This would be due to concurrent training, which improves the energy cost of locomotion [46]. Moreover, low to moderate strength training efforts with repetitions together with muscle failure avoidance may improve performance while also preventing the negative effects of muscle hypertrophy or fatigue [47]. In addition, isometric strength work is a good complement to the aforesaid type of training, as it increases strength without generating any major muscle fatigue [35]. The primary objective with strength training was not to maximize strength values but to reach acceptable levels to aid in injury prevention. The combination of various strength training methods may also have influenced the acquisition of optimal strength levels that minimize the occurrence of injuries [33].

Another possible reason for the low injury incidence values that are reported here may be the training load and the control of session development that took place over the course of the study. Training planning errors are a common cause of SI [48], therefore, maximizing the level of control that is exerted over the design and execution of the athletes' training plan is key to avoiding the overload that can lead to SI. The goal in this part of the HITP was not to exceed the maximum load tolerable while generating the greatest possible number of adaptations. Managing training loads based on both external and internal load data methods and mastering the intensity of training zones the athlete is familiar with can help to regulate the balance between training dose and training response. In addition, implementing identification systems of overtraining symptoms can help to prevent OI, e.g., by monitoring subjective fatigue values [49]. This latter strategy is all the more essential in periods of more intense efforts, such as in specific periods or competition periods [6]. Another key factor is regular work with the physiotherapist. Myofascial induction and sports massages have been proven to be effective methods to recover from fatigue and to prevent SI [20]. Therefore, working with a multidisciplinary team able to offer this service can greatly benefit the athletes' health and performance.

Despite its apparently positive OI prevention results, the HITP was not found to be effective at preventing TI. We did not find a statistically significant relationship between the athlete's experience of the HITP and the number of TIs that were incurred over the course of the study. This could point to the uncontrollable condition of TI [9]; despite working on cycling skills, athletes continue to suffer SI, mainly caused by bike segment falls. This phenomenon can also be observed among professional cyclists. Haberle et al. [28] recorded that during the 2010 to 2017 Tours de France, 53% of race dropouts were due to acute trauma and 47% to non-traumatic causes, such as OI or illness. In triathlon, the points where participants anticipate the most risk of traumatic injury are the cycling mount/dismount area and the cycling segment [6,50]. The less experienced the triathlete, the higher the risk of accidents in these sections [6,50]. Therefore, future studies should focus on developing accident prevention programs, perhaps including techniques such as imagery, which has been shown to be effective in other sports such as BMX [51].

As for gender differences, in this study, both sexes presented similar levels of injury occurrence. Although the percentage of athletes who suffered an injury between 2021 and 2023 was higher for males than it was for females, i.e., 55.6% and 30% for males and females, respectively, no significant differences were found. This finding is compatible with previous studies, which have shown the absence of a relationship between triathlon SI and gender [43,52]. However, TIs were more numerous and severe in men than in women ($p < 0.05$). This may be due to the higher speeds that are attained by men in the cycling segment, especially in competition, which can cause more severe TI if they suffer a fall [53]. However, although no statistically significant differences were found, OI IR was higher in women than in men. Women generally tend to suffer OI more frequently, possibly due to lower strength levels and hormonal causes [54]. Other studies have also pointed out that women tend to suffer more bone stress injuries than men [43]. Nevertheless, in the present study, women's IR was much lower than that reported by Hamilton et al. [55]. A possible explanation would be the preventive effect of the female-specific strength programming that was implemented in this study by increasing the women's strength training load compared to that of men, especially as regards that which was induced whilst doing the complementary and upper body exercises [41] (as illustrated in Figure 2).

This study has made a valuable contribution to the field, as for the first time, an injury prevention plan with potentially positive results has been proposed for triathletes. However, the work has several important limitations that should be considered when interpreting its results. The fact that we did not have a control group (either of matched high-performance athletes or of the same athletes, from before they underwent the HITP) limits the ability to directly attribute the observed injury outcomes to the HITP itself. Another important limitation of our study is the inability to identify which specific components of our training program might be most effective in reducing injury incidence. The training program was designed as a holistic approach, and the athletes who participated in it sustained low injury incidence. However, as this is a descriptive study, it does not allow for a definitive analysis of the causal relationships between program components and any observed reduction in injury occurrence or severity. Consequently, there is no concrete way to determine whether omitting certain elements of the program would result in the same or even better injury-related outcomes. The lack of uniformity in injury definitions and methodologies across existing studies also complicates direct comparisons with the published literature. This underscores the need for further research to isolate and examine the effects of specific training interventions within the holistic framework. Moreover, implementing an HITP of this nature presents significant logistical challenges. The complexity of the plan requires considerable investment in time and financial resources, which may not be feasible for all levels of triathletes.

Nonetheless, this study provides a concrete example of how an HITP minimizing injury incidence may be designed and implemented. We must remember, nevertheless, that injury etiology is multifactorial and such a program may not work in contexts other than the one that was here described. The question remains as to whether different approaches would improve the results.

Despite these limitations, our findings suggest that by applying appropriate adjustments and adaptations, the plan can potentially improve triathlete health and performance, offering a solid foundation for future research and practical applications in triathlon.

5. Conclusions

The present study presented a detailed triathlon HITP and the results of its implementation. Total SIs and severity reported were low, possibly due to the joint effect of strength training, load and session development control, and physiotherapy. A significant (but low) relationship was found between years of experience of the HITP and the number of OIs, but not of TIs, that were incurred. Though OI incidence was lower, TI did not appear to have been reduced despite the skills development work within the HITP that aimed to prevent or lessen it. In triathlon, external factors such as the course or competitor interaction make it more difficult to prevent TI. Men suffered more numerous and severe TIs than women, whose major cause of injury was overuse. There is also a need for new studies with control groups that can show what it is more effective in preventing SI in triathletes.

To our knowledge, this study is the first to present a detailed HITP proposal for a group of elite triathletes. As such, this study is particularly useful for coaches and athletes. This paper provides practical information on how to potentially minimize the occurrence of SI. Such information is important given that SI can potentially affect the health and performance of any age or level of triathlete.

Author Contributions: Conceptualization, S.S.-P. and H.A.-C.; methodology, R.C. and S.S.-P.; software, H.A.-C.; formal analysis, S.S.-P. and H.A.-C.; investigation, R.C. and H.A.-C.; resources, R.C.; data curation, H.A.-C.; writing—original draft preparation, H.A.-C.; writing—review and editing, S.S.-P.; visualization, R.C.; supervision, S.S.-P.; project administration, R.C. and S.S.-P.; funding acquisition, S.S.-P. All authors have read and agreed to the published version of the manuscript.

Funding: This study was supported by the "Conselleria de Educación, Cultura, Universidades y Empleo" in the grants to emerging research groups (ref. CIGE/2022/4).

Institutional Review Board Statement: All procedures used in this study were approved by the Alicante University Ethics Committee (UA-2023-10-27_2 expedient). The athletes gave their consent for their data to be published in this study. The whole data collection process followed the guidelines of the Declaration of Helsinki.

Informed Consent Statement: Informed consent was obtained from all subjects involved in the study.

Data Availability Statement: The data that support the findings of this study are available from the corresponding author upon reasonable request.

Acknowledgments: The authors want to thank the triathletes for their cooperation in the training process.

Conflicts of Interest: The authors declare no conflicts of interest.

References

1. ITU Olympic Triathlon—World Triathlon. Available online: https://triathlon.org/olympics (accessed on 19 May 2024).
2. Mujika, I. Olympic Preparation of a World-Class Female Triathlete. *Int. J. Sports Physiol. Perform.* **2014**, *9*, 727–731. [CrossRef]
3. Cejuela, R.; Selles-Perez, S. Training Characteristics and Performance of Two Male Elite Short-Distance Triathletes: From Junior to "World-Class". *Scand. J. Med. Sci. Sports* **2023**, *33*, 2444–2456. [CrossRef] [PubMed]
4. Åman, M.; Forssblad, M.; Henriksson-Larsén, K. Incidence and Severity of Reported Acute Sports Injuries in 35 Sports Using Insurance Registry Data. *Scand. J. Med. Sci. Sports* **2016**, *26*, 451–462. [CrossRef] [PubMed]
5. Vleck, V.; Caine, D.J.; Harmer, P.; Schiff, M. *Epidemiology of Injury in Olympic Sports. International Olympic Committee Encyclopaedia of Sports Medicine Series Triathlon*; Wiley-Blackwell: West Sussex, UK, 2009; pp. 294–320. [CrossRef]
6. Vleck, V.; Hoeden, D. Epidemiological aspects of illness and injury. In *Triathlon Medicine*; Springer Nature: Basel, Switzerland, 2019; pp. 19–41.
7. Vleck, V.; Millet, G.P.; Alves, F.B. The Impact of Triathlon Training and Racing on Athletes' General Health. *Sports Med.* **2014**, *44*, 1659–1692. [CrossRef]
8. Guevara, S.A.; Crunkhorn, M.L.; Drew, M.; Waddington, G.; Périard, J.D.; Etxebarria, N.; Toohey, L.A.; Charlton, P. Injury and Illness in Short-Course Triathletes: A Systematic Review. *J. Sport Health Sci.* **2024**, *13*, 172–185. [CrossRef]
9. Vleck, V.E.; Bentley, D.J.; Millet, G.P.; Cochrane, T. Triathlon Event Distance Specialization: Training and Injury Effects. *J. Strength Cond. Res.* **2010**, *24*, 30–36. [CrossRef]
10. Vleck, V.E.; Garbutt, G. Injury and Training Characteristics of Male Elite, Development Squad, and Club Triathletes. *Int. J. Sports Med.* **1998**, *19*, 38–42. [CrossRef]
11. Kennedy, M.D.; Knight, C.J.; Falk Neto, J.H.; Uzzell, K.S.; Szabo, S.W. Futureproofing Triathlon: Expert Suggestions to Improve Health and Performance in Triathletes. *BMC Sports Sci. Med. Rehabil.* **2020**, *12*, 1. [CrossRef] [PubMed]
12. Gosling, C.M.R.; Gabbe, B.J.; Forbes, A.B. Triathlon Related Musculoskeletal Injuries: The Status of Injury Prevention Knowledge. *J. Sci. Med. Sport* **2008**, *11*, 396–406. [CrossRef]
13. Vleck, V.; Alves, F.B. Triathlon Injury Review. *Br. J. Sports Med.* **2011**, *45*, 382–383. [CrossRef]
14. Edouard, P.; Ford, K.R. Great Challenges Toward Sports Injury Prevention and Rehabilitation. *Front. Sports Act. Living* **2020**, *2*, 56–63. [CrossRef]
15. Vleck, V. *Triathlete Training and Injury Analysis an Investigation in British National Squad and Age-Group Triathletes*, 1st ed.; VDM Verlag Dr. Müller: Saarbrücken, Germany, 2010.
16. Lauersen, J.B.; Andersen, T.E.; Andersen, L.B.; Lauersen, B. Strength Training as Superior, Dose-Dependent and Safe Prevention of Acute and Overuse Sports Injuries: A Systematic Review, Qualitative Analysis and Meta-Analysis. *Br. J. Sports Med.* **2018**, *52*, 1557–1563. [CrossRef] [PubMed]
17. Baldwin, K.M.; Badenhorst, C.E.; Cripps, A.J.; Landers, G.J.; Merrells, R.J.; Bulsara, M.K.; Hoyne, G.F. Strength Training for Long-Distance Triathletes: Theory to Practice. *Strength Cond. J.* **2022**, *44*, 1–14. [CrossRef]
18. Falk Neto, J.H.; Parent, E.C.; Vleck, V.; Kennedy, M.D. The Training Characteristics of Recreational-Level Triathletes: Influence on Fatigue and Health. *Sports* **2021**, *9*, 94. [CrossRef] [PubMed]
19. Gabbett, T.J. The Training-Injury Prevention Paradox: Should Athletes Be Training Smarter and Harder? *Br. J. Sports Med.* **2016**, *50*, 273–280. [CrossRef] [PubMed]
20. Gasibat, Q.; Suwehli, W. Determining the Benefits of Massage Mechanisms: A Review of Literature. *J. Rehabil. Sci.* **2017**, *2*, 58–67. [CrossRef]
21. Suarez-Arrones, L.; Nakamura, F.Y.; Maldonado, R.A.; Torreno, N.; Di Salvo, V.; Mendez-Villanueva, A. Applying a Holistic Hamstring Injury Prevention Approach in Elite Football: 12 Seasons, Single Club Study. *Scand. J. Med. Sci. Sports* **2021**, *31*, 861–874. [CrossRef]
22. Defi, I.R. Rehabilitation Role in Sport Injury. *Orthop. J. Sports Med.* **2023**, *11*, 23259671211S0083. [CrossRef]
23. Vriend, I.; Gouttebarge, V.; Finch, C.F.; van Mechelen, W.; Verhagen, E.A.L.M. Intervention Strategies Used in Sport Injury Prevention Studies: A Systematic Review Identifying Studies Applying the Haddon Matrix. *Sports Med.* **2017**, *47*, 2027–2043. [CrossRef]
24. Aicale, R.; Tarantino, D.; Maffulli, N. Overuse Injuries in Sport: A Comprehensive Overview. *J. Orthop. Surg. Res.* **2018**, *13*, 309. [CrossRef]
25. Pérez-Gómez, J.; Adsuar, J.C.; Alcaraz, P.E.; Carlos-Vivas, J. Physical Exercises for Preventing Injuries among Adult Male Football Players: A Systematic Review. *J. Sport Health Sci.* **2022**, *11*, 115–122. [CrossRef] [PubMed]
26. Andreoli, C.V.; Chiaramonti, B.C.; Buriel, E.; Pochini, A.D.C.; Ejnisman, B.; Cohen, M. Epidemiology of Sports Injuries in Basketball: Integrative Systematic Review. *BMJ Open Sport Exerc. Med.* **2018**, *4*, e000468. [CrossRef] [PubMed]

27. Wanivenhaus, F.; Fox, A.J.S.; Chaudhury, S.; Rodeo, S.A. Epidemiology of Injuries and Prevention Strategies in Competitive Swimmers. *Sports Health* **2012**, *4*, 246. [CrossRef] [PubMed]
28. Haeberle, H.S.; Navarro, S.M.; Power, E.J.; Schickendantz, M.S.; Farrow, L.D.; Ramkumar, P.N. Prevalence and Epidemiology of Injuries Among Elite Cyclists in the Tour de France. *Orthop. J. Sports Med.* **2018**, *6*, 1–5. [CrossRef] [PubMed]
29. Videbæk, S.; Bueno, A.M.; Nielsen, R.O.; Rasmussen, S. Incidence of Running-Related Injuries Per 1000 h of Running in Different Types of Runners: A Systematic Review and Meta-Analysis. *Sports Med.* **2015**, *45*, 1017–1026. [CrossRef] [PubMed]
30. McKay, A.K.A.; Stellingwerff, T.; Smith, E.S.; Martin, D.T.; Mujika, I.; Goosey-Tolfrey, V.L.; Sheppard, J.; Burke, L.M. Defining Training and Performance Caliber: A Participant Classification Framework. *Int. J. Sports Physiol. Perform.* **2022**, *17*, 317–331. [CrossRef] [PubMed]
31. Timpka, T.; Jacobsson, J.; Bickenbach, J.; Finch, C.F.; Ekberg, J.; Nordenfelt, L. What Is a Sports Injury? *Sports Med.* **2014**, *44*, 423–428. [CrossRef]
32. Issurin, V.B. Benefits and Limitations of Block Periodized Training Approaches to Athletes' Preparation: A Review. *Sports Med.* **2016**, *46*, 329–338. [CrossRef] [PubMed]
33. Llanos-Lagos, C.; Ramirez-Campillo, R.; Moran, J.; Sáez de Villarreal, E. Effect of Strength Training Programs in Middle- and Long-Distance Runners' Economy at Different Running Speeds: A Systematic Review with Meta-Analysis. *Sports Med.* **2024**, *54*, 895–932. [CrossRef]
34. Jidovtseff, B.; Harris, N.K.; Crielaard, J.M.; Cronin, J.B. Using the Load-Velocity Relationship for 1RM Prediction. *J. Strength Cond. Res.* **2011**, *25*, 267–270. [CrossRef]
35. Lum, D.; Comfort, P.; Barbosa, T.M.; Balasekaran, G. Comparing the Effects of Plyometric and Isometric Strength Training on Dynamic and Isometric Force-Time Characteristics. *Biol. Sport* **2022**, *39*, 189. [CrossRef]
36. Baxter, J.R.; Corrigan, P.; Hullfish, T.J.; O'Rourke, P.; Silbernagel, K.G. Exercise Progression to Incrementally Load the Achilles Tendon. *Med. Sci. Sports Exerc.* **2021**, *53*, 124–130. [CrossRef]
37. Riscart-López, J.; Rendeiro-Pinho, G.; Mil-Homens, P.; Soares-Dacosta, R.; Loturco, I.; Pareja-Blanco, F.; León-Prados, J.A. Effects of Four Different Velocity-Based Training Programming Models on Strength Gains and Physical Performance. *J. Strength Cond. Res.* **2021**, *35*, 596–603. [CrossRef] [PubMed]
38. Doma, K.; Deakin, G.B.; Schumann, M.; Bentley, D.J. Training Considerations for Optimising Endurance Development: An Alternate Concurrent Training Perspective. *Sports Med.* **2019**, *49*, 669–682. [CrossRef] [PubMed]
39. Ji, S.; Donath, L.; Wahl, P. Effects of Alternating Unilateral vs. Bilateral Resistance Training on Sprint and Endurance Cycling Performance in Trained Endurance Athletes: A 3-Armed, Randomized, Controlled, Pilot Trial. *J. Strength Cond. Res.* **2022**, *36*, 3280–3289. [CrossRef]
40. Fitzpatrick, D.A.; Cimadoro, G.; Cleather, D.J. The Magical Horizontal Force Muscle? A Preliminary Study Examining the "Force-Vector" Theory. *Sports* **2019**, *7*, 30. [CrossRef]
41. Miller, A.E.J.; MacDougall, J.D.; Tarnopolsky, M.A.; Sale, D.G. Gender Differences in Strength and Muscle Fiber Characteristics. *Eur. J. Appl. Physiol. Occup. Physiol.* **1993**, *66*, 254–262. [CrossRef]
42. Cardona, C.; Cejuela, R.; Esteve, J. *Resistance Sports Training Manual*, 1st ed.; Editorial Princesa: Madrid, Spain, 2019.
43. Crunkhorn, M.L.; Toohey, L.A.; Charlton, P.; Drew, M.; Watson, K.; Etxebarria, N. Injury Incidence and Prevalence in Elite Short-Course Triathletes: A 4-Year Prospective Study. *Br. J. Sports Med.* **2024**, *58*, 470–476. [CrossRef]
44. Collins, K.; Wagner, M.; Peterson, K.; Storey, M. Overuse Injuries in Triathletes. *Am. J. Sports Med.* **1989**, *17*, 675–680. [CrossRef] [PubMed]
45. Lauersen, J.B.; Bertelsen, D.M.; Andersen, L.B. The Effectiveness of Exercise Interventions to Prevent Sports Injuries: A Systematic Review and Meta-Analysis of Randomised Controlled Trials. *Br. J. Sports Med.* **2014**, *48*, 871–877. [CrossRef]
46. Berryman, N.; Mujika, I.; Bosquet, L. Concurrent Training for Sports Performance: The 2 Sides of the Medal. *Int. J. Sports Physiol. Perform.* **2019**, *14*, 279–285. [CrossRef]
47. Pareja-Blanco, F.; Rodríguez-Rosell, D.; Sánchez-Medina, L.; Sanchis-Moysi, J.; Dorado, C.; Mora-Custodio, R.; Yáñez-García, J.M.; Morales-Alamo, D.; Pérez-Suárez, I.; Calbet, J.A.L.; et al. Effects of Velocity Loss during Resistance Training on Athletic Performance, Strength Gains and Muscle Adaptations. *Scand. J. Med. Sci. Sports* **2017**, *27*, 724–735. [CrossRef] [PubMed]
48. Burns, J.; Keenan, A.M.; Redmond, A.C. Factors Associated with Triathlon-Related Overuse Injuries. *J. Orthop. Sports Phys. Ther.* **2003**, *33*, 177–184. [CrossRef]
49. Bales, J.; Bales, K. Training on a Knife's Edge: How to Balance Triathlon Training to Prevent Overuse Injuries. *Sports Med. Arthrosc. Rev.* **2012**, *20*, 214–216. [CrossRef]
50. Gosling, C.M.R.; Donaldson, A.; Forbes, A.B.; Gabbe, B.J. The Perception of Injury Risk and Safety in Triathlon Competition: An Exploratory Focus Group Study. *Clin. J. Sport Med.* **2013**, *23*, 70–73. [CrossRef] [PubMed]
51. Daneshfar, A.; Petersen, C.J.; Gahreman, D.E. The Effect of 4 Weeks Motor Imagery Training on Simulated BMX Race Performance. *Int. J. Sport Exerc. Psychol.* **2022**, *20*, 644–660. [CrossRef]
52. Egermann, M.; Brocai, D.; Lill, C.A.; Schmitt, H. Analysis of Injuries in Long-Distance Triathletes. *Int. J. Sports Med.* **2003**, *24*, 271–276. [CrossRef] [PubMed]
53. Figueiredo, P.; Marques, E.A.; Lepers, R. Changes in Contributions of Swimming, Cycling, and Running Performances on Overall Triathlon Performance Over a 26-Year Period. *J. Strength Cond. Res.* **2016**, *30*, 2406–2415. [CrossRef]

54. Zech, A.; Hollander, K.; Junge, A.; Steib, S.; Groll, A.; Heiner, J.; Nowak, F.; Pfeiffer, D.; Rahlf, A.L. Sex Differences in Injury Rates in Team-Sport Athletes: A Systematic Review and Meta-Regression Analysis. *J. Sport Health Sci.* **2022**, *11*, 104–114. [CrossRef]
55. Hamilton, B.; Targett, S. Ironman Triathlon: Medical Considerations. In *Sports Injuries*; Springer: Berlin/Heidelberg, Germany, 2015; pp. 1–7. [CrossRef]

Disclaimer/Publisher's Note: The statements, opinions and data contained in all publications are solely those of the individual author(s) and contributor(s) and not of MDPI and/or the editor(s). MDPI and/or the editor(s) disclaim responsibility for any injury to people or property resulting from any ideas, methods, instructions or products referred to in the content.

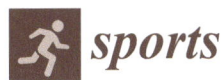

Article

Work, Training and Life Stress in ITU World Olympic Distance Age-Group Championship Triathletes

Veronica Vleck [1,*], Luís Miguel Massuça [2,3], Rodrigo de Moraes [3], João Henrique Falk Neto [4], Claudio Quagliarotti [5] and Maria Francesca Piacentini [5]

[1] CIPER, Faculdade de Motricidade Humana, Universidade de Lisboa, Cruz Quebrada, 1499-002 Lisbon, Portugal
[2] ICPOL, Instituto Superior de Ciências Policiais e Segurança Interna, 1300-663 Lisbon, Portugal; luis.massuca@gmail.com
[3] CIDEFES, Universidade Lusófona, 1749-024 Lisbon, Portugal; rodrigodemoraes2@gmail.com
[4] Athlete Health Lab., Faculty of Kinesiology, Sport and Recreation, University of Alberta, Edmonton, AB T6G 2R3, Canada; falkneto@ualberta.ca
[5] Department of Movement, Human and Health Sciences, University of Rome 'Foro Italico', 00135 Rome, Italy; claudruns@hotmail.it (C.Q.); mariafrancesca.piacentini@uniroma4.it (M.F.P.)
* Correspondence: vvleck@fmh.ulisboa.pt

Citation: Vleck, V.; Massuça, L.M.; de Moraes, R.; Falk Neto, J.H.; Quagliarotti, C.; Piacentini, M.F. Work, Training and Life Stress in ITU World Olympic Distance Age-Group Championship Triathletes. *Sports* 2023, *11*, 233. https://doi.org/10.3390/sports11120233

Academic Editors: G. Gregory Haff and Jon Oliver

Received: 4 April 2023
Revised: 25 May 2023
Accepted: 7 August 2023
Published: 24 November 2023

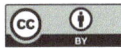

Copyright: © 2023 by the authors. Licensee MDPI, Basel, Switzerland. This article is an open access article distributed under the terms and conditions of the Creative Commons Attribution (CC BY) license (https://creativecommons.org/licenses/by/4.0/).

Abstract: We assessed the training, work and Life Stress demands of a mixed gender group of 48 top amateur short-distance triathletes using an online retrospective epidemiological survey and the Life Events Survey for Collegiate Athletes. On superficial inspection, these mainly masters athletes appeared to undergo all the types of training that are recommended for the aging athlete. However, there were significant scheduling differences between their weekday vs. their weekend training, suggesting that age-groupers' outside sports commitments may affect their training efficacy. The triathletes claimed to periodize, to obtain feedback on and to modify their training plans when appropriate—and some evidence of this was obtained. Over the year preceding the ITU World Age-Group Championships, they averaged 53%, 33% and 14% of their combined swim, cycle and run training time, respectively, within intensity zones 1, 2 and 3. Although the triathletes specifically stated that their training was focused on preparation for the ITU World Age-Group Championships, the way that they modified their training in the month before the event suggested that this aim was not necessarily achieved. Sports-related stress accounted for most—42.0 ± 26.7%—of their total Life Stress over the preceding year (vs. 12.7 ± 18.6% for Relationship-, 31.3 ± 25.9% for Personal- and 14.0 ± 21.1% for Career-related Stress). It affected most athletes, and was overwhelmingly negative, when it related to failure to attain athletic goal(s), to injury and/or to illness.

Keywords: Life Stress; polarization; monitoring; training efficacy; amateur triathlon

1. Introduction

The sport of triathlon involves sequential swimming, cycling and running under conditions that differ from those of its component single-sport events [1]. The triathlon swim, cycle and run are linked, within the same event, by (- in the case of a multi-lap swim- a possible swim–run–swim transition that by us is termed T0), a swim–bike transition (T1) and a bike–run (T2) transition. According to which of a range of possible distances are involved, triathlon competitions can be categorized as being either "short-distance" or "long-distance" events. Both types of event are competed in at either the "elite" level or at the "age-group" level [2,3]. Entry into elite-level competition is dependent on the individual athlete's national, regional and/or world ranking. In age-group competition, athletes compete against others who are within the same 5-year age band as themselves. Only short-distance triathlons, however, figure within the qualifying process for, and the actual, Olympic Games.

Millet, Bentley and Vleck [4] analyzed the evolution of the triathlon research literature from 1984 to 2006. They pointed out that the very fact of the triathlon becoming an Olympic sport had prompted researchers to investigate features (such as T2) that are specific to, and influence overall performance within, it. They also commented that coaches and athletes appeared to be benefiting from these studies, "first, because most of the leading scientists in the field have been athletes or coaches themselves... facilitating communication with their peers; second, (because), a good proportion of these studies have been conducted with national team athletes, and third, given the relative infancy of this sport and its multi-component nature, one might expect the empirical, field-based coaching knowledge to be more adaptable than in other endurance sports with a longer history and a more narrow range of skills". The same authors also highlighted the fact that triathlon can be, and indeed has been, used as a model to investigate the effects of both cross-training practice and training mode-specific adaptations. It is perhaps both surprising and unfortunate, therefore, that over the intervening 16 years since [4] was published, few additional data have emerged about how triathletes train. Moreover, much of the related physiology literature focuses on elites. It is not necessarily easy to directly apply what data have since been published to the improvement of the training practice of age-group triathletes in particular. Such age-group athletes actually make up the majority of the participants in the sport [5].

When it became an Olympic sport, the focus of elite short-distance triathlon training changed from non-drafting- to draft-legal- competition. Draft-legal triathlons have very different physiological demands from those of amateur triathlons. The latter have remained non-drafting [2,3,6,7]. The following quote, from Sperlich, Treff and Boone [8], could just as well apply to elite and amateur triathlons: they "display strikingly different characteristics related to metabolic stress (i.e., magnitude of aerobic and anaerobic energy contribution), biomechanical loading (...), psychological challenges (...), environmental factors, competition features (duration, pacing, drafting and format) and also the timing and duration of the competitive season. Therefore, the performance defining factors are specific to the discipline and to the season and as such will strongly affect the training characteristics".

Triathlon training can be characterized in terms of training intensity distribution (TID). This is the proportion of time that is spent within each of three training intensity zones [9], namely, zone 1, at or below the first ventilatory threshold ($<VT_1$); zone 2, between the first and the second ventilatory thresholds (VT_1-VT_2); and zone 3, at or beyond the second ventilatory threshold ($>VT_2$) [10]. A few studies of the training of highly performing elite, full-time, triathletes have been published (e.g., [11,12]). Such athletes appear, from these few data, to generally follow a polarized training model. They spend a high percentage of their training time within zone 1. They also spend greater percentages of their training time within zone 3 than they do within zone 2. This polarization may be combined with a pyramidal TID distribution, in which case a higher relative percentage of total training time is spent in zone 2. The actual percentages of training time that are spent in each zone will, of course, vary, depending on which part of the training year is involved. The problem is, as mentioned before, that these findings about elites essentially relate to "a different sport" within triathlon. They are also case studies. Case studies reflect personal coaching/athlete signatures rather than general or evidence-based practice. Not necessarily that much information can be gained from them as regards how to optimize *amateur* triathlon training practice. This is not least because the "off training stressors" of "full-time" (elite) and "part-time" (amateur) athletes will obviously differ. Such off training stressors can include training other than swimming, cycling and running, which themselves can considerably alter TID proportions [13]. There are also simply insufficient data in the current literature to allow for an informed judgement to be made on the extent to which the published training-related data for elite triathletes can be extrapolated to that of amateurs.

To date, the most detailed examination of triathlon training that relates its characteristics to *the extent of* ensuing maladaptation, in a *group* of short-distance specialists, that exists in the literature is *still* Vleck's 1996 longitudinal prospective study of British National Squad athletes. The study lasted seven months and was published in full in [14]. Importantly, the data collection for the study predated the funding injection into British triathlon that led to more of its athletes being able to both focus on the global race circuit and to "go full-time". As such, the research covered the preparation of amateur athletes for *non-drafting* National- and European Championship-level triathlon competition. This means that the training (and the TID) data that were obtained by the study likely more closely approximate those of the top age-groupers, as opposed to those of the professional triathletes, of today.

All of the subjects who took part in Vleck's study were top-50 finishers at their National Olympic distance (OD) Championships, either within the year of, or within the year prior to, the study. The athletes' (1.5/40/10 km) OD performance times are commensurate with, and still even perhaps slightly faster than, those that are currently achieved by (age-matched) top-level amateurs. The usual length of their competitive seasons and their training focus appear to be similar. That is, the training of both groups was built around National, Continental, (and then World) Championship level age-group competition. These facts underscore the potential interest of the data that were collected within Vleck's prospective study to those who are looking to optimize age-group training. However, Vleck's study purposely excluded athletes who were over 35 years old. Such "masters" triathletes are now of increasing research interest, for two reasons. Firstly, masters athletes account for the majority of amateur triathletes. Secondly, on superficial inspection, the multi-disciplinary endurance-based, high-intensity and resistance exercise training that is involved in preparing for a triathlon appears to comply with most, if not all, of the most recently published exercise guidelines for the aging athlete [15]. Applied research into the efficacy of training practice in age-group masters-level triathletes thus provides an opportunity to explore the appropriateness of the aforesaid guidelines. Unfortunately, no training *and* maladaptation data of an equivalent depth and study duration to that which Vleck [14] obtained for under-35-year-olds exist for older triathletes who are preparing for non-drafting, OD triathlon competition. It is unclear, therefore, to what extent the training practice of such masters triathletes may actually be optimal.

Fairly recently, Falk Neto et al. [16] prospectively assessed the training and maladaptation of nine recreational triathletes. They did so over the 6 weeks that led up to, and for 2 weeks after, an OD triathlon that was a key event of the athletes' competitive season. Falk Neto et al. used the session rating of perceived exertion method to monitor their athletes' daily training load. They also administered the Daily Analysis of Life Demands, the Training Distress Scale and the Alberta Swim Fatigue and Health questionnaires to the athletes every week. They found no discernable pattern in the athletes' swim, bike and run training load within the five weeks leading up to the race. They also reported high variability in training load over the entire study duration. The triathletes spent an average of 47% of their training time in zone 1. More than half of their training, i.e., 25% and 28% percent, respectively, was spent in zones 2 and 3. In only 2 out of the 8 weeks of the study was a greater amount of training time spent in zone 1 than was spent in zones 2 and 3 combined. The authors concluded that, with their "large spikes in training load and a high overall training intensity", their age-group sample had *not* apparently followed what is generally considered to be ideal endurance training practice [17]. Certainly, large spikes in training load have been linked to increased risk for injury and illness in triathletes. So, too, has combined, weighted, higher-intensity bike and run training [18,19]. However, although two out of the nine won their age-group, most of Falk Neto et al.'s subjects were neither particularly experienced, nor particularly successful, triathletes. The fact that their performance levels were heterogenous limits our capacity to make specific inferences about age-group triathlon training practice from their data. We do not know to what extent those athletes who compete at the *top* level of the amateur triathlon may exhibit similar (potential) "training mistakes". Given that qualification for the World Age-Group Championships is performance-based, being on the start list for it could be used as an appropriate subject selection criterion for such individuals.

We do note that Falk Neto's athletes did not manifest adverse effects from their apparent "departure" from general training guidelines. But, as the study was only 8 weeks long, this finding was not unexpected. The small number of study participants might also be why, out of all of those that were used, only the Alberta Swim Health Questionnaire flagged up symptoms of fatigue. The overall academic literature cannot be easily grouped into that which deals with elite vs. that which deals with age-group triathletes [14]. What it does say about the injury- and illness-related consequences, and the impact to general health, of triathlon training and racing was reviewed by [2,20,21], the consensus being that, as long as certain limits are respected, triathlon participation is fairly safe for the well-trained athlete [22]. However, said academic literature has barely examined the *psychological* effects of triathlon participation [23]. Emerging evidence also suggests that in amateurs, this effect is largely positive. Parsons-Smith et al. [24] observed, on the basis of the k-cluster of pre-performance scores, only 1.5% (out of a sample of 592) age-group triathletes to exhibit the "inverse Everest" profile—which is associated with elevated risk of psychopathology—on the Brunel Mood Scale. This 1.5% prevalence of the inverse Everest Profile in age-group triathletes is strikingly lower than the 5% prevalence of the general population. Even so, practically zero information exists in the academic literature on how the amateur triathlete's mental and physical health are influenced by lifestyle and morbidity factors, or vice versa.

We again draw the reader's attention to the fact that "age-groupers" are, by definition, not full-time triathletes. How the best age-groupers manage to fit training around their professional and other non-sports-related commitments is unclear. This issue is important because it will clearly have an impact on training quality. The relative levels of sports, relationship, career and personal stress that top age-groupers experience [25] are also insufficiently investigated. We know that people who participate in swimming, cycling and running can exhibit lower levels of psychological distress scores than those who walk or do no physical activity [26]. We also know that difficulty in balancing their training and other life commitments may lead recreational triathletes to experience high levels of negative stress [27]. However, we do not know what the major contributors to this negative stress are in this athlete group, which of these risk factors are potentially the most easily modifiable, nor how such risk factors potentially interact with each other. For example, mainly club-based training may mean that older triathletes experience less social loneliness. But, if the training that is provided by it is not triathlon-specific and does not take training in all the individual triathlon disciplines into account, club-based activity may not have a wholly positive impact on injury risk. We also know little of the degree to which triathlon training efficacy is monitored by or in age-groupers [2,14]. Nor has the extent to which top amateurs exhibit training flexibility, and respond to changes in their circumstances by taking positive action to minimize the risk of subsequent training maladaptation, been examined. Logically, such issues are of research interest.

Therefore, we analyzed the work, training and racing habits, and associated Life Stress, of top age-group triathletes who were both on the start line of, and indicated that the main goal that they had focused their training towards was, International Triathlon Union (ITU) World Age-Group Championship-level, OD competition. Both because this was an exploratory study and to increase subject numbers, we used a retrospective study design. Such a design is less sensitive than the longitudinal prospective one that was implemented by [14,16]. However, the training volume and intensity distribution were, in this case, examined across successive training blocks, rather than across successive weeks, of the entire year leading up to the 2013 ITU World Age-Group Championships. Where possible, we looked for divergence from accepted "training norms". We also examined the data for the possible existence of/lack of relationships between potential "training"-related factors and failures. Our aim, in so doing, was to be able to suggest potential directions for future applied research into how to optimize training and maximize performance in age-group triathletes.

2. Materials and Methods

2.1. Subjects

Overall, 4348 athletes were registered to race in the 2013 ITU Triathlon World Elite and Age-Group Championships over the Team Relay, Sprint and Olympic Distance events. The event also included an Open race (i.e., one that did not require prior race performance-based qualification). Of the athletes who were on the Race Director's contact list, 602 gave their written informed consent and participated in a mostly retrospective epidemiological survey. They did so after having received an emailed request to that effect. Each subject who requested it was emailed a signed copy of a confirmation of data confidentiality form. He or she was then sent an individualized link to an online training, injury, illness and stress-related questionnaire. The survey opened for completion three days after the 2013 ITU World OD Age-Group Championships. It closed one month after the event.

This paper reports data for those age-group triathletes who were on the start list for the ITU World Championships who (i) specifically stated that their training over the previous year was focused on preparation for OD competition and (ii) answered the section of the online survey that dealt with their training intensity distribution over the previous year *in full*. They accounted for 48 out of the 602 athletes who had provided written informed consent to participate.

2.2. Survey Content

Both the survey and the study were approved to proceed, before the race took place, by the Institutional Ethics Committee of Faculdade de Motricidade Humana, University of Lisbon. The survey covered the athlete's medical history, sporting background, performance level, level of coaching support and training feedback, work commitments, the general structure of his/her training week, and his/her injury and illness history. Said questions were updated from, and built on the results of, previous research surveys that were conducted by the lead author. These investigations into triathlon training and maladaptation had been conducted successively over a period of approximately 30 years. They are listed within the bibliographies of [2,20,21]. The Life Events Stress for Collegiate Athletes (LESCA) [28] was included in the survey, with Professor Petrie's permission. Brief details of both are provided below.

2.2.1. Medical History

The athletes indicated whether they had personal/familial cardiovascular issues, a history of fainting/dizziness/loss of consciousness while/not while exercising, asthma/exercise-induced asthma, allergies and/or were suffering from serious illness/condition(s) that could affect the ability to exercise. They could also indicate which medication(s) they were on (if any) and why, if they chose to do so.

2.2.2. Sporting Background/Performance

The age-groupers indicated their years of training and racing experience in both triathlon and its component sports. Usual times over the previous year and over the most common triathlon race distances were also provided. The athletes differentiated between whether such times had been recorded for individual swim, cycle or run time trials, or within triathlon competition. The athletes confirmed which event(s) and category they raced in at the ITU World Championships. They provided self-assessments both of their individual prowess in each of triathlon's component disciplines (including both the swim–bike and the bike–run transitions) and of their current training status. These data were used, in conjunction with data from other sections of the survey, to assess the extent to which self-identified/potential weakness(es) (Sections 2.2.3–2.2.5) were being identified or not. They were also used to identify whether active action was subsequently being taken by the athletes to address their weaknesses.

2.2.3. Support and Commitments

The extent to which athletes trained with single-sport athletes and clubs, the type of coaching that they received and the extent to which their technique in each of the sections of a triathlon was usually analyzed were reported. We also asked about whether the athletes were in part/full time work/study or self-employed, about their average weekly number of working hours and whether (such) work was full-time or shift-based. Details (with session times) of how each athlete fitted swim, bike, run and weight training sessions around his/her work and other commitments were obtained. So, too, was information on the extent to which the athletes considered their training to be polarized, implemented goal setting, and modified their training as a result of failure(s) to attain their goals, injury and/or illness.

2.2.4. Training Duration, Frequency and Intensity Distribution

Moreover, for each of the so-called training phases (i.e., the Endurance Base-EB, Pre-Competition-PC, Competition-C, Taper-T and Off-Season-Off) of their training year, the athletes self-reported their usual weekly training durations and frequencies for swimming, swim–cycle training, cycling, cycle–run training, running, weight training and other sport/exercise modes. Weekly training durations and frequencies were also obtained for the types of sessions that Vleck's studies [14,18,20,29,30] have previously specifically examined with regards to their potential associated overuse injury risk (i.e., for swim–bike transition, "long bike", "hill reps bike", "speed work bike", bike–run transition, "other bike", "long run", "hill reps run", "speed work run" and "other run" sessions). For swimming, cycling and running training only, average weekly training times within each of five exercise intensity levels, of which level five was the highest [14,18], were also recorded for each training block. Details of how each such exercise intensity level related to various physiological markers, to the Borg CR-10 scale of perceived exertion and to the "talk scale" were provided to the athletes. The triathletes were also given examples of both the types of work to rest ratios that exercising within each intensity level would involve for swimming, cycling and running, and example training sessions for them (Table 1).

Table 1. The explanations of training intensity levels that were provided within the Vleck (2013) training and injury survey *.

	Training Intensity Level
1	Intensity: low, well under lactate threshold (LT), 60–70% HRmax. RPE easy, 1–3. Rest: little or none. Energy source: fats. Examples: Easy workouts/recovery sets, warm up/cool down.
2	Intensity: 1–2 mM below LT, 70–75% HRmax. Easy to moderate. RPE 2–4. Rests 05–15 s. Energy source: fats with marginal CHO. Examples: Swim long intervals with very short rests (3 × 800 m w/15 s, 5 × 400 m w/10 s, 12 × 200 m w/5 s), continuous swims. Bike: 1.5–3 h of continuous riding. Long, easy 1–2 h runs.
3	Level of exertion: moderate. RPE 4–6. Rest 10–30 s. Energy source: CHO with some fat. Examples: Swim long intervals with short rest (5 × 500 m w/20 s, 3 × 800 m w/20 s, 8 × 250 m w/15 s, 20 × 100 m w/10 s), continuous (1500–3000 m) swims. Bike: 30–90 min continuous riding. Straight brick sessions (bike: run). Short rest intervals, e.g., 2 × 20 min w/2 min, 3 × 12 min w/1 min, 4 × 8 min w/30 s. Run: 20–30 min continuous. Straight brick running.
4	Level of effort: moderate to hard maximal steady-state training. RPE 6–8. Rest 15–45 s. Energy source: CHO with marginal fat. Examples: Swim moderate intervals with moderate rest (12 × 100 m). Volume range usually 1000–2000 m. Bike brick intervals; moderate length intervals with moderate rest (6 × 5 min w/2 min, 3 × 8 min w/4 min, 8 × 3 min w/1 min); time trials (10–20 miles) and races. Run brick intervals; moderate length intervals with moderate rests (e.g., 5 × 3 min w/1.5 min, 4 × 4 min w/2 min, 3 × 8 min w/4 min, etc.), or races.
5	Level of effort: hard-maximal and near maximal quality training, speech impossible. RPE 9–10. Energy source: CHO. Work to rest ratio 1:2 to 1:4. Examples: Swim short reps with long rests (e.g., 10 × 50 m odd easy, even-FAST; 6 × 75 m building by 25's w/1 min, 12 × 25 m sprints leaving on 30 s), at or near maximum pace. Volume range usually 400–1000 m. Bike hill repeats using hills that take 2–3 min to climb at a fast sustained pace; or short intervals with long rests (8 × 1 min w/2 min, 12× 1.5 min w/1 min etc.). Run hill repeats (200–400 m length) or repeats with long rest (e.g., 8 × 400 w/2 min, 5 × 800 w/4 min or 12 × 200 w/1 min).

Key: CHO, carbohydrate; %HRmax, percentage of (sport-specific) maximum heart rate; LT, lactate threshold; m, metres; max, maximum; min, minutes; Mm, millimolar; reps, repetitions; RPE, rating of perceived exertion (10-point Borg scale); s, seconds; w/, with rest/recovery of. * More details of what the various intensity levels equated to were given in Vleck (2010)—where they were termed "L1, L2, L3 easy (extensive anaerobic threshold), L3 hard or intensive anaerobic threshold (i.e., 40 km bike and 5–10 km run race intensity), and Level 4 (intensity very high, 2–6 mM above LT)".

Said information was based, with permission, on previously published United States Olympic Committee athlete training guidelines for swimming, cycling and running. These guidelines are detailed in [14]. They had been cross-checked and their suitability for triathletes agreed to by three British National Triathlon Squad coaches before they were first used within Vleck's longitudinal study [14]. Training intensity levels 1 and 2 together, level 3, and levels 4 and 5 together were, for the purposes of this paper, classed as being synonymous with training intensity zone 1 (z1), with zone 2 (z2) and with zone 3 (z3), respectively. As such, they were thus considered to broadly correspond to the following exercise intensities: (i) $<VT_1$; (ii) VT_1-VT_2; and (iii) $>VT_2$, respectively. All the training duration-related data that were collected from the athletes were estimated to the nearest half hour. This was the case, whatever the specific session type that the information related to.

The athletes who took part in the survey originated from various countries around the globe. The ITU World Age-Group OD Championships took place in late September in London, England. This meant that the event did not necessarily fall within the competitive phase of the racing season of an individual athlete's country of residence. Therefore, each competitor also reported whether the month leading up to the World Championships fell within the Endurance-Base, Pre-Competition, Competition, Taper or Off-Season phase of his/her training year. They also reported whether and how their amount of recovery and number of races within said month differed from what was customary for them for that type of training phase. They gave the same information regarding their weekly training frequencies, total weekly training times and individual training session durations for each swim, cycle and run intensity level.

2.2.5. Life Stress

The athletes also completed "The Life Events Survey for Collegiate Athletes", or LESCA [28]. This survey was used with the author's permission. The LESCA has previously been shown to possess good content validity. It also provides a stable measure of Life Stress. Scores on the LESCA have also been shown to be a better predictor of athletic injury than those that are obtained from the Social and Athletic Readjustment Rating Scale [28]. The LESCA involves an 8-point Likert scale. This allows individuals to not only rate the degree of stress (from 1 to 4, that is, from minor to major), but also the type of stress impact (i.e., beneficial/positive or detrimental/negative) that has been experienced by them over the previous year.

Three different Life Stress scores were obtained from the athletes' ratings on the LESCA. Negative Life Stress and Positive Life Stress scores were derived by summing the impact scores of those events that were rated as undesirable (negative) and desirable (positive), respectively. A Total Life Stress score was obtained by adding the absolute values of the negative and positive scores. Total, positive and negative stress values were also calculated for the following sub-components of Life Stress variables: (i) Sport; (ii) Relationship; (iii) Career; and (iv) Personal Stress. These were derived from the scores from questions whose original number in Petrie's LESCA paper were as follows (i) for Sport Stress: 15–16, 24, 33–35, 42, 44–57, 63–64 and 67; (ii) for Relationship Stress: 1, 8–10, 12–14, 17–18, 29–31, 39–40 and 60; (iii) for Career Stress: 11, 19, 21, 23, 25, 32, 58 and 61–62; and (iv) for Personal Stress: 2–7, 20, 27–28, 36, 38, 40–41, 43 and 66–68.

2.2.6. Injury and Illness

Finally, injury and illness data both for the year and for the month prior to completion of the survey were obtained. This was in addition to the reporting of injury and/or illness that occurred *at* the World Championships. The definitions and methods of data collection for the online survey-based injury-related data were those that have been consistently implemented by Vleck [14,18,20,29,30], as reviewed by Vleck and Hoeden [20]. They included details of the anatomical location, the severity and the recurrence of both overuse and traumatic injury. The survey explicitly stated that "here an injury is defined as any musculoskeletal problem that caused you to stop training for at least one day, reduce mileage, take medicine or seek medical aid. Traumatic injuries are those caused by hazard encounters such as hitting a car or falling off your bike and overuse injuries are those that you would consider to have been caused by repetitive strain. The following definitions of severity also apply, both for injury and for illness: Minor: '1–4 days lost', Moderate: '5–14 days lost', Severe: '15 or more days lost', Out of season: resulted in your entire season being affected, regardless of where the injury or illness occurred in the season. Recurring injury: an injury that occurs more than once, with an interval of at least 7 days between successive recurrences." Where, when and why the injury or illness was considered by the athlete to occur were also noted. Details of the degree, timing and type of clinical/non-clinical support for injury and/or illness that was sought/obtained by each individual, both during and after the ITU World Championships, were collected. Medical tent/team-based clinical injury and illness data were also collected over the duration of the ITU World Championships. None of the athletes who featured in this particular analysis presented for such clinical assistance. Therefore, no such clinically diagnosed on-site injury/illness data were available for this specific paper.

During the data collection period and for each of the above-named individual survey sections, the athletes were encouraged to add personal comments/explanations of their replies. They did so extensively. The athletes were also encouraged to request clarification from the lead author where necessary.

2.3. Statistical Analysis

The level of coaching specificity that the athletes received was compared between the three triathlon disciplines using the Chi-squared test. All the training data that were obtained were scatter-plotted. In almost no cases were the athletes' training data normally distributed. Levene's test for homogeneity of variance was conducted before any demographic data were compared.

With regards to the analysis of the athletes' "work sports balance", (i) the Wilcoxon signed-rank test was used to study the differences between weekday vs. weekend training, and (ii) the Friedman two-way analysis of variance by ranks was used to examine the differences between swim vs. bike vs. run vs. weights vs. other, the differences in the weekly training frequency and training time by exercise mode (i.e., swim vs. swim–bike vs. bike vs. bike–run vs. run vs. weights vs. other) and by training block (i.e., EB vs. PC vs. C vs. T vs. Off) and the differences in the (frequency and training time per mode related) details of the athletes' swim, bike and run training sessions. Where significant differences were revealed by the Friedman test, a post hoc test with Bonferroni correction was then used to identify which specific training data pairs differed from each other.

In order to identify whether the training durations within each of the five exercise intensity zones varied significantly from each other during each phase of the periodization, Friedman's two-way analysis of variance by ranks and post hoc tests with Bonferroni corrections were again used. The same tests were used to check whether there were significant differences in time, or in percentage of time, in each training intensity, between the five phases of the training year (i.e., EB, PC, C, T and Off).

Student's *t*-test for independent variables was also used to check for significant differences between the time spent at each level of training intensity, for each type of training block, of the 10 fastest and the 10 slowest performers in the World Age-Group Championships in the group.

The 'Statistics Package for the Social Sciences' (SPSS, High Wycombe, UK), version 28.0, was used throughout the analyses. We set the 95% confidence limit as the level of statistical significance. Given the large number of analyses that were involved in the preparation of this paper, and in the interests of decluttering, some statistical data have been omitted from its training data-related Tables and Figures. In such cases, the data that *are* provided in this paper are given in exactly the same format (i.e., as means ± standard deviation SD) as they have been provided in the majority of the triathlon literature. This allows for direct comparisons to be made between the data in this paper and those from the previously published studies that employed an identical data collection methodology (as reported within [14,29,30]). The relevant median, interquartile ratio, mean rank data, etc. are available from the first author.

3. Results

3.1. Subject Characteristics

Forty-eight age-groupers, competing at ITU World OD Age-Group Championship level, fulfilled the subject criterion for this study. These 21 males and 27 females were spread across the age-groups from 20–24 up to 65–69 years old (Table 2). Overall, 68.7% of the study participants were 35 years of age or older.

Table 2. Age-groups and gender distribution of the study subjects.

Age-Group	20–24	25–29	30–34	35–39	40–44	45–49	50–54	55–59	60–64	65–69
N (of whom M)	2 (1)	5 (2)	8 (3)	5 (3)	3 (2)	4 (1)	7 (3)	6 (3)	4 (2)	4 (1)

Key: N, number; M, males.

The athletes possessed an average training and (in brackets) racing background of (mean ± SD) 10.2 ± 6.2 (9.0 ± 6.2) years in triathlon, 13.3 ± 7.2 (9.6 ± 7.9) years in swimming, 10.6 ± 5.8 (6.5 ± 5.9) years in cycling, 18.9 ± 8.0 (16.2 ± 7.5) years in athletics and 16.0 ± 7.4 (13.7 ± 7.2) years in other sports. They placed from 2nd to 122th (averaging 36.5 ± 26.9 th) within their respective age-groups at the 2013 ITU World Age-Group Championships. Their average times for Olympic distance triathlon competition were 2:13:25 ± 0:16:07 (1:58:55–3:00:00) hh:mm:ss for the males and 2:32:57 ± 18:26:46 (2:11:56–3:18:00) hh:mm:ss for the females. Detailed (single-sport time trial, as well as triathlon-specific) performance-related data for each age-group that was represented in this study are also available from the first author on request. So are self-assessed rankings of each of the individual athlete's relative swim, swim–bike transition, bike, bike–run transition and running ability within triathlon competition.

3.2. Training Support

Almost half of the athletes in the group (47.9%) were regularly training with single-sport specialists. Those who sometimes did so and those who never did so accounted for 31.3% and 20.8%, respectively, of these top age-groupers. The type of coaching that the athletes received differed between the three triathlon disciplines. More often than not, the athletes received club-based coaching (Table 3). More athletes were swimming club or triathlon club members (50.0% and 58.3%) than were members of cycling or athletics clubs (27.1% and 25.0%), other clubs (6.3%) or not in any sports club (10.4%). In only approximately a third of cases, whatever the exercise mode, did the athlete consider his/her club-based coaching to be triathlon-specific. Of the athletes who were coached, other than self-coached, and whose coaching was geared towards triathlon: 27.1% had the same coach overseeing their training for all three triathlon disciplines "all the time"; 20.1% had it for "most of the time"; 12.5% had it "sometimes"; and 25.0% "never" received that level of support.

Table 3. Coaching and its specificity—% of athletes *.

Type of Coaching	Swim	Bike	Run
None	4.2	14.6	10.4
Self-coached	16.7	31.3	25.0
Club-based coaching	39.6	18.8	29.2
Internet-based coaching	6.3	4.2	4.2
Other type of coaching	33.3	-	-
Triathlon specific	37.5	37.5	35.4
Single-sport specific	18.8	6.3	8.3

* The level of coaching specificity that the athletes received was shown to be significantly associated, at the $p < 0.01$ level, with which of the three triathlon disciplines it was being provided within, by the Chi-squared test. Key: -, no reply.

Almost all (95.8%) of the group indicated that they had "set goals" for the 2013 season. In all such cases, these goals were specifically stated to have been to beat a specific competition time, to qualify for the World Championships, to compete in the World Championships or a combination of the aforesaid goals. Seventy-eight percent of individuals also indicated that they had a periodized training plan for the season. This plan had been worked out either by themselves or together with their coach, and was based around their aforementioned goals.

3.3. Life–Sports Balance and Load

3.3.1. Balance between Training and outside Sports Commitments

For the majority (62.5%) of the athletes, their training plan was built around working at a full-time job. Just over a third (31.3%) of the group were part-time workers, and 8.3% were self-employed. Half of the triathletes worked fixed hours, while 12.0% did shift work. On top of working/studying 7.6 ± 2.5 h per day, these top age-groupers trained 1.7 ± 0.5 (min–max, 0.57–3.0) times every day. They did so irrespective of whether the day in question was a weekday or fell over a weekend. We did not assess time spent looking after family members (and children, in particular) within the survey. Nonetheless, some athletes commented that had it not been possible to share such responsibilities with a partner, they would potentially have had a detrimental impact on their training. The athletes' training schedules were fairly variable, but were clearly influenced by their weekday commitments. Both the proportion of their total number of weekly training sessions that were planned within it and the type and the timing of said sessions differed between weekday- and weekend-based training (Table 4).

Table 4. The scheduling of "working week" vs. weekend-based training in top short-distance amateur triathletes (mean ± SD).

		Swim (S)	Bike (B)	Run (R)	Weights (W)	Other (O)
		\multicolumn{5}{c}{During the Week}				
Sessions (over 5 days) [a]		2.7 ± 1.0 ***	2.1 ± 1.3 ***	2.2 ± 1.1 ***	1.0 ± 1.3 ***	0.3 ± 0.6 *
As % of within week total	Before 9 a.m.	29.8 ± 38.9	28.7 ± 41.3	22.0 ± 38.4	16.7 ± 35.4	16.7 ± 35.4
	9 a.m.–12 p.m.	14.3 ± 32.0 ***	16.9 ± 32.4 ***	12.0 ± 29.9	25.9 ± 43.4	25.9 ± 43.4
	12 p.m.–3 p.m.	6.2 ± 15.7	15.2 ± 28.1	12.0 ± 29.9	3.7 ± 11.1	3.7 ± 11.1
	3 p.m.–6 p.m.	21.4 ± 31.9 ***	16.9 ± 34.0 *	30.7 ± 46.1	15.0 ± 33.7	15.0 ± 33.7
	6 p.m.–10 p.m.	28.4 ± 34.4	27.7 ± 42.5 ***	24.0 ± 41.1	37.0 ± 48.4	37.0 ± 48.4
		\multicolumn{5}{c}{At Weekends}				
		Swim (S)	Bike (B)	Run (R)	Weights (W)	Other (O)
Sessions (over 2 days) [b]		0.4 ± 0.6	1.3 ± 0.7	1.3 ± 0.8	0.1 ± 0.3	0.0 ± 0.3
as % of weekly total		11.3 ± 19.8	44.6 ± 26.0	36.9 ± 19.3	9.3 ± 22.9	10.0 ± 31.6
As % of weekend total	Before 9 a.m.	48.9 ± 50.2	34.4 ± 46.2	28.4 ± 43.9	0	0
	9 a.m.–12 p.m.	17.8 ± 37.5	51.5 ± 48.3	50.9 ± 48.2	0	0
	12 p.m.–3 p.m.	26.7 ± 45.8	8.5 ± 24.0	14.9 ± 31.7	60.0 ± 54.8	0
	3 p.m.–6 p.m.	6.7 ± 25.8	3.3 ± 16.5	3.5 ± 12.9	40.0 ± 54.8	100
	6 p.m.–10 p.m.	0	0	2.3 ± 15.2	0	0

Note (statistics): Wilcoxon test (week vs. weekends): ***, $p < 0.001$; *, $p < 0.05$. Friedman's test (swim vs. bike vs. run vs. weights vs. other): [a], $X^2(4) = 103.084$, $p < 0.001$, N = 47; [b], $X^2(4) = 131.649$, $p < 0.001$, N = 47. Post hoc tests, after Bonferroni correction, significant at $p < 0.001$, during the week, for S-W, S-O, B-W, B-O, R-W, R-O, and during the weekend, for S-B, S-R, B-W, B-O, R-W, R-O.

Over 88% of the athletes' 3.1 ± 1.1 scheduled weekly swim training sessions took place within the working week. A total of 52% of them were fitted in before 0900 h, and 28.3% of them took place between 1800 and 2200 h. That is, the majority of the swims were performed before or after what are usually considered to be normal working hours. During weekends, no one reported swimming within the 1800–2200 h slot. The situation as regards the usual timing of the athletes' 3.4 ± 1.2 weekly bike training sessions was less clear-cut. Over half of them were performed during the week. Most (45.8%) of the athletes did none of their within-week bike training sessions before 9 am. Less than a third (27.1%) did between a third and half of such sessions before 9 am. Only 12.5% did all of their weekday bike training before 9 am. Those who did none, 1/3–1/2 and all of their "work week" bike sessions between 0900 h and midday accounted for 41.7%, 16.8% and 10.4% of the group, respectively. As for the "lunchtime" slot of between 1200 and 1500 h, 75% of the group did none and 8.4% did 1/3–1/2 of their weekday bike sessions in it. Between 1500 and 1800 h, 18.9% of the athletes did 1/3–1/2 of their bike sessions, but 66.7% of them did none of them. In total, 54 %, 41.9% and 10.4% of athletes, respectively, did none, 1/3–1/2 and 25% of their weekday sessions after normal working hours, i.e., between 1800 and 2200 h. Within weekends, the way the athletes' cycle training was scheduled changed. A far larger proportion of this training was performed before midday than occurred during the week. As for running training, the athletes' normal training plan involved 3.6 ± 1.6 such sessions per week. Of these runs, 2.2 ± 1.1 were carried out over the Monday–Friday period. A further 1.3 ± 0.8 runs were performed over the weekend. Of the five weekday run "time-slots" that we assessed, the one that accounted for the largest proportion of scheduled runs was the one before 0900 h. In fact, 18.8% and 14.7% of athletes did all or between 40% and 66%, respectively, of their weekday runs before 9 am. Overall, 25% of the group did between 25% and all of such runs between 1200 and 1500 h, 20.9% did between a third and all of them between 1500 and 1800 h, and 38.9% did between a quarter and all of them between 1800 and 2200 h. Then, again, the way that scheduling of this training occurred changed during the weekends. Finally, the athletes' weight training sessions, of which 1.1 ± 1.4 were normally scheduled per week, were also mostly performed during the working week. This swimming, biking, running and weight training was not all the training that the athletes were doing, however. The triathletes reported themselves to also be normally doing 0.3 ± 0.7 weekly training sessions in other sports.

3.3.2. Training and Racing Load

The athletes competed in an average of 3.2 ± 4.4 (range 25) 5 km runs, 1.0 ± 1.2 (range 5) 10 km runs, 0.7 ± 1.0 (range 4) half marathons and 0.2 ± 0.5 (range 2) marathons over the year leading up to the World Championships. They also took part in 1.4 ± 2.0 (range 9) 10-mile cycle time-trials and 0.9 ± 1.9 (range 10) 40 km cycle time trials. On average, they competed in 2.3 ± 2.2 (range 9) Sprint distance triathlons, 3.5 ± 1.7 (range 8) Olympic distance triathlons, 0.1 ± 02 (range 1) middle-distance triathlons, 0.1 ± 0.4 (range 1) Half Ironman distance triathlons and no Ironman distance triathlons. The time that the athletes estimated that they had spent racing over the same year was calculated as 17.5 ± 7.0 h on average (min–max, 5.5–35.5). The latter value was arrived at when what were presumably rogue values that were given by 4 athletes (of 532, 600–650, 550–600 and 20 h racing per week over 12 months) were ignored.

Table 5. Weekly training frequencies and total training time in h (mean, SD), by training phase.

		EB	PC	C	T	Off
Swim (S)	Frequency	3.6 ± 1.2	3.9 ± 1.1	3.9 ± 0.9	3.2 ± 0.9	2.9 ± 1.1
	Total time (h)	6.6 ± 3.7	7.0 ± 3.6	6.7 ± 3.2	4.9 ± 2.5	4.8 ± 3.1
Swim–Bike (SB)	Frequency	1.2 ± 0.5	1.6 ± 0.9	1.6 ± 0.6	1.4 ± 0.6	1.0 ± 0.2
	Total time (h)	1.2 ± 1.3	1.7 ± 1.9	1.9 ± 1.7	1.2 ± 1.1	1.3 ± 1.5
Bike (B)	Frequency	3.6 ± 0.9	4.0 ± 1.1	4.1 ± 1.1	3.4 ± 1.0	2.9 ± 1.3
	Total time (h)	9.9 ± 4.6	10.5 ± 5.0	10.1 ± 4.8	6.8 ± 3.7	6.8 ± 4.4
Bike–Run (BR)	Frequency	1.7 ± 0.8	2.2 ± 0.9	2.3 ± 0.8	1.8 ± 0.8	1.2 ± 0.5
	Total time (h)	2.4 ± 2.3	3.4 ± 3.1	3.6 ± 2.9	2.3 ± 2.2	0.9 ± 0.8
Run (R)	Frequency	4.2 ± 1.1	4.1 ± 1.1	4.1 ± 1.0	3.5 ± 1.1	3.6 ± 1.1
	Total time (h)	7.1 ± 3.2	7.0 ± 3.0	6.5 ± 2.9	4.8 ± 2.5	5.8 ± 2.8
Weights (W)	Frequency	2.4 ± 1.1	2.1 ± 1.1	4.7 ± 0.9	1.3 ± 0.6	2.1 ± 1.3
	Total time (h)	3.0 ± 2.4	2.6 ± 2.2	1.9 ± 1.5	1.5 ± 1.1	2.6 ± 2.3
Other (O)	Frequency	1.9 ± 1.3	1.6 ± 1.3	1.5 ± 1.3	1.4 ± 1.2	2.4 ± 1.6
	Total time (h)	2.4 ± 2.9	1.7 ± 1.8	1.5 ± 1.7	1.4 ± 1.7	2.8 ± 2.8

Key: EB, Endurance Base; PC, Pre-Competition; C, Competition; T, taper; Off, Off-Season; freq, frequency.

Statistics related footnote to Table 5 (Friedman's test)[a]: (i) Differences in total training time—h-per mode (i.e., swim vs. swim–bike vs. bike vs. bike–run vs. run vs. weights vs. other): EB, $X^2(6) = 186.583$, $p < 0.001$, N = 48; PC, $X^2(6) = 195.227$, $p < 0.001$, N = 48; C, $X^2(6) = 195.659$, $p < 0.001$, N = 48; T, $X^2(6) = 192.794$, $p < 0.001$, N = 48; Off, $X^2(6) = 143.654$, $p < 0.001$, N = 48; (ii) Differences in total training time—h-per training block (i.e., EB vs. PC vs. C vs. T vs. Off): Swim, $X^2(4) = 75.129$, $p < 0.001$, N = 48; Swim–Bike, $X^2(4) = 37.409$, $p < 0.001$, N = 48; Bike, $X^2(4) = 79.030$, $p < 0.001$, N = 48; Bike–Run, $X^2(4) = 71.583$, $p < 0.001$, N = 48; Run, $X^2(4) = 75.362$, $p < 0.001$, N = 48; Weights, $X^2(4) = 65.685$, $p < 0.001$, N = 48; Others, $X^2(4) = 39.307$, $p < 0.001$, N = 48; (iii) Differences in frequency: EB, $X^2(6) = 186.583$, $p < 0.001$, N = 48; PC, $X^2(6) = 195.227$, $p < 0.001$, N = 48; C, $X^2(6) = 195.659$, $p < 0.001$, N = 48; T, $X^2(6) = 192.794$, $p < 0.001$, N = 48; Off, $X^2(6) = 143.654$, $p < 0.001$, N = 48. Post hoc tests, EB vs. C, for time: *** BR; for freq: *** BR, W; * SB; for EB vs. T, for time: *** S, SB, B, R; for freq: *** SB, BR; for EB vs. Off, for time: *** S, B, * BR, R; for PC vs. T, for time: *** S, B, R, * BR; for freq: *** SB; for PC vs. Off, for time: *** S, B, BR, R, for freq: *** BR, W; for C vs. T, for time: ** S, B, BR, R; for C vs. Off, for time: *** S, B, BR, * SB; for freq: *** BR, * R, for freq:, *** W; for T vs. Off, for time: *** R; for freq: *** BR, * W. *** $p < 0.01$, ** $p < 0.02$, $p < 0.05$. [a] Significance values were adjusted by Bonferroni correction.

What these top OD age-groupers considered to be their own normal training, per 7-day week, is presented in Table 5 (above). A more detailed breakdown of their training frequency data is shown in Table 6. The aforesaid data are expressed in terms of swim, bike and run "speed", "long", "hill rep" sessions, etc. (as per [15,29,30]). Details of the athletes' weight training are also provided in the same Table. The male and female training-related data are not reported separately because a prior analysis of 124 (Sprint, OD and team relay) age-group competitors who were competing at the same ITU World Championships [31] did not reveal any notable differences in training practice between the two genders.

Table 6. Swim, bike and run training weekly session frequency and total time (h): details (mean ± SD).

Variable			EB	PC	C	T	Off
Swim-Bike Transition (T1)		Frequency	1.2 ± 0.7	1.4 ± 0.7	1.5 ± 0.8	1.3 ± 0.6	1.1 ± 0.4
		Total time (h)	1.1 ± 0.3	1.5 ± 0.9	1.6 ± 0.9	1.4 ± 0.8	1.0 ± 0.0
Long Bike (LB)		Frequency	2.3 ± 0.7	2.2 ± 0.6	2.1 ± 0.7	1.3 ± 0.4	1.7 ± 0.8
		Total time (h)	7.1 ± 3.0	6.6 ± 3.2	5.3 ± 2.7	2.8 ± 2.2	4.5 ± 3.1
Hill Reps Bike (HRB)		Frequency	1.5 ± 0.6	1.7 ± 0.6	1.7 ± 0.6	1.2 ± 0.4	1.2 ± 0.4
		Total time (h)	2.0 ± 1.3	2.6 ± 1.3	2.5 ± 1.4	1.4 ± 0.9	1.3 ± 0.7
Speed Work Bike (SWB)	Field	Frequency	1.3 ± 0.5	1.8 ± 0.6	2.0 ± 0.7	1.7 ± 0.6	1.1 ± 0.4
	T/T	Frequency	1.8 ± 0.7	1.6 ± 0.6	1.4 ± 0.5	1.3 ± 0.5	1.4 ± 0.6
	Both	Total time (h)	2.5 ± 1.5	3.5 ± 1.4	3.7 ± 1.6	2.7 ± 1.2	1.8 ± 1.2
Bike–Run Transition (T2)		Frequency	1.4 ± 0.6	1.8 ± 0.9	1.9 ± 0.8	1.7 ± 0.9	1.0 ± 0.2
		Total time (h)	1.6 ± 1.1	2.2 ± 1.5	2.5 ± 1.4	1.9 ± 1.1	1.1 ± 0.4
Other Bike (OB)		Frequency	1.6 ± 0.7	1.7 ± 1.0	1.7 ± 1.0	1.6 ± 0.7	1.9 ± 0.9
		Total time (h)	3.0 ± 2.7	2.8 ± 2.6	2.8 ± 2.6	2.4 ± 2.1	2.9 ± 2.3
Long Run (LR)		Frequency	2.1 ± 0.5	2.0 ± 0.6	1.8 ± 0.8	1.3 ± 0.5	1.8 ± 1.0
		Total time (h)	4.7 ± 2.0	4.1 ± 2.3	3.6 ± 3.0	2.0 ± 1.2	3.3 ± 1.9
Hill Reps Run (HRR)		Frequency	1.5 ± 0.5	1.5 ± 0.6	1.4 ± 0.5	1.1 ± 0.3	1.2 ± 0.5
		Total time (h)	1.8 ± 1.1	2.0 ± 1.1	1.7 ± 1.0	1.3 ± 0.8	1.5 ± 1.0
Speed Work Run (SWR)		Frequency	1.9 ± 0.7	2.2 ± 0.6	2.3 ± 0.6	1.9 ± 0.6	1.5 ± 0.6
		Total time (h)	2.5 ± 1.3	3.2 ± 1.5	3.5 ± 1.5	2.4 ± 1.0	1.6 ± 0.9
Other Run (OR)		Frequency	2.0 ± 1.2	1.9 ± 1.2	1.8 ± 1.1	1.8 ± 1.0	2.1 ± 1.2
		Total time (h)	3.3 ± 2.7	3.2 ± 2.5	3.1 ± 2.5	2.7 ± 2.2	3.0 ± 2.4

Key: EB, Endurance Base; PC, Pre-Competition; C, Competition; T, Taper; Off, Off-Season; T/T, turbo trainer; total time (in h, not hh:mm, because the question only asked for data to the nearest half hour).

Statistics related footnote to Table 6 (Friedman's test, note that not all the athletes provided these data in full) [a]: Differences between time used in training modes during training blocks, i.e., (i) EB, $X2(9) = 115.666$, $p < 0.001$, $N = 26$; PC, $X2(9) = 89.839$, $p < 0.001$, $N = 26$; C, $X2(9) = 78.428$, $p < 0.001$, $N = 26$; T, $X2(9) = 45.654$, $p < 0.001$, $N = 25$; Off, $X2(9) = 75.545$, $p < 0.001$, $N = 26$; and (ii) frequency: EB, $X2(10) = 85.772$, $p < 0.001$, $N = 33$; PC, $X2(10) = 58.160$, $p < 0.001$, $N = 32$; C, $X2(10) = 63.225$, $p < 0.001$, $N = 31$; T, $X2(10) = 64.605$, $p < 0.001$, $N = 32$; Off, $X2(10) = 78.405$, $p < 0.001$, $N = 31$. Post hoc tests, EB vs. PC: for freq: *** SWB, * for field SWB, for time: * both SWB; for EB vs. C, for freq: *** SWB, ** T2; for time: *** T2; for EB vs. T, for freq: *** LB, LR; ** HRR; for time: *** LB, LR; for EB vs. Off, for both time and freq: *** LB; for PC vs. T, for freq: *** LB, HRB, LR; for time: *** LB, HRB, both SWB, LR, SWR; for PC vs. off, for time: *** LB, HRB, both SWB, T2, SWR; for freq: *** field SWB, T2, SWR; for PC vs. Off, for time: *** LB, HRB, SWR, * LR; for freq: *** LB, HRB; for C vs. Off, for time: *** both SWB, SWR; ** T1; for freq *** field SWB, T2, SWR, ** HRB; for T vs. Off, for time, *** LR; * T2; for freq *** field SWB, T2, ** LR. ***, $p < 0.01$, ** $p < 0.02$, * $p < 0.05$. [a] Significance values were adjusted by Bonferroni correction.

3.3.3. Changes in Training Intensity across the Training Year

The overall average weekly total (swim, bike and run) training time that was spent within each of the three training intensity zones z1–3 changed with the training phase (z1, $F(4,239) = 3.478$, $p = 0.009$; z2, $F(4,239) = 9.222$, $p < 0.001$; z3, $F(4,239) = 16.163$, $p < 0.001$) (Table 7 and Figures 1 and 2). Within the Endurance-Base, Pre-Competitive, Taper and Off-Season phases, the training time that was spent in z1 exceeded that spent within z2 and z3. Within the Competition phase, z2 was the training zone in which the highest proportion of swim training time was spent. Most of the triathletes' training time was spent cycling, regardless of what training macrocycle type or intensity zone they were in.

Table 7. Weekly self-reported usual training time in three intensity zones and five types of training blocks (mean hh:mm ± SD).

	Intensity Level (Zone in Brackets)			ANOVA		Post Hoc Test [a]		
	L1–2 (z1)	L3 (z2)	L4–5 (z3)	$F_{(2,143)}$	Sig.	z1–z2	z1–z3	z2–z3
				Endurance-Base				
Swim	1:30:37 ± 1:16:40	1:00:37 ± 0:44:24	0:30:37 ± 0:36:52	14.073	<0.001	0.027	<0.001	0.027
Bike	2:43:07 ± 2:05:45	1:28:07 ± 0:55:50	0:46:52 ± 0:54:58	22.784	<0.001	<0.001	<0.001	ns
Run	2:06:15 ± 1:11:53	1:05:37 ± 0:57:36	0:31:15 ± 0:29:39	14.943	<0.001	<0.001	<0.001	ns
Total	6:19:59 ± 4:34:18	3:34:21 ± 2:37:50	1:48:44 ± 2:01:29	27.969	<0.001	<0.001	<0.001	ns
				Pre-Competition				
Swim	1:08:45 ± 0:53:56	1:08:07 ± 0:36:59	0:55:37 ± 0:42:25	1.299	ns	ns	ns	ns
Bike	2:21:52 ± 1:56:33	1:51:52 ± 1:03:56	1:13:07 ± 0:49:28	8.502	<0.001	ns	<0.001	ns
Run	1:46:15 ± 1:03:24	1:11:15 ± 0:52:44	0:50:00 ± 0:35:43	6.136	0.003	0.009	0.009	ns
Total	5:16:52 ± 3:53:53	4:11:14 ± 2:33:39	2:58:44 ± 2:07:36	7.354	0.001	ns	0.001	ns
				Competition				
Swim	0:54:22 ± 0:47:47	1:08:07 ± 0:39:58	0:55:37 ± 0:42:25	1.465	ns	ns	ns	ns
Bike	2:05:37 ± 1:54:13	1:53:07 ± 1:10:37	1:21:52 ± 1:03:38	3.311	0.039	ns	0.041	ns
Run	1:30:00 ± 0:59:59	1:07:30 ± 0:48:08	0:54:22 ± 0:42:16	2.951	ns	ns	ns	ns
Total	4:29:59 ± 3:41:59	4:08:44 ± 2:38:43	3:11:51 ± 2:28:19	2.494	ns	ns	ns	ns
				Taper				
Swim	0:57:30 ± 0:50:35	0:48:45 ± 0:34:14	0:35:37 ± 0:33:42	3.586	0.030	ns	0.026	ns
Bike	1:46:15 ± 1:50:31	1:16:52 ± 1:00:36	0:43:44 ± 0:38:37	8.101	<0.001	ns	<0.001	ns
Run	1:14:22 ± 0:55:20	0:43:07 ± 0:28:57	0:28:45 ± 0:34:25	9.886	<0.001	0.001	0.001	ns
Total	3:58:07 ± 3:36:26	2:05:37 ± 2:03:47	1:48:06 ± 1:46:44	9.934	<0.001	0.026	<0.001	ns
				Off-Season				
Swim	1:22:30 ± 1:20:48	0:44:22 ± 0:39:37	0:20:37 ± 0:42:29	15.183	<0.001	0.001	<0.001	ns
Bike	2:14:59 ± 1:52:35	0:55:37 ± 0:59:40	0:16:52 ± 0:27:36	30.713	<0.001	<0.001	<0.001	ns
Run	1:51:52 ± 1:08:16	0:48:44 ± 0:50:30	0:19:22 ± 0:31:51	19.566	<0.001	<0.001	<0.001	ns
Total	5:29:21 ± 4:21:39	2:28:43 ± 2:29:47	0:56:51 ± 1:41:56	43.692	<0.001	<0.001	<0.001	ns

Key: [a], with Bonferroni correction; L1–2, intensity levels 1 and 2; L3–4, intensity levels 3 and 4; L3, intensity level 3; z1, zone 1; z2, zone 2; z3, zone 3; Sig., significant; ns, non-significant.

The athletes' low-intensity (z1) swim or cycle training time did not vary significantly across training phases. This was not the case as regards their time spent doing higher-intensity work (i.e., swimming-z2, $F_{(4,239)}$ = 16.506, $p < 0.001$; swimming-z3, $F_{(4,239)}$ = 7.367, $p < 0.001$; cycling-z2, $F_{(4,239)}$ = 12.650, $p < 0.001$; cycling-z3, $F_{(4,239)}$ = 13.585, $p < 0.001$). Run z1, z2 and z3 training time did differ with training phase (z1, $F_{(4,239)}$ = 4.710, $p = 0.001$; z2, $F_{(4,239)}$ = 3.166, $p = 0.015$; z3, $F_{(4,239)}$ = 8.618, $p < 0.001$).

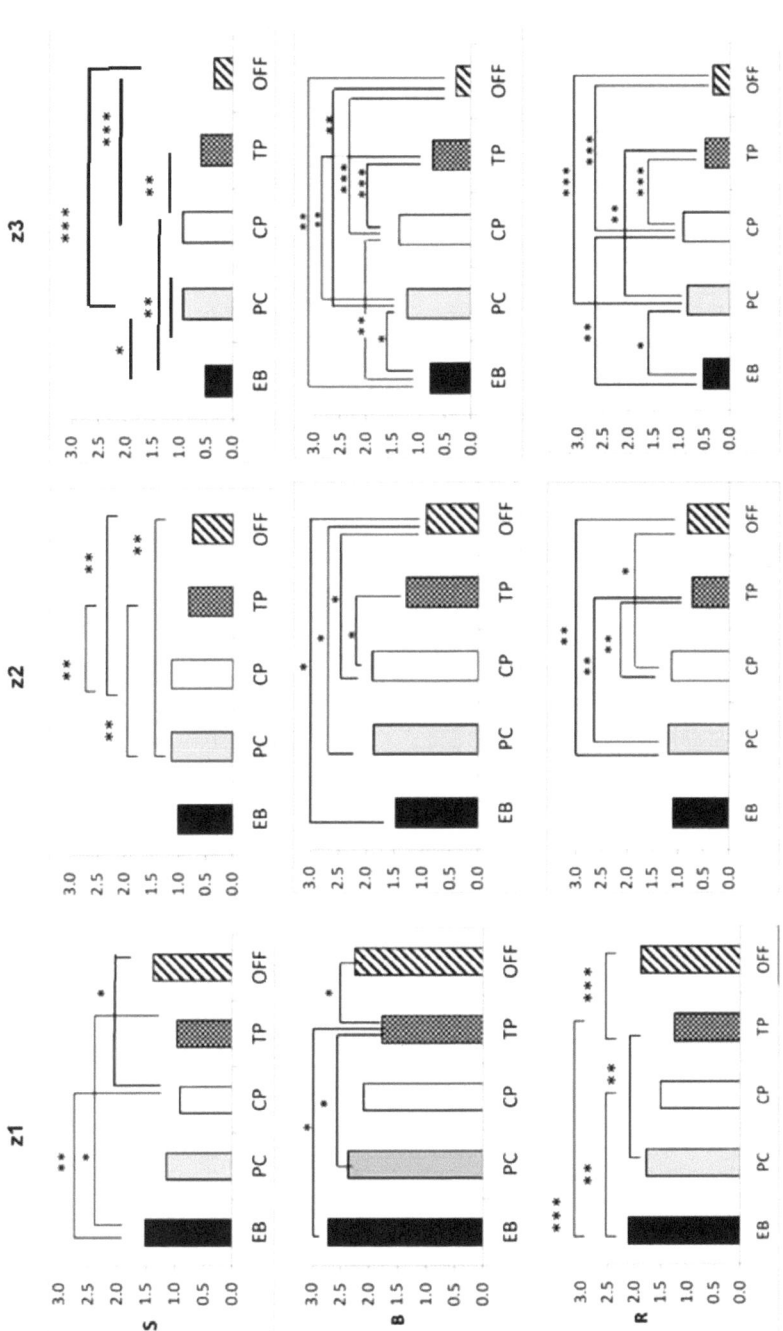

Figure 1. Average weekly training time (h) in each intensity zone, by discipline, by training phase. Key: EB, Endurance Base phase; PC, Pre-Competition phase; CP, Competition phase; TP, Taper phase; Off, Off-Season; S, swim; B, bike; R, run; z1, training intensity zone 1; z2, training intensity zone 2; z3, training intensity zone 3; * $p < 0.05$, ** $p < 0.02$, *** $p < 0.01$.

Training phase-based differences in the time that was spent exercising within each intensity zone were seen (i) for swimming, within each of the Endurance-Base, Taper and Off-Season periods; (ii) for cycling, within all five training cycles; and (iii) for running, within every phase, apart from within the Competition phase. The total swim, bike and run (SBR) training time that was spent within z1, z2 and z3 also differed within all the assessed training phases, apart from the Competition phase. Examples of this include (i) for the Endurance-Base phase, between z1 and z3 ($p < 0.001$), between z1 and z2 ($p = 0.015$) and between z2 and z3 ($p < 0.001$); (ii) for the Pre-Competition phase, between z1 and z3 ($p < 0.001$) and between z2 and z3 ($p < 0.001$); (iii) for the Competition phase, between z2 and z3 ($p = 0.021$); (iv) for Taper, between z1 and z3 ($p < 0.001$) and between z2 and z3 ($p = 0.006$); and (v) for the Off-Season phase, between z1 and z3 ($p < 0.001$) and between z1 and z2 ($p = 0.001$), as well as between z2 and z3 ($p = 0.001$).

From the data that the athletes themselves provided, it appears that the average percentage of their combined weekly swim, cycle and run training time that they normally spent within z1, z2 and z3, respectively, was 53%, 33% and 14%, respectively (Table 6, Figure 2). In no individual macrocycle or discipline did the average proportion of reported swim, cycle and run training that the athletes spent in z1 exceed 56%. The actual percentage of training time that was spent in z1 steadily dropped from the Endurance-Base phase through the Pre-Competition to the Competition periods. Training time within z1 was higher within the Taper and Off-Season phases than it was in other phases. Conversely, the relative proportion of training time that was spent in z3 generally progressively increased over the Endurance-Base to the Pre-Competition through to the Competition periods. It only did not do so when Taper work—which would normally immediately precede important races—was being performed. The training time that was spent within z2 varied by a maximum of 8% over the same periods.

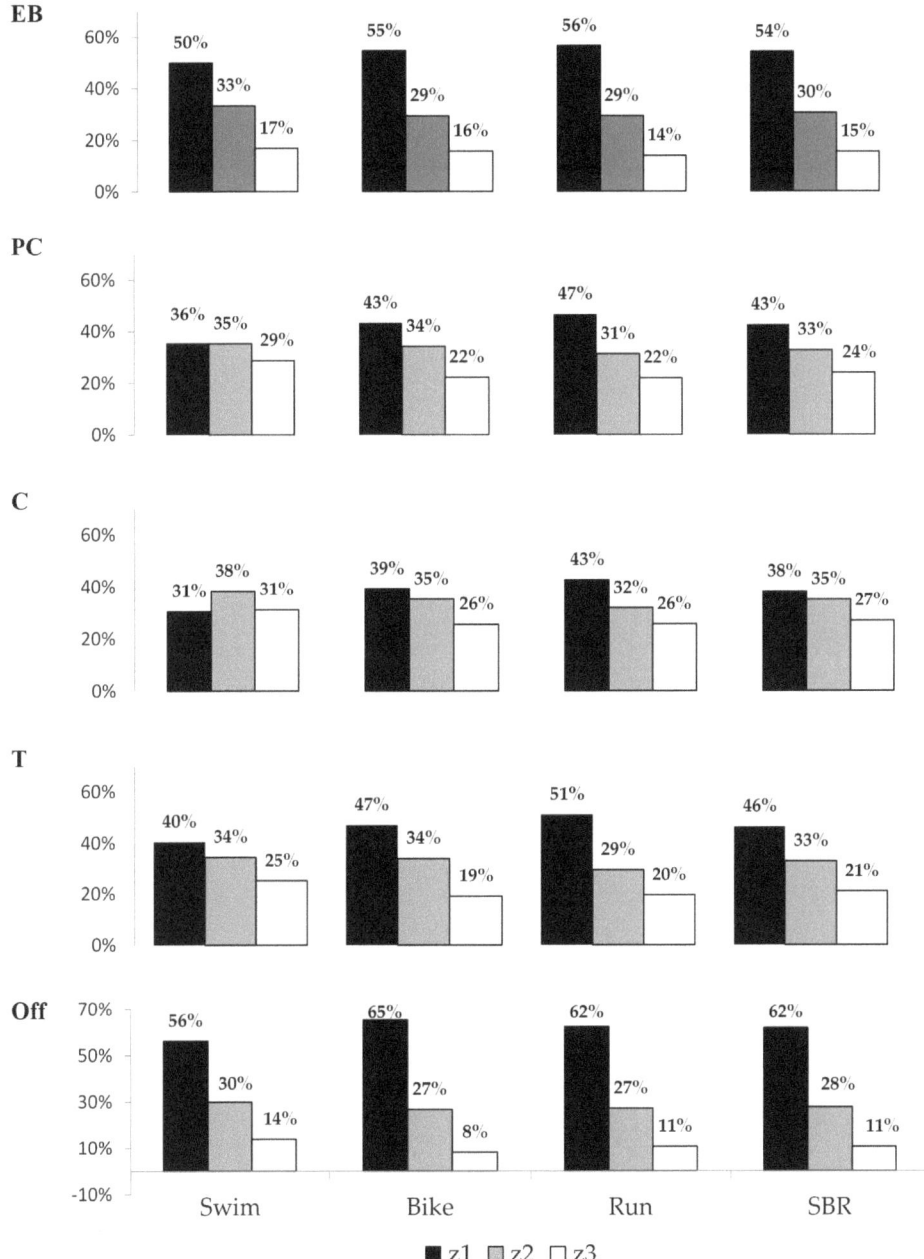

Figure 2. Percentage of training time spent in exercise intensity zones z1, z2 and z3, both overall and in swimming, cycling and running, within the Endurance-Base (EB), Pre-Competition (PC), Competition (C), Taper (T) and Off-Season (Off) phases of the year leading up to the World Championships. Key: SBR Combined swim, bike and run training.

We also compared the training of the fastest 10 and the slowest 10 triathletes in our subject group of 48. No significant differences were seen between the two sub-groups in either changes in training intensity across the training year or in TID. The data are not shown here. We note that the way the study participants' finishing positions were spread across their age-group field was not perfectly matched between the different age-groups that featured in this study. This, our sample size and the fact that the number of athletes within the competition varied between the individual age-groups that featured in this study meant that we were unable to adjust the analysis for the fact that triathlon performance changes with age.

3.3.4. Training Feedback and Adjustment

Most of the group (70.8%) indicated that they were receiving feedback on the aforesaid exercise training from a coach. This is a far larger proportion of the subject group than those who were receiving feedback from a physiotherapist (35.4%), from a general (medical) practitioner (4.2%), from a sports medicine doctor (8.3%), from lab testing (12.5%), from training camps (16.7%), from an online training diary (20.8%), from their heart rate monitor (47.9%), from the academic literature (16.3%), from the world wide web (39.6%) or from other sources (12.5%).

The regularity with which feedback on their swim, bike, run, swim–bike transition or bike–run transition technique was received, however, varied widely among individuals. Some individuals obtained such feedback after almost every training session, while others almost never obtained it. Technique feedback was consistently most often obtained for swimming and running. It was given less regularly for cycling, almost never for the bike–run transition and even less regularly for swim–bike transition training. There were also only low, non-significant correlations between the individual athlete's self-assessment of their relative ability in swimming, the swim–bike transition, cycling, the bike–run transition and running and the regularity with which they received technique-related feedback for it.

3.3.5. Changes from Normal Training in the Immediate Lead-Up to Worlds

The 48 athletes who took part in this study represented different countries and continents. None of the athletes indicated that these World Championships fell within the competition period of their training year. Only 6.3% of the subjects reported that the event fell within their Pre-Competition period. The World Championships fell within the Endurance-Base period and within the Pre-Competition period in 45.8% and 47.9% of the group, respectively. How the athletes considered themselves to have altered their training over the month leading up to the event from what they considered to be their normal training for that period of the training year is illustrated in Figure 3.

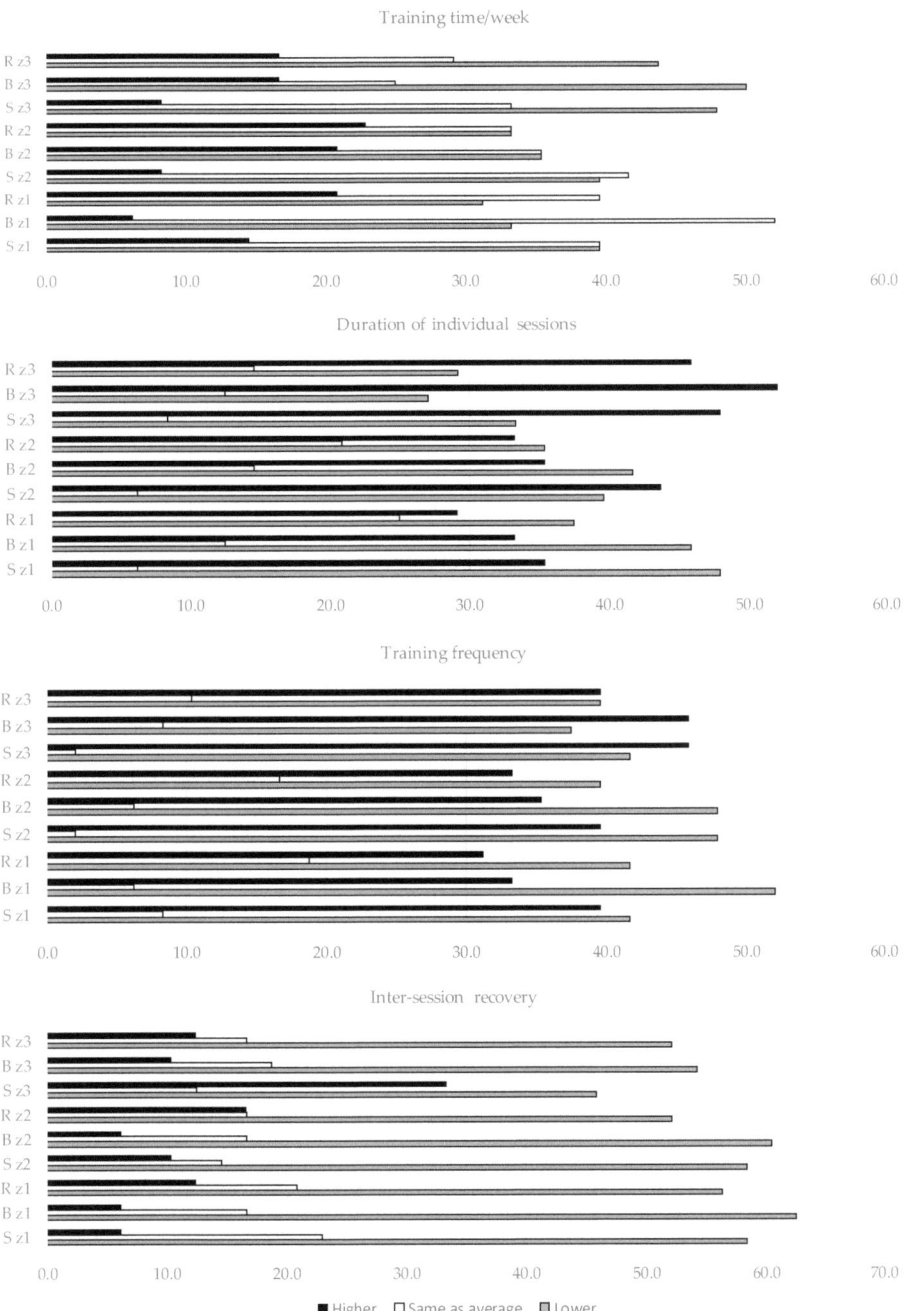

Figure 3. Proportion of the athletes who did/did not modify their training in the month leading up to the ITU Age-Group World Championships from that which was customary for them for the training phase within which it fell. Key: S, swim; B, bike; R, run; z1, zone 1; z2, zone 2; z3, zone 3.

Neither these changes nor their potential cause were particularly clear-cut. What stood out, however, was that, apart from as regards weekly training time, those athletes who did not change their training from what they themselves had recorded as normal for themselves appeared to be in the minority. Most of the athletes deemed their levels of inter-training session recovery to have been lower than normal within the month leading up to the World Age-Group Championships. However, a similar proportion of the group considered themselves to have lowered their training frequency in the higher run and bike intensity levels as deemed themselves to have increased it. Although more athletes than not increased their session duration in these same levels, the majority of the group indicated their total overall training volume in the month leading up to Worlds to have been less than customary. As for the number of races that the athletes competed in within the month leading up to Worlds, this was less than normal in 47.9% of the group, the same as normal in 45.8% of the group and more than normal in 6.3% of the group. Overall recovery times between sessions were thought to be less than, the same as and more than normal in 10.4%, 52.1% and 37.5% of the athletes, respectively.

This training modification was presumably at least partly schedule-related. It was performed in addition to the updating of goals and subsequent training that was implemented "at the end of each macrocycle", "after each major race" and "after illness, injury and/or unexplained performance decrement" by 25.0%, 47.9% and 37.5% of the athletes, respectively. We note, however, that 22.9% of the group stated that they had not updated their goals and subsequent training from what had been set at the onset of the season, at any point within that season, when they finished the survey.

3.4. Health Status

Those who reported themselves to be affected by injury over the preceding year accounted for 16.7%, and over the month prior to survey completion, for 29.2% of the group. Overall, 12.5% of the athletes were injured at the World Championships. Injury prevalence at the exact moment of survey completion was 33.3%. A further 2.1% of the group were, at that point, as yet unsure as to whether they were injured or not. The details of these injuries shall be reported in a separate paper. Overall, the proportions of the group who were ill over the month prior to Worlds, and within the event, were 16.7% and 4%, respectively. All the illness cases that occurred within the month leading up to Worlds were related, by the athletes, to cold/virus/bronchitis, "a bug" and/or to flu-like symptoms. One athlete also contracted food poisoning. One had a concurrent ear/eye infection. At the point of survey completion, 4.2% of the group were ill. On the same occasion, i.e., inside one month of racing in the ITU World OD Age-group Championships, more of the athletes (39.6%) considered their state of training to be "good" than anything else. This compares to the 4.2% of the study participants who thought their training status to be very, very good; 18.8% who thought it to be very good; 20.8% who considered it neither good nor poor; and 16.7% who reported it as poor.

However, 22.9% of the group had competed while knowing—and 6.3% while unsure—that they had a family history of cardiovascular disease. The proportion of our subject group who had raced the World Championships with current cardiovascular issues or breathing difficulties was 10.4% (Table 8). In total, 9 out of the 48 (i.e., 18.8%) indicated themselves to have previously suffered or be suffering from a serious illness or condition that could affect their ability to exercise. In three individuals (6.3%), this limitation was at least partly due to their having suffered (training-related) traumatic injury. Moreover, 39.6% and 2.1% of the athletes reported themselves as suffering or possibly suffering from allergies, respectively. These allergies were mostly attributed to food/stings/dust/animals/selected medications. In one case, the cause of allergy was unknown to the individual, despite it previously having caused anaphylactic shock.

Table 8. Proportion of the athletes who went into the race with pre-existing morbidity factors, injury and/or illness.

Percentage Affected (with % Who Were Unsure in Brackets)			
Family History of CV Disease	22.9 (6.3)	Asthma	14.6 (2.1)
Current CV problems	10.4	Ex-induced asthma	14.6 (2.1)
Ever fainted, blacked out or had dizzy spells	27.1	Hay fever	22.9
Ever experienced loss of consciousness or fainting with exercise	8.3	Allergies	39.6 (2.1)
Have/had serious illness or condition that could affect current ability to exercise			18.8

Key: CV, cardiovascular; Ex-induced, exercise induced.

3.5. Stress Levels

Over the year leading up to the ITU World Age-Group Championships, the athletes reported themselves as having incurred Total Life stress, negative Life Stress and positive Life Stress scores of 19.1 ± 20.7 (min–max, 0–89), -19.3 ± 20.7 (0–64) and 7.3 ± 8.9 (0–36) units, respectively. Overall, $39.7 \pm 33.1\%$ of their Total Life Stress was considered to be positive and $60.4 \pm 3.7\%$ to be negative. Sports-, Relationship-, Personal- and Career-related Stress was held accountable for $42.0 \pm 26.7\%$, $12.7 \pm 18.6\%$, $31.3 \pm 25.9\%$ and $14.0 \pm 21.1\%$ of the athletes' Total Life Stress, respectively. That is, most of the stress that the athletes reported via the Life Stress Questionnaire was Sports-related Stress. The relative proportions of positive and negative stress that were reported were (i) $39.7 \pm 33.1\%$ vs. $60.4 \pm 37.1\%$ for Sport Stress; (ii) $26.8 \pm 37.6\%$ vs. $73.2 \pm 37.65\%$ for Relationship Stress; (iii) $39.6 \pm 37.1\%$ vs. $60.4 \pm 37.2\%$ for Personal Stress; and (iv) $40.1 \pm 41.6\%$ vs. $59.4 \pm 41.6\%$ for Career Stress. Sports-related Stress affected most athletes and was overwhelmingly negative when it pertained to injury, illness and/or the individual's failure to attain his/her sporting goal(s). These findings are shown in Figures 4 and 5.

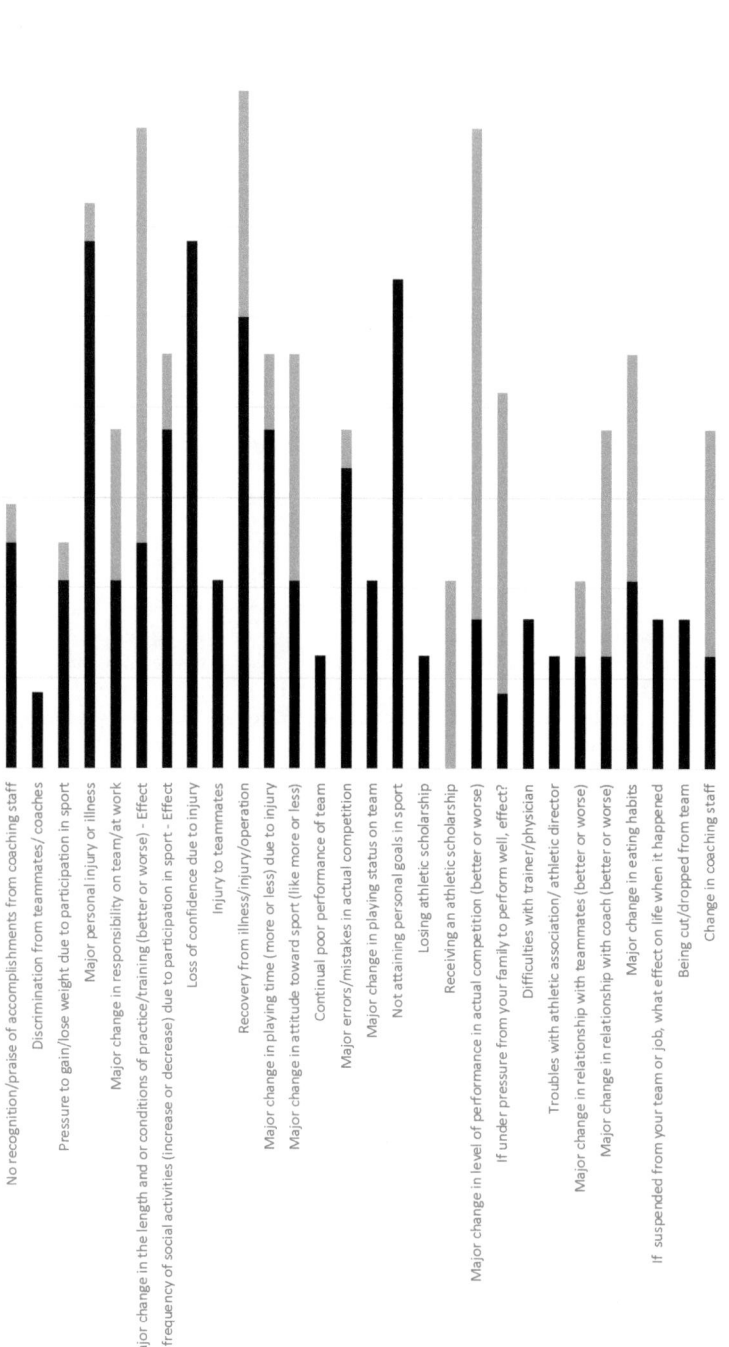

Figure 4. The proportions of top age-group triathletes who were affected by selected positive and negative sports-related Life Stressors in the lead up to the ITU World OD Age-group Championships.

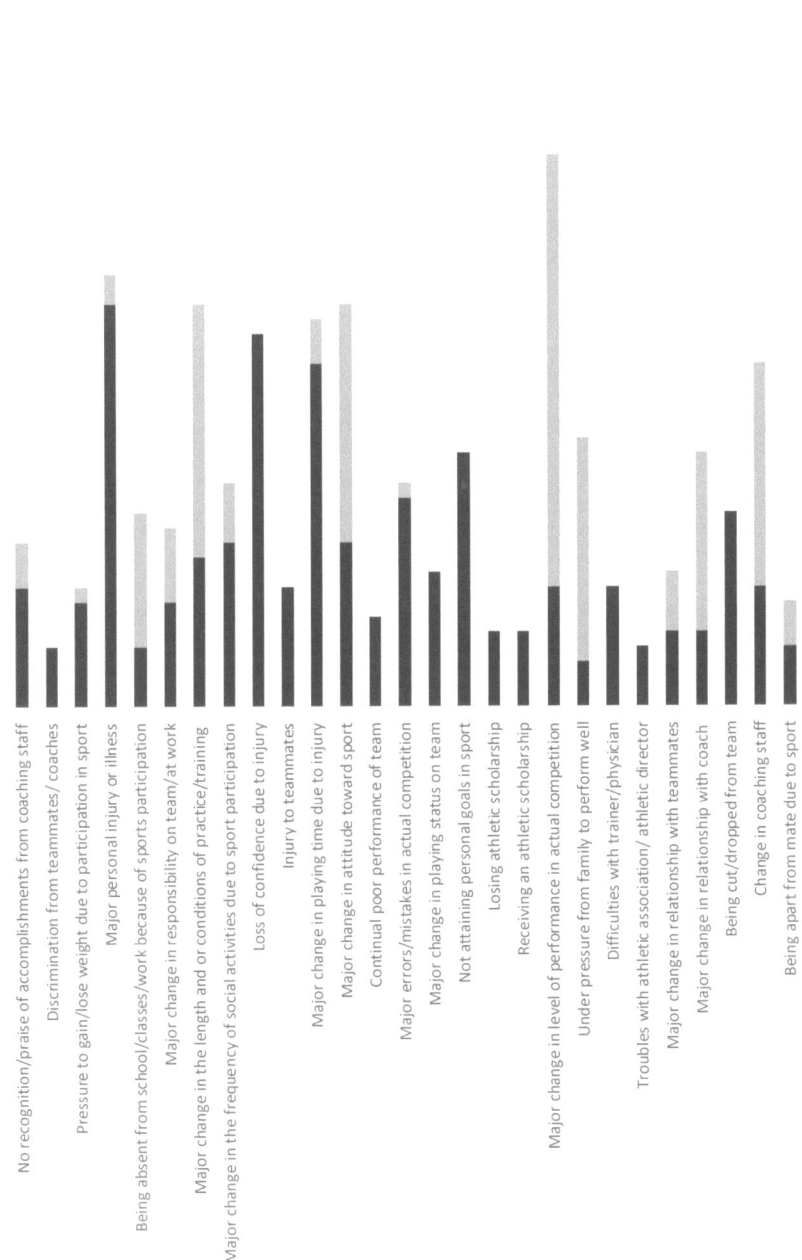

Figure 5. Sports-related Life Stress scores for the year leading up to the ITU World OD Age-Group Championships (arbitrary units).

4. Discussion

This study aimed to obtain a global overview of the training, work and Life Stress of top amateur short-distance triathletes. It also involved a preliminary assessment of the extent to which the training structure, monitoring and flexibility of such athletes may or may not be optimal. Our goal in so doing was to pinpoint potentially useful directions for research with the potential to be translated into improvement in the training practice of this athlete sub-group. We remind the reader that the survey was mainly retrospective, and that the 48 athletes whom it involved represented a small proportion of the total number of age-group athletes who were competing at the World Championships. Both issues have implications for the ability to generalize our findings beyond our sample population. We recommend, therefore, that our observations first be confirmed via a "proof of pilot" retrospective survey that itself involves a sufficiently large number of athletes for it to have adequate statistical power. The ensuing findings should then be checked via a prospective longitudinal "proof of principle" epidemiological study. Its limitations notwithstanding, however, this "pilot study" has yielded important findings.

Most of the athletes whom we surveyed were fitting their triathlon training around fixed-hour full-time work. The triathletes claimed to implement goal setting within, to periodize, to obtain feedback on and to modify their training plans when appropriate. Some evidence to support such claims was obtained. The athletes' key focus for the season in question, in 95.8% of cases, was qualification for/performance within the ITU World Age-Group Championships [32]. However, both the timing of the placement of the Championships within the athletes' normal training year and the way that they modified their training within the month leading up to the event suggested that the actual training that the athletes achieved was not necessarily fully commensurate with the aforementioned sporting goal. This may partly explain why Sports-related Stress accounted for the majority of the total Life Stress that the athletes reported themselves as having experienced over the year leading up to the ITU World Age-Group Championships.

Before discussing our results, it is necessary to first place the level of the age-group athletes whose data we have analyzed in context with the relevant academic literature. All of our mostly masters athletes individual and triathlon-specific personal best competition times were somewhat slower than those of the elite (but not professional) under-35-year-olds of the same sex who participated in Vleck's prospective training diary study [14]. The latter had also been preparing for draft-legal OD competition. The OD triathlon personal best times of our males were, nonetheless, faster than those of the athletes who participated in Falk Neto et al.'s prospective study of age-group-level OD training [16]. They were also faster (at 2:13:25 ± 0:16:07 vs. 2:12:24 ± 0:02:54; in hh:mm:ss) than Aoyagi et al.'s (2021) nine younger "faster" well-trained males [6].

We mention Aoyagi's work because it is the *only* existing report of the exercise intensities at which age-group athletes *race* the non-drafting OD competition that their training preparation is based around of which we are aware. Their 17 males raced the swim, cycle and run legs at 89.8 ± 3.7%, 91.1 ± 4.4% and 90.7 ± 5.1% of HRmax, respectively. The proportion of competition time that was spent below the aerobic threshold (HRz1), between the aerobic and the anaerobic threshold (HRz2) and above the anaerobic threshold (HRz3) was 1.5 ± 2.3%, 6.6 ± 15.0% and 91.9 ± 16.3%, respectively, for the 1.5 km swim. It was 2.8 ± 8.0%, 18.4 ± 24.0% and 78.8 ± 28.1%, respectively, for the 40 km cycle. For the 10 km run, it was 4.1 ± 10.6%, 39.9 ± 38.5% and 56.0 ± 42.1%, respectively. We note that when the athletes were split into a faster and slower group, the mean %HRmax and intensity distribution during swimming and cycling was similar in both groups. However, the faster athletes in the group spent relatively more of their running time in intensity zones z2 and z3. Thus, although our athletes, as well as being faster, also had at least four times (and in some cases double) the equivalent training/racing experience in triathlon's component sports of Aoyagi et al.'s (younger) athletes, Aoyagi's data give us a rough idea of what kind of *race* exercise intensity distributions the *training* data that we collected here (as shown in Tables 4–7 and Figures 1 and 2) likely related to.

This observation (despite being somewhat labored) could open up new avenues of applied research into triathlon training efficacy. There are some issues with comparing the training-related data that were obtained by the various studies, however. The most important of these is likely the fact that the various author groups did not use identical means of ascribing training intensity zones. Aoyagi et al. used laboratory-based, measurement to set zones. With Vleck's method (Table 1), the athletes themselves set the intensity levels—albeit doing so on the basis of multiple criteria that included laboratory-derived measures. This "indirect" setting was implemented because—as was the case here—laboratory testing was not necessarily an option that was available to the athletes. Vleck's triathletes did not record which combination(s) of the criteria for the setting of exercise intensity that are outlined in Table 1 they used. Nor did they note what proportion of this combination was derived from laboratory-based measures. In Vleck's original study [14], however, this same method of ascribing training intensity levels (and then zones) was to some extent validated, by the athletes who took part in it, against the actual race times that they achieved over the course of the study. The same method was also part validated, in other athletes, against the results of laboratory-based incremental lactate and cardiorespiratory tests [31]. Since this is potentially highly relevant to training diary-based research into training-related maladaptation, we suggest that more detailed examination be carried out into the extent to which the method of self-ascribing training zones that was used in both Vleck's original study and by this research (Table 1) both yield comparable results to laboratory-derived measures [33] and could be improved.

Our data may, additionally, be somewhat skewed by the fact that we asked for training duration estimations to be made to the nearest half hour. This is why we have only reported total overall training durations across and within all the sports that the athletes were doing when/where such information was obtained via direct questioning, and have not calculated total training loads. Adding up values that have been rounded up or down, from multiple questions, yields misleading numbers. Even so, however, the proportion of training time that each of our top age-groupers were spending in intensity zones z1, z2 and z3 was clearly *not* around the 75–80%, 5% and 15–20% values, respectively, that are commonly recommended, in terms of eventual performance yield, to be undertaken within each of the triathlon's component sports [34]. The average percentage of combined swim, cycle and run training time that the entire athlete group reported itself to normally spend within z1, z2 and z3 was 53%, 33% and 14%, respectively. In no individual training block or individual triathlon discipline did the average proportion of swim, cycle and run training that the athletes spend in zone 1 exceed 56%. Falk Neto et al. [16], whose intensity zones were set via RPE and guidelines in the literature and whose training data were prospective, reported that their slower age-group athletes spent 47% of training time in z1, 25% in z2 and 28% in z3. Vleck (2010) [14,35], using the same method of ascribing training intensity level as was used in this study, but over 30 weeks of prospective longitudinal data collection, reported that their 8 faster triathletes spent 70.4%, 6.1% and 9.1% of their overall training time in their intensity levels 1–2, 3 and 4–5, respectively, i.e., in z1, z2 and z3, respectively.

It would be easy to assume, given the direction of change of the proportions of training time that were spent in each zone from the slowest to the fastest athletes in these studies, that the TID data from these three studies support Seiler's model. This would likely be a supposition too far. We do not yet have the data to support the making of an explicit link between the proportion of training time that was spent in each intensity level by these various ability groups and their performance level (as opposed to anything else). Vleck, for example, did not compare the periodization of better vs. worse performers in the athletes who took part in her larger prospective survey. The athletes also differed on other measures that have been shown to differ among different ability levels of OD triathletes. For example, the athletes in this study possessed considerably more years of triathlon training and racing experience than Falk Neto's similarly aged athletes (at 10.2 ± 6.2 and 9.0 ± 6.2 years, respectively, vs. 4.5 years). In an initial retrospective study, competitive experience (as well as "desire to achieve", "stress" levels being "tense/anxious", total mood disturbance and "can't cope") was shown by Vleck to differ with athlete ability level in the same group of OD athletes from which their prospective study participants were drawn [14]. It is not clear, however, seeing as they were younger, whether the athletes in Vleck's prospective study were relatively more experienced. What is probable, given their ages, is that that they had less-demanding work commitments.

Most, but not all, the athletes in this study had full-time jobs, with fairly "normal" working hours. On average, they worked 7.6 ± 2.5 h every day. The number of times they trained per week stayed fairly constant over the year. There were some expected fluctuations from this when the triathletes were tapering or in their Off-Season (see Tables 5 and 6). Most of the group were fitting their training around work. It seems logical that their total weekly training hours would stay fairly constant over the year, while the makeup of said training changed. As was expected, the athletes fitted the majority of their weekday training sessions in before or after what are usually considered to be normal working hours. They also did some "lunchtime" training. This is the first time that actual data, rather than anecdotal reports (as described in [14]), have been obtained regarding this point. We did not specifically ask to what extent the athletes cycled or ran to and from work. Nor—although we did obtain details of the frequency, individual and overall weekly duration of "long" and "speed" sessions in each discipline—did we inquire about how the cycling of low-, medium- and high-intensity training work was organized over an average week. This was unfortunate. It is also unfortunate that we did not inquire as to whether said training was conducted "indoors" or "outdoors". Both issues should be followed up.

Not unexpectedly, the proportion of the athletes' training sessions that were conducted, in each discipline, within specific time slots definitely differed between weekday- and weekend-based training (Table 4). This situation can potentially affect the extent to which recovery and adaptation might occur between the athletes' training sessions. The degree of inherent injury risk that a given athlete was exposed to, given the timing of his/her training, could vary accordingly. For example, far more weekday than weekend based bike training was conducted in the evenings. We do not know the extent to which this training was conducted outside when daylight might be waning, or inside on a turbo trainer. Both of the latter situations might augment injury risk, but to *different extents*. Nor can we calculate the probability that, given that, it may be that the simplest reason for why these athletes are not fulfilling the recommended proportions of $z1$, $z2$ and $z3$ training was simply because they found it difficult to fit their training in around their other commitments. Z1 training takes longer to complete. The possibility that (e.g., employment-related) limitations in their training time leads these athletes to do high amounts of higher-intensity training than they might otherwise have chosen to do was raised by McCormick [27]. Although the sample numbers were too small for the authors to be sure, McCormick's point appears to have been supported by Falk Neto's unpublished data [36]. These age-groupers were doing at least some of their training in organized group/club sessions, which are unlikely to have included much z1 training.

Certainly, club-related socialization may have had some positive repercussions in terms of the athletes' general mental and social health. Most of our subjects were enrolled in single-sport- rather than in triathlon-specific clubs, however. They were not, therefore, necessarily receiving training that took what they were doing in the other triathlon disciplines into account while in that environment (Table 3). Indeed, in answer to the question "if you are coached (other than self-coached), and your training is geared towards triathlon, do you have the same coach overseeing all three disciplines", only 27.1% of the group answered "always." Even so, some level of training periodization among the Endurance-Base, Pre-competition, Taper and Competition phases of the training year, as well as in the Off-Season, was demonstrated in the athletes' replies to the online survey. They achieved this periodization across training phases within each individual triathlon discipline. They also periodized their overall swim, bike and run training (as shown in Tables 5–7 and Figures 1 and 2). We saw similar results regarding the periodization that occurred both within and across training phases and disciplines when we extended the number of athletes in the training-related dataset up to 124. We did so by adding the data for those athletes for whom up to 3 out of 45 training intensity-related replies were missing into the existing dataset [31]. Nonetheless, our data that specifically related to how the athletes trained within the one-month lead up to the World Age-Group Championships indicate that the extent to which these age-groupers modified their training intensity distribution, racing load *and inter-session recovery* in the light of external factors (Figure 3) may not always have been ideal. We observed that, as the athletes were representing multiple countries (and time zones of origin), "Worlds" did not necessarily fall within the competition period of each individual athlete's training year. It was certainly unclear from the data that we obtained—which examined how their training for that month was modified from what was normal for them for the macro-cycle in question—to what extent the athletes took this issue into account.

The level of feedback that the athletes were receiving on their training in relation to their perceived ability also supports the premise that their training adjustment process could, nonetheless, perhaps be improved. The data that we obtained regarding the extent to which these age-groupers acted in response to the failure of that training (i.e., injury, illness or unexplained performance decrement) support this assertion. So, too, does the extent to which such failure occurred, as exemplified by the injury prevalence values that we obtained. We further highlight the fact that 40% of the athletes in this study self-identified themselves as allergy sufferers. Similar observations were made for the larger 602-athlete sample from which this group was drawn [31]. Although we could find no comparative data for amateur triathletes to compare this to in the academic literature, Teixeira et al. [37] observed allergy symptoms in 54.2% of a mixed sample of 59 elite triathletes and runners. This observation may point to an adverse, potentially training-related, immune status in at least some amateur triathletes. The results that are reported here in age-group triathletes are clearly worth following up on with at least the Allergy Questionnaire for Athletes [37], if not more [38].

We consider it highly noteworthy, moreover, that the majority of the Life Stress that the athletes reported was Sports-related Stress. Outstanding personal achievement and a major change in performance in actual competition, recovery from illness/injury and a major change in academic/work activity were the triathletes' main sources of Life Stress over the year leading up to the World Championships. The LESCA does not directly enquire about stress accruing from difficulties in maintaining what the athlete perceives to be the appropriate life work/sports balance. Nonetheless, the fact that a major change in work/academic activity was a source of stress could indicate work/sports balance to be an important issue. We note that the issues that were identified as directly sports-related were the ones that caused the most negative stress (as illustrated in Figures 4 and 5). They included not attaining personal goals in sports, major personal injury or illness, a major change in playing (i.e., training) time due to injury, recovery from injury/illness/operation and loss of confidence due to injury, as well as a lack of recognition of the athlete's accomplishments from coaching staff. As we only assessed 48 athletes here, there were not enough of such injury/illness data to bother assessing what they were linked to. Given the level of detail that the athletes provided on the etiology of any injury/illness that they sustained for that month (far more so than for the other time periods that we assessed), we reserve such an analysis for our larger 602-athlete sample. It is perhaps a pity, however, that the LESCA data were (also) not obtained over the same one-month time frame. This will limit the extent to which they can be linked to injury in particular.

5. Conclusions and Future Directions

We feel that the scheduling, completion, TID distribution and possible efficacy of this group's training may be linked to the "work/life/sport" scheduling conflicts that are associated with being "part-timers." The minimal sociocultural data that exist for triathletes thus far have suggested them to be generally well-educated individuals who also excel in their business lives. They have also, however, been reported to exhibit less (sports-related) harm avoidance behavior than their single-sport counterparts [39]. We recommend that systematic examination of both the benefits and barriers that are experienced by age-group triathletes in combining their sports, academic and/or professional careers be carried out. We also recommend that the impact that such issues can have on the physical and mental health and well-being of such athletes be assessed [40].

This wide-ranging study has highlighted just how much research into training and adaptation in age-group triathletes still needs to be conducted before its results can easily be translated into improvement in training practice. Given that it was retrospective and involved a small percentage of the total number of athletes who took part in the event, we firstly need to examine the extent to which the findings of this study may be extrapolated to the wider subject population. We saw that the TID of these amateur triathletes is not apparently what has been considered to be best practice for *single-discipline* endurance sports. But, the TID values that we calculated were based on retrospective data. They also do not account for the athletes' weight training, for their training in other sports or for their off-training activity. Moreover, the triathlon has repeatedly been acknowledged to be more than the sum of its single-sport counterparts. Its cycle training and run training have certainly already been shown to have synergistic, cumulative effects [18,41]. Perhaps the most important question here, therefore, is not so much the holistic one of "is classic polarized training ideal for triathlon?" As Sperlich et al. [8] recently pointed out: "it may be questionable if a general best-practice or "optimal" TID exists at all, and if so, the replication of TID will not be feasible in the long run". The far more pressing question to be addressed is surely a far more individualistic one. It is "what is the best training practice that a given age-group athlete can feasibly achieve, given his/her work and other commitments?" This study revealed significant differences between weekday- and weekend-based training in the timing of, and therefore, in the recovery/training adaptation periods between, successive training sessions. As triathlon coaches, we make decisions on the timing and order of our athletes' successive swim, cycle, bike and weight training sessions that are based more on our personal experience than on any available scientific evidence. Swimming, for example, is generally considered to have less impact than running. It is often chosen over running, for that reason, to follow a high-intensity turbo training session. Examination, in top age-groupers, of the order in which they cycle high-, medium- and low-intensity work across the (four,- including weight training) triathlon disciplines may prove useful. So, too, may investigation into how top amateurs adjust this type of periodization in view of their work demands. The dual careers literature may prove to be helpful to investigators in this regard.

The second logical follow-up to these studies is an investigation of how exactly their "within" and "outside" training stressors may have influenced maladaptation in the larger retrospective study of 602 triathletes—for which sufficient injury and illness data appear to be available to do this—of which they formed a part. How these influenced training needs to be followed up. So, too, do the possible explanations of why said training diverged from either accepted or the individual athlete's norms. Far more athletes reported their inter-session recovery to be *less* (as opposed to the same as or higher) than normal during the month-long lead up to the World Championships, for example. They did so, even though they had confirmed that the World Championships were the focus of their entire training year. Did the same finding occur in the larger sample of 602 athletes? If so, why? What might have influenced this departure from accepted training wisdom? What research questions need to be addressed for us to be able to use the answers to improve training practice?

Of additional interest are the average weekly number of (swim, cycle, run and resistance) training sessions that the triathletes did, regardless of when the athletes were in their training year, and how these data relate to the most recently published updated exercise training guidelines for masters athletes [15]. "A combination of exercise stresses (endurance, sprint, and strength) is likely required to optimally maintain physical capacity into older age... Athletes should do only one to two threshold or high-intensity training sessions per week, interspersed with two to four long slow distance sessions per week, depending on their training history. They should also factor in one or two strength training sessions per week." Investigation of how variable "normal" athlete training within each of the various triathlon age-groups is, and how such "normal" training varies from one age-group to another, in tandem with examination of how this is reflected by decreases in actual performance, would be the logical follow-up to this observation. For such research to be successful, far larger sample sizes are needed than we utilized in this first exploratory study. Research into how the risk factors that have already specifically been linked to the occurrence of overuse injury in triathletes [2,20,21,29,30] differ across age-groups, and change across the athlete's life span, is also likely to yield results that could have important implications for the improvement of training practice in age-group triathletes.

Author Contributions: Online survey design, implementation and funding, V.V.; training data analysis only of 48 athletes, L.M.M., R.d.M. and V.V.; further data analysis for the same 48 athletes, V.V.; cross-checking of study findings against the results of analyses involving larger athlete sample sizes, V.V.; writing—original (Portuguese) draft preparation of section dealing with TID distributions only, L.M.M. and R.d.M.; writing of the complete paper, V.V.; review and revisions resulting in the submission, V.V., L.M.M., M.F.P., J.H.F.N. and C.Q. R.d.M. analyzed the distribution of exercise intensity data in partial fulfillment of the requirements for the award of a Master's degree from the Universidade Lusófona, POR. L.M.M. and V.V. were principal and secondary supervisors, respectively, for De Moraes' dissertation (entitled "Quantificação da distribuição da intensidade do treino dos triatletas participantes no Campeonato do Mundo de 2013 [Training intensity distribution in triathletes competing in the 2013 ITU World Championships])". All authors have read and agreed to the published version of the manuscript.

Funding: CIPER—Centro Interdisciplinar para o Estudo da Performance Humana (unit 447) acknowledges the support of the "Fundação para a Ciência e Tecnologia", as expressed by Grant UIDB/00447/2020. The first author thanks Professor Sanjay Sharma and St George's Medical School, London, for funding her travel costs to the 2013 ITU World Championships- where she carried out an associated medical tent-based study.

Institutional Review Board Statement: The study was conducted according to the guidelines of the Declaration of Helsinki. Both the study and the survey were approved to proceed, before the study took place, by the Institutional Ethics Committee of Faculdade de Motricidade Humana, University of Lisbon. The final Ethics Committee report, number 18/2014, was emitted on 30 May 2014.

Informed Consent Statement: Informed consent was obtained from all the subjects who were involved in this study.

Data Availability Statement: The dataset contains private medical information. It is not publicly available.

Acknowledgments: We thank Robert Püstow, Upsolut Sports UK Ltd.; Jasmine Flatters O.B.E., the ITU and Race Technical Delegate; Sanjay Sharma and the athletes, coaches, technical and medical staff of the 2013 ITU World Championships for their invaluable support of the data collection process. The first author again especially thanks Sanjay Sharma for giving her the exceptional opportunity to witness, at first-hand, how top-class race medical support is conducted. She also thanks Trent Petrie for kindly allowing her to use his LESCA questionnaire.

Conflicts of Interest: None of the authors are aware of any conflict of interest associated with or proceeding from this study.

References

1. Bentley, D.J.; Millet, G.P.; Vleck, V.E.; McNaughton, L.R. Specific aspects of contemporary triathlon. *Sports Med.* **2002**, *32*, 345–359. [CrossRef] [PubMed]
2. Vleck, V.; Millet, G.P.; Alves, F.B. The impact of triathlon training and racing on athletes' general health. *Sports Med.* **2014**, *44*, 1659–1692. [CrossRef] [PubMed]
3. Walsh, J.A. The rise of elite short-course triathlon re-emphasises the necessity to transition efficiently from cycling to running. *Sports* **2019**, *7*, 99. [CrossRef] [PubMed]
4. Millet, G.P.; Bentley, D.J.; Vleck, V.E. The relationships between science and sport: Application in triathlon. *Int. J. Sports Physiol. Perform.* **2007**, *2*, 315–322. [CrossRef] [PubMed]
5. Rios, L. 2016 USA Triathlon Membership Survey Report. Colorado Springs, Colorado. USA Triathlon. 2017. Available online: https://www.teamusa.org/USA-Triathlon/News/Articles-and-Releases/2017/December/18/USA-Triathlon-Membership-Survey-Report (accessed on 11 January 2023).

6. Aoyagi, A.; Ishikura, K.; Nabekura, Y. Exercise intensity during Olympic-distance triathlon in well-trained age-group athletes: An observational study. *Sports* **2021**, *9*, 18. [CrossRef]
7. Piacentini, M.F.; Bianchini, L.A.; Minganti, C.; Sias, M.; Di Castro, A.; Vleck, V. Is the bike segment of modern Olympic triathlon more a transition towards running in males than it is in females? *Sports* **2019**, *7*, 76. [CrossRef]
8. Sperlich, B.; Treff, G.; Boone, J. Training intensity distribution in endurance sports: Time to consider sport specificity and waking hour activity. *Med. Sci. Sports Exerc.* **2022**, *54*, 1227–1228. [CrossRef]
9. Stöggl, T.; Sperlich, B. Polarized training has greater impact on key endurance variables than threshold, high intensity, or high volume training. *Front. Physiol.* **2014**, *5*, 33. [CrossRef]
10. Skinner, J.S.; McLellan, T.H. The transition from aerobic to anaerobic metabolism. *Res. Q. Exerc. Sport* **1980**, *51*, 234–248. [CrossRef]
11. Mujika, I. Olympic preparation of a world-class female triathlete. *Int. J. Sports Physiol. Perform.* **2014**, *9*, 727–731. [CrossRef]
12. Cejuela, R.; Sellés-Pérez, S. Road to Tokyo 2020 Olympic Games: Training characteristics of a world class male triathlete. *Front. Physiol.* **2022**, *13*, 835705. [CrossRef] [PubMed]
13. Treff, G.; Leppich, R.; Winkert, K.; Steinacker, J.M.; Mayer, B.; Sperlich, B. The integration of training and off-training activities substantially alters training volume and load analysis in elite rowers. *Sci. Rep.* **2021**, *11*, 17218. [CrossRef] [PubMed]
14. Vleck, V. *Triathlete Training and Injury Analysis—An Investigation in British National Squad and Age-Group Triathletes*; Verlag Dr Mueller: Saarbrucken, Germany, 2010; ISBN-10: 3639212053; ISBN-13: 978-3639212051.
15. Borges, N.R.; Del Vecchio, L. Exercise recommendations for masters athletes. In *Exercise and Physical Activity for Older Adults*; Bouchard, D.R., Ed.; Human Kinetics: Champaign, IL, USA, 2021.
16. Falk Neto, J.H.; Parent, E.C.; Vleck, V.; Kennedy, M.D. The training characteristics of recreational-level triathletes: Influence on fatigue and health. *Sports* **2021**, *9*, 94. [CrossRef]
17. Seiler, S. What is best practice for training intensity and duration distribution in endurance athletes? *IJSPP* **2010**, *5*, 276–291. [CrossRef]
18. Vleck, V.; Bessone Alves, F. Cross-training and injury risk in British Olympic distance triathletes. *BJSM* **2011**, *45*, 382. [CrossRef]
19. Halson, S.L. Monitoring training load to understand fatigue in athletes. *Sports Med.* **2014**, *44* (Suppl. S2), S139–S147. [CrossRef]
20. Vleck, V.; Hoeden, D. Epidemiological aspects of illness and injury. In *Triathlon Medicine*; Springer Nature: Basel, Switzerland, 2019; pp. 19–41.
21. Vleck, V.E. Triathlon. In *Epidemiology of Injury in Olympic Sports*; Caine, D.J., Harmer, P., Schiff, M., Eds.; International Olympic Committee Encyclopaedia of Sports Medicine Series; Wiley-Blackwell: West Sussex, UK, 2010; pp. 294–320.
22. Dallam, G.M.; Jonas, S.; Miller, T.K. Medical considerations in triathlon competition: Recommendations for triathlon organisers, competitors and coaches. *Sports Med.* **2005**, *35*, 143–161. [CrossRef]
23. Vleck, V. The changing relationship between multidisciplinary (triathlon) exercise and health across the lifespan. In *Movimento Humano, Cultura e Saúde: Situação Atual e Abordagem Educacional (Human Movement, Culture and Health)*; Lisbon University Press: Lisbon, Portugal, 2018.
24. Parsons-Smith, R.L.; Barkase, S.; Lovell, G.P.; Vleck, V.; Terry, P.C. Mood profiles of amateur triathletes: Implications for mental health and performance. *Front. Psychol.* **2022**, *13*, 925992. [CrossRef]
25. Fawkner, H.J.; McMurray, N.E.; Summers, J.J. Athletic injury and minor life events: A prospective study. *J. Sci. Med. Sport* **1999**, *2*, 117–124. [CrossRef]
26. Hamer, M.; Stamatakis, E.; Steptoe, A. Dose-response relationship between physical activity and mental health: The Scottish Health Survey. *BJSM* **2009**, *43*, 1111–1114. [CrossRef]
27. McCormick, A.; Meijen, C.; Marcora, S. Psychological demands experienced by recreational endurance athletes. *Int. J. Sport Exerc. Psychol.* **2018**, *16*, 415–430. [CrossRef]
28. Petrie, T.A. Psychosocial antecedents of athletic injury: The effects of life stress and social support on female collegiate gymnasts. *Behav. Med.* **1992**, *18*, 127–138. [CrossRef] [PubMed]
29. Vleck, V.E.; Garbutt, G. Injury and training characteristics of male Elite, Development Squad, and club triathletes. *Int. J. Sports Med.* **1998**, *19*, 38–42. [CrossRef] [PubMed]
30. Vleck, V.E.; Bentley, D.J.; Millet, G.P.; Cochrane, T. Triathlon event distance specialization: Training and injury effects. *J. Strength Cond. Res.* **2010**, *24*, 30–36. [CrossRef]
31. Vleck, V. (CIPER, Faculdade de Motricidade Humana, Universidade de Lisboa, Lisbon, Portugal). Unpublished work.
32. Lamont, M.; Kennelly, M. A qualitative exploration of participant motives among committed amateur triathletes. *Leis. Sci.* **2012**, *34*, 236–255. [CrossRef]
33. Bellinger, P.; Arnold, B.; Minahan, C. Quantifying the training-intensity distribution in middle-distance runners: The influence of different methods of training-intensity quantification. *Int. J. Sports Physiol. Perform.* **2019**, *15*, 319–323. [CrossRef]
34. Seiler, K.S.; Kjerland, G.O. Quantifying training intensity distribution in elite endurance athletes: Is there evidence for an "optimal" distribution? *Scand. J. Med. Sci.* **2006**, *16*, 49–56. [CrossRef]
35. Vleck, V.E.; Lepers, R.; Bessone Alves, F.; Millet, G.P. Is elite triathletes' training polarized? In Proceedings of the First International Triathlon Union World Conference on Science in Triathlon, Alicante, Spain, 24-26 March 2011.
36. Falk-Neto, J.H.; University of Alberta: Edmonton, AB, Canada. Personal communication, 2022.
37. Teixeira, R.; Leite, G.d.S.; Bonini, M.; Gorjão, R.; Agondi, R.; Kokron, C.M.; Carvalho, C.R.F. Atopy in elite endurance athletes. *Clin. J. Sport Med.* **2018**, *28*, 268–271. [CrossRef]

38. Bonini, M.; Braido, F.; Baiardini, I.; DEL Giacco, S.; Gramiccioni, C.; Manara, M.; Tagliapietra, G.; Scardigno, A.; Sargentini, V.; Brozzi, M.; et al. AQUA: Allergy questionnaire for athletes. development and validation. *Med. Sci. Sports Exerc.* **2009**, *41*, 5, 1034–1041. [CrossRef]
39. Clingman, J.M.; Hilliard, D.V. Some personality characteristics of the super-adherer: Following those who go beyond fitness. *J. Sport Behav.* **1987**, *10*, 123–136.
40. An, B.; Sato, M.; Harada, H. Grit, leisure involvement, and life satisfaction: A case of amateur triathletes in Japan. *Leis. Sci.* 2021. [CrossRef]
41. Millet, G.P.; Vleck, V.E.; Bentley, D.J. Physiological differences between cycling and running- lessons from triathletes. *Sports Med.* **2009**, *39*, 179–206. [CrossRef] [PubMed]

Disclaimer/Publisher's Note: The statements, opinions and data contained in all publications are solely those of the individual author(s) and contributor(s) and not of MDPI and/or the editor(s). MDPI and/or the editor(s) disclaim responsibility for any injury to people or property resulting from any ideas, methods, instructions or products referred to in the content.

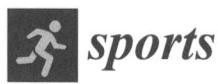

Article

Gender Effect on the Relationship between Talent Identification Tests and Later World Triathlon Series Performance

Alba Cuba-Dorado [1,*], Veronica Vleck [2], Tania Álvarez-Yates [1] and Oscar Garcia-Garcia [1]

[1] Laboratory of Sport Performance, Physical Condition and Wellness, Faculty of Education and Sport Sciences, University of Vigo, Campus A Xunqueira s/n, 36005 Pontevedra, Spain; tanalvarez@uvigo.es (T.Á.-Y.); oscargarcia@uvigo.es (O.G.-G.)

[2] Centre for the Interdisciplinary Study of Human Performance (CIPER), Faculdade de Motricidade Humana, University of Lisbon, Estrada da Costa, Cruz Quebrada-Dafundo, 1499-002 Lisbon, Portugal; vvleck@fmh.ulisboa.pt

* Correspondence: acuba@uvigo.es; Tel.: +34-986-801-772

Abstract: Background: We examined the explanatory power of the Spanish triathlon talent identification (TID) tests for later World Triathlon Series (WTS)-level racing performance as a function of gender. Methods: Youth TID (100 m and 1000 m swimming and 400 m and 1000 m running) test performance times for when they were 14–19 years old, and WTS performance data up to the end of 2017, were obtained for 29 female and 24 male "successful" Spanish triathletes. The relationships between the athletes' test performances and their later best WTS ranking positions and performance times were modeled using multiple linear regression. Results: The swimming and running TID test data had greater explanatory power for best WTS ranking in the females and for best WTS position in the males (R^2a = 0.34 and 0.37, respectively, $p \leq 0.009$). The swimming TID times were better related to later race performance than were the running TID times. The predictive power of the TID tests for WTS performance was, however, low, irrespective of exercise mode and athlete gender. Conclusions: These results confirm that triathlon TID tests should not be based solely on swimming and running performance. Moreover, the predictive value of the individual tests within the Spanish TID battery is gender specific.

Keywords: elite; testing; prediction; triathlete; talent; gender

Citation: Cuba-Dorado, A.; Vleck, V.; Álvarez-Yates, T.; Garcia-Garcia, O. Gender Effect on the Relationship between Talent Identification Tests and Later World Triathlon Series Performance. *Sports* **2021**, *9*, 164. https://doi.org/10.3390/sports9120164

Academic Editor: Michael Duncan

Received: 14 October 2021
Accepted: 1 December 2021
Published: 6 December 2021

Publisher's Note: MDPI stays neutral with regard to jurisdictional claims in published maps and institutional affiliations.

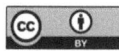

Copyright: © 2021 by the authors. Licensee MDPI, Basel, Switzerland. This article is an open access article distributed under the terms and conditions of the Creative Commons Attribution (CC BY) license (https://creativecommons.org/licenses/by/4.0/).

1. Introduction

Triathlons involve sequential swimming, cycling and running. Only athletes with around a top 150 world ranking may compete in the World Triathlon Series (WTS), i.e., the highest level of competition below the Olympic Games. The annual WTS circuit involves up to nine races over the Olympic (OD) (1.5 km swim, 40 km bike, 10 km run) and Sprint (0.75 km swim, 20 km bike and 5 km run) distances, plus a (more highly scored) Grand Final over the OD. The final WTS season ranking equates to a world championship ranking. Climatic conditions permitting, at any given event, both sexes compete over the same race distances. Within-competition analyses [1–3] have, however, demonstrated that gender differences exist in the relative importance of individual swimming, cycling and running performance to the overall race result in elite triathlon.

The running discipline makes the most decisive contribution to finishing position in World Cups [3,4], World Championship/WTS Grand Finals and the Olympic Games, but more so for males. Swimming performance affects final race position less [1,3]. Vleck et al. [4] reported World Cup performance to relate both to average swimming speed and position at the swim exit. Slower swimmers must reduce their time gap to the leading bike pack(s) by the run start. Swimming speed more strongly affects finishing position in females, however [1,3]. Because of their differences in speed and performance density, cycling performance can become more important in females [2]. Females form more, smaller, cycle packs and are likely less able to bridge gaps between such packs [3].

Pacing strategy also affects elite performance. In both genders, speed up to the first buoy of a one-lap World Cup swim was associated with finishing position. The top 50% of males swam this faster than the bottom 50%. Thereafter, swimming speeds were similar [3]. Elites also reportedly adopt a positive or a reverse J-shaped pacing strategy out of the bike–run transition (T2), running faster within the first kilometer and, when faced with direct opponents, over the final 400 m or less of the run [3–6]. Because they generally exit T2 in larger groups, and have similar 10 km times, this ability to do an "end spurt" may prove to be especially important in males.

To date, only one race analysis [2] has exclusively focused on WTS events. It examined the relative influence of the three triathlon disciplines on WTS performance, across two Olympic cycles, in 1670 males and 1706 females. Competitors were grouped by finishing position (G1: 1st–3rd place; G2: 4th–8th place; G3: 9th–16th place and G4: ≥17th place). The main effects of years and rank groups were compared. For females, swim and bike segment differences existed only between G4 and the other groups (p = 0.001–0.029). Each group differed from the other for the run (p < 0.001). For males, swimming performance differed only between G4 and the other groups (p = 0.001–0.039). Although running was where differences existed between all the groups (p < 0.001), it was apparently important for success that a good runner be positioned with the first cycling pack. Bike splits did not differ, however, between the different male groups, for whom "the bike leg seemed to be a smooth transition towards running" [2]. Only the first 16 women had similar bike splits, however. Even at the WTS level, females likely divide up into more bike groups, further apart, and may therefore be more affected by residual fatigue at the run start than males [2].

These gender differences in the relative extent to which performance in its component disciplines influences triathlon performance [2,3] may have important consequences for talent identification (ID). The extent to which talent ID test results relate to adult performance is used to justify the resources that are allocated to it. This then can markedly impact the selected athletes' likelihood of sporting success. To date, however, most triathlon talent ID research has either involved mixed-gender groups or just males. "While . . . we know very little about predictors of talent in elite sport, we know even less about predicting talent in female athletes. Given the often-unique development systems for high-performance female athletes, this discrepancy might limit our ability to gain a deeper understanding of talent, and . . . lead to potentially harmful consequences for the female athlete population" [7].

We do not know the extent to which the individual predictive capacities of the tests within the Spanish Triathlon Federation (FETRI) battery differ with gender. Although they were previously reported to have little predictive capacity [8] (in that case for National Championship-level performance), the study sample was of mixed gender. The extent to which FETRI talent ID test results separately relate to male and female WTS performance is unknown. Therefore, the aim of this study was to explore, as a function of gender, the extent to which the FETRI talent ID test results predicted the later WTS performance of Spanish triathletes.

2. Materials and Methods

2.1. Study Design

An explanatory transverse study design was used to establish the relationship between the FETRI talent ID test results (Table 1), and later WTS performance, of both males and females (Table 2). Two independent analyses were carried out: (1) for best end-season WTS ranking (RankWTS) and (2) for best WTS individual event position (PositionWTS).

2.2. Participants

Our subjects were considered "the successful products" of the FETRI talent ID process because they either obtained a final WTS ranking or raced at the WTS level in 2009–2017.

Table 1. FETRI scoring system for performance of the individual components of the Spanish triathlon ID test battery.

Age	Points	Females				Males			
		R400	R1000	S100	S1000	R400	R1000	S100	S1000
14 years	3	1:19.0	3:55.0	1:17.0	14:10.0	1:07.0	3:14.0	1:09.0	13:30.0
	10	1:12.0	3:20.0	1:10.0	13:00.0	1:00.0	2:46.0	1:02.0	12:20.0
	12	1:10.0	3:10.0	1:08.0	12:40.0	0:58.0	2:40.0	1:00.0	12:00.0
16–17 years	2	1:19.0	3:55.0	1:17.0	14:10.0	1:07.0	3:14.0	1:09.0	13:30.0
	10	1:11.0	3:15.0	1:09.0	12:50.0	0:59.0	2:43.0	1:01.0	12:10.0
	11	1:10.0	3:10.0	1:08.0	12:40.0	0:58.0	2:40.0	1:00.0	12:00.0
18–19 years	1	1:19.0	3:55.0	1:17.0	14:10.0	1:07.0	3:14.0	1:09.0	13:30.0
	10	1:10.0	3:10.0	1:08.0	12:40.0	0:58.0	2:40.0	1:00.0	12:00.0

Athlete's age was determined by their age on 31 December in the year of the tests. Performance times are given in mm:ss.s. S100: 100 m freestyle swimming test, S1000: 1000 m freestyle swimming test. R400: 400 m running test; R1000: 1000 m running test.

Table 2. Performance times achieved within the FETRI talent identification test battery; best seasonal WTS rankings, best seasonal finishing positions within an individual WTS event achieved by "successful" Spanish triathletes (mean ± SD).

Talent ID Test Performances	Females			Males		
	N	Time (min:ss.s ± s)	4R (%)	N	Time (min:ss.s ± s)	4R (%)
S100	29	01:05.82 ± 2.56	93.28 ± 4.15	24	01:00.81 ± 3.52	90.04 ± 5.30
S1000	29	12:53.07 ± 42.01	89.64 ± 16.46	24	12:27.38 ± 55.54	89.38 ± 6.71
R400	28	01:10.96 ± 3.99	88.78 ± 7.41	22	00:58.51 ± 2.92	92.95 ± 4.27
R1000	29	03:17.72 ± 9.64	93.90 ± 5.80	23	02:46.26 ± 9.98	93.57 ± 4.23
WTS Results	Females			Males		
	N	Mean ± SD	Min-Max	N	Mean ± SD	Min-Max
Rank	26	100 ± 44	44–159	24	83 ± 53	1–165
Position	21	36 ± 14	18–58	19	24 ± 18	1–55

N: number of triathletes; F: females, M: males, 4R: percentage of the best ever times within the talent identification test, S100: 100 m freestyle swimming test, S1000: 1000 m freestyle swimming test. R400: 400 m running test; R1000; 1000 m running test. WTS: World Triathlon Series; Rank: best ranking position obtained by the triathletes within the WTS (i.e., RankWTS), Position: best position obtained by the triathlete within an individual WTS race (i.e., PositionWTS).

2.3. Procedures

From 2009 to 2016, 3502 fourteen to nineteen year-olds underwent the FETRI test battery. This comprised two freestyle swimming tests (i.e., S100: a 100 m time trial; S1000: a 1000 m time trial) in a 25 m pool, and two running track tests (i.e., R400: a 400 m time trial; R1000: a 1000 m time trial). Each test performance time (in seconds, T) was scored, up to a maximum of 12 points, using a proprietary FETRI age- and sex-specific scale (Table 1) [8–10]. Those who scored 8 or more points in each of at least three tests were then separated into age- and gender-specific subgroups. One-year age groups, as opposed to category (e.g., "junior" or "cadet") groupings, were used to offset relative age effect(s) [11]. Each individual's total test performance time was then expressed as a percentage of the fastest ever summated four (swim and run) test times for their age subgroup (variable 4R).

The World Triathlon results database (see www.triathlon.org accessed on 1 april 2021) was then used to identify the "successful" 24 males and 29 females to which this study pertains before their talent ID data were obtained from FETRI.

The research protocol was both in accordance with the Declaration of Helsinki and approved by the local University Ethics committee.

2.4. Statistical Analysis

Sufficient sample size was calculated using G * Power v3.1.9.4 for Windows (Heinrich-Heine-Universität Düsseldorf, GER), resulting in an N of 48 being considered appropriate (effect size = 0.36; α error probability = 0.05; power = 0.95). Sample normality, linearity and homoscedasticity were assumed after carrying out the Kolmogorov–Smirnov test. Pearson's bivariate correlation coefficient was used to determine the inter-relationships between test times. The relationships between the successful athletes' talent ID test results and their RankWTS and PositionWTS data were modeled using step-by-step multiple linear regression. The degree of data independence was calculated using the Durbin–Watson test (and assuming independence of values between 1.5 and 2.5). Variance inflation factor (VIF) values above 10 were taken to indicate multicollinearity. The 95% confidence level was considered statistically significant. All the analyses were performed with the Statistics Package for the Social Sciences (SPSS version 19.0 for Windows, SPSS Inc., Chicago, IL, USA).

3. Results

The athletes' swimming and running test times (Table 3) were positively intercorrelated in the males. The correlation coefficients were large for between S100 and S1000 (r = 0.853, p = 0.001), and moderate for between S100 and R400 (r = 0.431, p = 0.045), S100 and R1000 (r = 0.431, p = 0.045), S1000 and R1000 (r = 0.552, p = 0.006) and R1000 and R400 (r = 0.742, p = 0.001). In the females, only R400 and R1000 (r = 0.836, p = 0.001), and S100 and S1000 (r = 0.750, p = 0.001) were significantly intercorrelated.

Table 3. Summary of the linear regression models for the best seasonal WTS ranking position and best seasonal finishing positions within an individual WTS event achieved by "successful" Spanish triathletes.

		WTS Performance Predictors						
		Predictors	R^2	R^2_a	R	Error	Sig	D-W
Rank	All	$4R_{R1000}$, T_{S100}, $4R_{S1000}$	0.346	0.303	0.588	40.710	0.000	1.16
	F	$4R_{R1000}$, TS100, $4R_{S1000}$	0.415	0.336	0.645	35.479	0.007	1.73
	M	T_{R400}, $4R_{S1000}$	0.391	0.326	0.625	44.863	0.009	1.56
Position	All	$4R_{R1000}$, T_{S100}, T_{S1000}	0.415	0.365	0.644	13.577	0.000	2.10
	F	T_{S1000}, $4R_{S100}$	0.342	0.268	0.584	11.977	0.023	1.13
	M	T_{S1000}, T_{S100}	0.442	0.372	0.664	14.351	0.009	1.69

R: Multiple linear regression; R^2: R Square; R^2_a: adjusted R2; Error: standard error; D-W: Durbin–Watson test. F: females, M: males, 4R: percentage of the best ever times within the talent identification test, S100: 100 m freestyle swimming test, S1000: 1000 m freestyle swimming test. R400: 400 m running test; R1000; 1000 m running test. WTS: World Triathlon Series; Rank: best ranking position obtained by the triathletes within the WTS (i.e., RankWTS), Position: best position obtained by the triathlete within an individual WTS race (i.e., PositionWTS).

Table 3 also presents the linear regression models for the relationships between talent ID test results and both RankWTS and PositionWTS. For the values obtained with the Durbin–Watson test (with the exception of "all cases" in the response to RankWTS and "females" in the response to PositionWTS) independence of the residuals was assumed. As no VIF values exceeded 3.5, multicollinearity was not considered to be a problem.

The females' talent ID test results best explained their best WTS ranking. According to the value of the adjusted coefficient of determination (R^2_a) ($p \leq 0.007$), 33.6% of the total variance in best female ranking at the end of the season was explained by $4R_{R1000}$, T_{S100} and $4R_{S1000}$. The regression equation was:

$$\text{Female RankWTS} = -960.306 + 7.060 \times 4R_{S1000} - 2.852 \times 4R_{R1000} + 10.285 \times T_{S100} \quad (1)$$

The males' talent ID test results, however, better explained best individual WTS race position than best male season-end WTS rankings. The corresponding R^2_a ($p \leq 0.009$) indicated that 37.2% of the total variance in male PositionWTS was explained by S100 and S1000 performance times:

$$\text{Male PositionWTS} = -101.692 - 0.315 \times T_{S1000} + 5.933 \times T_{S100} \quad (2)$$

4. Discussion

Few data relating to the accuracy of early talent decisions exist [7]. "High-quality scientific research is needed in order to (a) determine the reliability and validity of talent identification and selection initiatives, (b) inform evidence-based models of athlete development, and (c) identify gaps in current understanding and directions for future work. Ineffective or inaccurate decisions have important repercussions for all stakeholders involved (e.g., dropout, decreased motivation, misplaced resources, and investment)" [12].

Baker et al. [12] stated that it is "imperative to better understand factors related to female-specific talent development." Although their review of the talent-related literature indicated over thirty such triathlon studies to have taken place thus far, we believe this to be the first one to examine the accuracy of talent decisions for expert male and female triathletes. FETRI test performance poorly predicted WTS performance in both genders. In our "successful" females, talent ID results explained 33.6% of the variance in best end-season WTS ranking (i.e., the more important of the two variables) and 26.8% of the variance in best individual WTS race placing. In "successful" males, the corresponding values were 32.6% and 37.2%. In our results, when both genders were analyzed together (Table 3), the explanatory power of the tests dropped (from 33.65% in females and 32.6% in males) to 30.3% overall for best end-season WTS ranking and to 36.5% for best individual WTS event position. This is both unsurprising, given that the constraints and developmental models of females differ from those of males, and confirms that the predictive capacity of the battery FETRI talent ID test is gender specific.

The explanatory power of the *individual* FETRI tests for best WTS performance also differed with gender. Again, this finding, given the gender differences in the relative importance of performance within each triathlon discipline that exists at the WTS level, was expected, since the "disciplines that precede the triathlon run appear to have more impact on overall race performance in females than they do in males. In males, where the performance density is better, the ability to complete a fast, sprint type, run finish can be definitive" [2].

However, we did not set out to predict WTS performance *per se*. Rather, we explored how much of the variance in male and female WTS performance could be explained by performance in each of the FETRI swim and run tests. The prognostic validity of these predictors for draft-legal OD triathlon performance is unconfirmed, nor are the optimal pacing strategies within the WTS competition yet known. However, the (44 race) analysis that was conducted by Piacentini et al. [2] found differences in swim times, bike times and run times between podium (G1), 4th and 8th place (G2), 9th and 16th place (G3), and ≥17th place (G4) female WTS finishers. Within males, these differences occurred only for swimming and running. No difference in swimming segment times was noted, in both sexes, between the first three such groups. It was clearly important to overall WTS performance that good runners were able to position themselves within the first cycling packs to reach T2.

Piacentini's study population would have included our males and females, classing them as G1–G4 and G4 triathletes, respectively. In males, therefore, we expected to see significant relationships between the swim and run FETRI test results and performance. Piacentini et al. [2] observed that for males, exiting the water and exiting T2 close to the leader, with a fast running split, appeared to be major determinants of success. In females, both the T1 and T2 exits were important, as was a very fast run split. In males, G1 also differed from G2 to G4 as regards entry into T1 and exit from T2. Entry into T1 was less important than exit from T2, and run sprinting ability was likely more important, in males. In females, position out of T2 was likely more important for overall performance than was sprinting ability.

The 1000 m swim test featured in all our models, as did the 100 m swim test, in all cases apart from the males' best RankWTS. As regards the running tests, when both genders were analyzed together, the 1000 m featured in both the RankWTS and the PositionWTS models. When we analyzed each sex separately, the 1000 m run only had predictive power for the females' best RankWTS. In males, the 400 m run test predicted best WTS finishing place. Again, our results broadly agree with Piacentini et al. [2]. The triathlon run is a more decisive contributor than the swim and the bike to the race result, at multiple levels of elite competition. Observed correlation coefficients between triathlon swim and run performance, and overall finishing position, of −0.36–0.42 vs. 0.88–0.94 for males and −0.47–0.49 vs. r = 0.71–0.85 for females, respectively, support this [1–3]. However, the FETRI swim tests explained more variance in WTS performance than the run tests did. Some possible reasons why this was the case, aside from the relative heterogeneity that existed in the performance levels of our two gender groups, are detailed below.

The S100 and S1000 tests that our triathletes underwent in the FETRI talent ID battery are thought to be largely anaerobic and aerobic, respectively. To *some* extent, they reflect the reality of elite competition, "for which the ability to start fast . . . and then maintain a steady swim pace below 90% of . . . maximal speed could be seen as a preferred pacing strategy" [6]. World-Cup-level triathletes have been noted to swim faster up to the first swim buoy and then to sustain a relatively slower pace over the rest of (each) swim lap [3,4]. This first buoy is normally *250–350 m* from the shore/pontoon. How fast the speeds over the first 100 m, compared to the rest, of that 250–350 m are is unknown, however. No "surge" data are available for these intermediate sections, nor do we know to what extent elites speed up just before the swim–land transition(s). Yet, it seems appropriate that the talent ID test battery includes both a short and a longer swim. However, we do not know which of the various test distances used by different federations (e.g., the 200 m and 400 m of Italy that Bottoni et al. [13] reported vs. the 100 m and 1000 m of Spain) is the optimal combination.

Perhaps, however, the potential relevance of the shorter swim test is increasing over time. The 2017/2018 WTS season included more sprint distance events [6]. The best WTS triathletes from a given country are fairly likely to also represent it at the Olympic Games, not only over in the OD but also within the mixed team relay (MTAR). MTAR competitors do a 300 m swim, a 6.6 km cycle and *a 1 km* run before handing over to a teammate, in the given order of female–male–female–male. Sharma and Periard [5] reported that Australian athletes competing at the 2014 MTAR World Championships also implemented positive swim pacing, "likely due to a desire to be at the head of the swim group and avoid being disrupted (i.e., stroke mechanics, breathing, "fighting" for position) by swimming in a large group." It makes sense that the ability to make a fast start at the very onset of the swim may become increasingly important in elites, although insufficient data are yet published relating to this point.

As for running, the 400 m and 1000 m run tests that our triathletes performed as part of the FETRI talent ID battery have a marked anaerobic component. Although the triathlon run was traditionally thought to be predominantly aerobic, the situation in elite draft-legal races is more nuanced [5]. This may partly be because of the common athlete tactic, which for the OD seems to contradict physiological principles, of a fast start out of T2. Within-race analyses usually report this fast start to occur over the first *1000 m*, i.e., over the same distance as the longer FETRI run test, but researchers traditionally position their cameras at 1 km from T2. Etxebarria et al. [14] also examined (only male) pacing over 2.5 km sections of the 10 km run after 2016. They did this over 14 World Cup and WTS events, over three years and 726 race outcomes. The 171 males ran "the first lap of the standard four lap circuit substantially faster than laps 2 (~7%), 3 (~9%) and 4 (~12%)."

We are unaware of any speed data relating to between when an athlete racks their bike and perhaps trying to avoid "getting stuck in a traffic jam" [15]) when he/she gets out on to earlier parts of the run. However, "at the speeds run by elite male triathletes drafting may have some benefit on oxygen consumption and therefore performance; as such triathletes may want to adopt a faster start to keep up with leading runners. Additionally, triathletes present in the front group and thus in contention for the victory could have a psychological advantage over chasing athletes and therefore perform better . . . " However, balancing the benefits of drafting against the physiological cost of a faster start would be a key consideration, with the potential for specific athletes (i.e., those with " ... higher anaerobic tolerance qualities to target an aggressive pacing strategy") [5].

The athletes, particularly males, as, historically, they have greater performance density, who can do this *and* then do a "kick" or spurt over the last *400 m or less* of the 10 km, *when/if needed,* are likely to possess a competitive advantage over those who cannot. Interestingly, Sharma and Periard [5] demonstrated that fast run starts also occur within the MTAR. It is unknown to what extent they occur in Sprint distance WTS races, but these can account for approximately a quarter of WTS events [2]. Such information is therefore relevant to future talent ID and development.

We expected our low predictive power of the FETRI data for WTS performance. Talent ID tests generally possess low predictive power [7,16]. Moreover, Cuba-Dorado et al. [8] already found this, albeit in a mixed-gender sample, in relation to the draft-legal Spanish National OD Championships performance of the same year. Piacentini et al. [2] already demonstrated smaller time differences to exist between groups and athletes at the WTS level than have been previously recorded for lower-tier elite events. Obviously, differentiating between individuals who are at the same level of participation is particularly challenging at the top level [12]. The low predictive power shown by our results notwithstanding, it is heartening that the FETRI test battery predicted better WTS rankings than it did best individual WTS event placings. Rankings are both a measure of performance consistency and (partly) circumvent the problem of triathlon not having standardized course lengths or course difficulty ratings. The WTS ranking is by far the more important of the two variables.

We note that the predictive power of the talent ID tests for the WTS ranking was slightly better in females. A clear relative age effect (RAE), even for one-year groupings, was reported in males on this *same* test battery. It is less evident in females, which may partly explain the gender difference [11]. Despite the fact that an RAE was demonstrated for the male triathletes who competed in the 2012 Olympic Games [17], none of the investigations of the Spanish test set to date (including this one) seem to have adequately accounted for the physical maturity levels of the individual athletes at the time of its administration. Basing the 4R data around one-year athlete groups, as opposed to the two-year performance categories that exist in Spain, only does so to some extent. At least in males, the RAE has been demonstrated even within these one-year age categories [11]. This study did not account for the time interval between the athletes doing the talent ID tests and their WTS results, although Cuba-Dorado et al. [8] also reported that the length of the time interval between the administration of the Spanish talent ID tests and the competition under investigation affected the explanatory power of the tests for said competition results. Deliberate sports practice over a long period of time has certainly been shown to influence the difference in performance between experts and novices. This is especially so for running [18].

However, given *how* low the explanatory power of the FETRI battery is (and the advent of the MTAR as an Olympic event), in both genders, it may be worthwhile re-evaluating how it is made up. Our results confirm, for the WTS, what Bottoni et al. [13] wrote a decade ago, i.e., that triathlon talent ID test batteries should not exclusively focus on evaluating swimming and running performance. Bottoni et al. [13] made that assertion on the basis of comparative retrospective data, dating back to when their subjects were 14 years of age, for sixty-six top 5 male World Cup, World Championship and Olympic Games finishers over the period 2000–2008 vs. top 15 Italian males. The data indicated that cognitive/psychological assessment [13,19], and assessing the athlete's level of physiological and psychological maturity [20] are good ideas. So too is the collection of data on the athlete's previous performance/training history [7].

We emphasize that talent identification should focus on recognizing athletes who have the *potential* for future excellence [21], because early entry into the talent ID system and its associated benefits can be a crucial factor in talent development [22]. It remains important that the scoring criteria for identifying athletes via the existing FETRI tests are not too restrictive. This would allow enough triathletes to continue within the talent identification program and, later on, be assessed both on their rates of improvement [13] and more specific aspects of elite performance such as their technical and tactical skills [22].

In addition to being accused of relying "on a relatively small number of heavily weighted variables measured in isolation from the sport context," many talent ID batteries stand accused of "adopting testing batteries that do not accurately represent the sport demands" [16]. Johnston and Baker's comment is definitely pertinent to the sport of triathlon, which *must be seen to be more than the sum of the sports of which it is made up* [23]. Using the 4R variable, which partly accounts for performance across shorter and longer distances of each of two of the three triathlon disciplines, measured separately, is not enough to do this. A key reason for this likely is that the triathlete's cycling ability, which can to some extent compensate for a poor position, relative to the leading bike packs, at the swim exit, and affect how fresh they are at the run start [24], is ignored.

It is logical that once an athlete has been selected via the initial talent ID process, a more detailed assessment of their potential to achieve elite-level performance be conducted [5,6]. Said assessment should include measurement of the universally acknowledged key triathlete ability of starting each discipline with minimal residual fatigue from the preceding disciplines. This could be done by a cycle–run-specific transition test, at least three lab-based versions and two field-based versions of which exist [25]. The five tests all assess the extent to which the triathlon run start is influenced by residual fatigue from the bike section. They perhaps vary in their suitability of application for different scenarios and different athlete groups.

We draw the reader's attention to the fact that both laboratory and anecdotal race data suggest that the athletes who are less well adjusted at the run start exhibit decreased stride lengths. "Athletes with longer running contact times may produce the same impulse for a lower metabolic cost than their stiff ... and/or fast twitch counterparts" [26]. It may be that the athletes who exhibit a higher stride frequency at the run start *may then pay for this by not subsequently being able to exert a "kick" or speed spurt, if it is needed, at the run finish*. The extent to which the athlete exhibits a less efficient running style, and their pacing over the rest of the race, may be related to their cycle: anaerobic power reserve (APR) [27] and/or run-specific anaerobic speed reserve (ASR) [28]. These are typically defined as the difference between maximal sprint power output and power output at maximum oxygen uptake (VO_2max) and the difference between maximal sprinting speed and running speed at VO_2max, respectively. We note that, although the study had methodological issues, when the performances of senior and junior males on the Spanish bike–run field test (i.e., a 30 min steady-state cycle plus a self-paced 3 km run) [29] were compared, they were found to differ in run pacing style. Because having a good APR/ASR may differentiate between athletes who are relatively homogenous as regards other, commonly measured, markers, and because APR/ASR development relates to both developmental and training levels, it may be a useful longitudinal marker. Cycle and run field tests for it exist [27,30]. The ability to recover from cycle surges will of course affect the athlete's fatigue at the run start. This may then compound the negative effects of positive run pacing. Since "a lower anaerobic capacity leads to an inability to accelerate at the end of the race, which can accrue because of a reliance on anaerobic energy to maintain pace in an athlete of inferior running economy" [28], the higher the athlete level, the more relevant APR/ASR testing may become.

"Parameters which differentiate athletes at one competition level may not be as valuable as athletes' progress" [20]. Variability in the extent to which the performance in the same component of the test battery contributes to successful performance across different levels of competition is also something to explore. It would be interesting to study, on a longitudinal basis, whether monitoring the factors that are perhaps then identified as distinguishing "expertise" from "eminence" (e.g., between being able to achieve a top 50 placing at National Triathlon Championships vs. obtaining a high enough world ranking to be competing at the WTS level) [16] could be used to distinguish between triathletes with differing capabilities of sustaining a given pacing strategy, and then to train this capacity [19].

Given all of the above, it can be considered both a strength and a limitation of our study that it focused specifically on the extent to which the *Spanish* talent ID test battery explained later WTS-level performance. It is only because Spain has been one of the top-performing countries in the world for triathlon that we were able to achieve such high numbers of "successful" elites, of both genders, for our regression analysis. Had we been able, however, to extend this analysis to involve the "successful" athletes from other countries as well, we would probably have been able to gain better insight into exactly which of the different talent ID test distance combinations that are implemented by such countries best explains the variance in top-level triathlon performance.

5. Conclusions

We confirmed, at the WTS level, the finding that "retrospective analysis of running and swimming performance outcomes *only* is not an appropriate method for predicting future triathlon success" [13]. However, as research into the efficacy of talent selection decisions, particularly that which compares the two sexes, is rare [7,19], our demonstration of clear gender differences in the explanatory power of the individual tests within the talent ID battery for WTS performance is noteworthy. So too are the clear corollaries between these gender differences and how males and females were actually performing in the WTS-level competition.

Author Contributions: Conceptualization, A.C.-D. and O.G.-G.; methodology, A.C.-D. and O.G.-G.; software, A.C-D. and O.G.-G.; validation, A.C.-D. and O.G.-G.; formal analysis, A.C.-D. and O.G.-G.; investigation, A.C.-D. and O.G.-G.; resources, A.C.-D. and O.G.-G.; data curation, A.C.-D.; writing—original draft preparation, A.C.-D., T.A and O.G.-G.; writing—discussion, V.V., writing—review and editing, A.C.-D., V.V., T.Á.-Y. and O.G.-G.; supervision, V.V. and O.G.-G. All authors have read and agreed to the published version of the manuscript.

Funding: This research received no external funding.

Institutional Review Board Statement: The study was conducted according to the guidelines of the Declaration of Helsinki and approved by the Ethics Research Committee of the Faculty of Education and Sports Sciences of the University of Vigo (Protocol Code: 02-2501-17 and approved 25 January 2017).

Informed Consent Statement: Not applicable.

Data Availability Statement: Data of the talent ID test battery and the National Sports Development Program scoring scales were obtained from the FETRI website (see www.triatlon.org accessed on 1 April 2021). World Triathlon Series performance was extracted from the World Triathlon results database (see www.triatlon.org accessed on 1 April 2021).

Acknowledgments: We thank the Spanish Triathlon Federation for giving us their written permission to publish their 2015 Talent Scoring Scales (Federación Española de Triatlón 2019a, b), as well as all the athletes and support staff who took part in this project. V.V. acknowledges the support of the Fundação para a Ciência e Tecnologia, as expressed by Grant UIDB/00447/2020 to CIPER-Centro Interdisciplinar para o Estudo da Performance Humana (unit 447).

Conflicts of Interest: The authors declare no conflict of interest.

References

1. Cejuela, R.; Cortell-Tormo, J.M.; Mira-Chinchilla, J.J.; Pérez-Turpin, J.A.; Villa, J.G. Gender differences in elite Olympic distance triathlon performances. *J. Hum. Sport Exerc.* **2012**, *7*, 434–445. [CrossRef]
2. Piacentini, M.F.; Bianchini, L.A.; Minganti, C.; Sias, M.; Di Castro, A.; Vleck, V. Is the bike segment of modern Olympic triathlon more a transition towards running in males that it is in females? *Sports* **2019**, *7*, 76. [CrossRef] [PubMed]
3. Vleck, V.E.; Bentley, D.J.; Millet, G.P.; Bürgi, A. Pacing during an elite Olympic distance triathlon: Comparison between male and female competitors. *J. Sci. Med. Sport* **2008**, *11*, 424–432. [CrossRef] [PubMed]
4. Vleck, V.E.; Burgi, A.; Bentley, D.J. The consequences of swim, cycle, and run performance on overall result in elite Olympic distance triathlon. *Int. J. Sports Med.* **2006**, *27*, 43–48. [CrossRef]

5. Sharma, A.P.; Periard, J.D. Physiological requirements of the different distances of triathlon. In *Triathlon Medicine*; Migliorini, S., Ed.; Springer: Berlin/Heidelberg, Germany, 2020; pp. 5–17. [CrossRef]
6. Walsh, J.A. The rise of elite short-course triathlon re-emphasises the necessity to transition efficiently from cycling to running. *Sports* **2019**, *7*, 99. [CrossRef]
7. Johnston, K.; Wattie, N.; Schorer, J.; Baker, J. Talent identification in sport: A systematic review. *Sports Med.* **2018**, *48*, 97–109. [CrossRef]
8. Cuba-Dorado, A.; García-García, O.; Morales-Sánchez, V.; Hernández-Mendo, A. The explanatory capacity of talent identification tests for performance in triathlon competitions: A longitudinal analysis. *J. Hum. Kinet.* **2020**, *75*, 185–193. [CrossRef] [PubMed]
9. Federación Española de Triatlón (2019a). Baremos PNTD natación 2015 [National Sports Development Programme—Swimming Scale-2015]. Available online: https://triatlon.org/wp-content/uploads/2019/10/Baremacion-2015-natacion.pdf (accessed on 5 May 2021).
10. Federación Española de Triatlón (2019b). Baremos PNTD Carrera a pie 2015. [National Sports Development Programme—Running scale-2015]. Available online: https://triatlon.org/wp-content/uploads/2019/10/NUEVA-Baremacion-2015-carrera-a-pie.pdf (accessed on 5 May 2021).
11. Ortigosa-Márquez, J.M.; Reigal, R.E.; Serpa, S.; Hernández-Mendo, A. Relative age effect on national selection process in triathlon. *Rev. Int. Med. Cienc. Act. Fís. Deporte* **2018**, *18*, 199–211. [CrossRef]
12. Baker, J.; Wilson, S.; Johnston, K.; Dehghansai, N.; Koenigsberg, A.; Steven de Vegt, S.; Wattie, N. Talent Research in Sport 1990–2018: A Scoping Review. *Front. Psychol.* **2020**, *11*, 607710. [CrossRef]
13. Bottoni, A.; Gianfelici, A.; Tamburri, R.; Faina, M. Talent selection criteria for Olympic distance triathlon. *J. Hum. Sport Exerc.* **2011**, *6*, 293–304. [CrossRef]
14. Etxebarria, N.; Wright, J.; Jeacocke, H.; Mesquida, C.; Pyne, D.B. Running your best triathlon race. *Int. J. Sports Physiol. Perform.* **2021**, *16*, 744–747. [CrossRef]
15. Millet, G.P.; Vleck, V.E. Physiological and biomechanical adaptations to the cycle to run transition in Olympic triathlon: Review and practical recommendations for training. *Br. J. Sports Med.* **2000**, *34*, 384–390. [CrossRef]
16. Johnston, K.; Baker, J. Waste reduction strategies: Factors affecting talent wastage and the efficacy of talent selection in sport. *Front. Psychol.* **2020**, *10*, 2925. [CrossRef]
17. Werneck, F.Z.; Lima, J.R.; Coelho, E.F.; Matta, M.D.; Figueiredo, A.J. Efeito da idade relativa em atletas Olímpicos de triatlo [Effect of relative age on Olympic triathlon athletes]. *Rev. Bras. Med. Esporte* **2014**, *20*, 394–397. [CrossRef]
18. Macnamara, B.N.; Hambrick, D.Z.; Oswald, F.L. Deliberate practice and performance in music, games, sports, education, and professions: A meta-analysis. *Psychol. Sci.* **2014**, *25*, 1608–1618. [CrossRef] [PubMed]
19. Baker, J.; Wattie, N.; Schorer, J. A proposed conceptualization of talent in sport: The first step in a long and winding road. *Psychol. Sport Exerc.* **2019**, *43*, 27–33. [CrossRef]
20. Mitchell, L.G.; Rattray, B.; Saunders, P.U.; Pyne, D.B. The relationship between talent identification testing parameters and performance in elite junior swimmers. *J. Sci. Med. Sport* **2018**, *21*, 1281–1285. [CrossRef]
21. Vaeyens, R.; Lenoir, M.; Williams, A.M.; Philippaerts, R.M. Talent identification and development programmes in sport: Current models and future directions. *Sports Med.* **2008**, *38*, 703–714. [CrossRef] [PubMed]
22. Koopmann, T.; Faber, I.; Baker, J.; Schorer, J. Assessing technical skills in talented youth athletes: A systematic review. *Sports Med.* **2020**, *50*, 1593–1611. [CrossRef]
23. Vleck, V. Triathlon. In *Epidemiology of Injury in Olympic Sports*; Caine, D.J., Harmer, P.A., Schiff, M.A., Eds.; Blackwell Publishing: Chichester, UK, 2010; pp. 294–320. [CrossRef]
24. Etxebarria, N.; Anson, J.M.; Pyne, D.B.; Ferguson, R.A. Cycling attributes that enhance running performance after the cycle section in triathlon. *Int. J. Sports Physiol. Perform.* **2013**, *8*, 502–509. [CrossRef]
25. Vleck, V.; Alves, B. Triathlon transition tests: Overview and recommendations for future research. *RICYDE* **2011**, *7*, 1–3. [CrossRef]
26. Sandford, G.N.; Kilding, A.E.; Ross, A.; Laursen, P.B. Maximal sprint speed and the anaerobic speed reserve domain: The untapped tools that differentiate the world's best male 800 m runners. *Sports Med.* **2019**, *49*, 843–852. [CrossRef] [PubMed]
27. Sanders, D.; Heijboer, M. The anaerobic power reserve and its applicability in professional road cycling. *J. Sports Sci.* **2019**, *37*, 621–629. [CrossRef]
28. Mercier, Q.; Aftalion, A.; Hanley, B. A model for world-class 10,000 m running performances: Strategy and optimization. *Front. Sports Act. Living* **2021**, *2*, 226. [CrossRef] [PubMed]

29. Díaz, V.; Peinado, A.B.; Vleck, V.E.; Alvarez-Sánchez, M.; Benito, P.J.; Alves, F.B.; Calderón, F.J.; Zapico, A.G. Longitudinal changes in response to a cycle-run field test of young male national "talent identification" and senior elite triathlon squads. *J. Strength Cond Res.* **2012**, *26*, 2209–2219. [CrossRef] [PubMed]
30. Sandford, G.N.; Rogers, S.A.; Sharma, A.P.; Kilding, A.E.; Ross, A.; Laursen, P.B. Implementing anaerobic speed reserve testing in the field: Validation of VO2max prediction from 1500-m race performance in elite middle-distance runners. *Int. J. Sports Physiol. Perform.* **2019**, *14*, 1147–1150. [CrossRef]

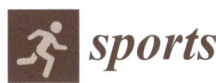

Article

The Training Characteristics of Recreational-Level Triathletes: Influence on Fatigue and Health

João Henrique Falk Neto [1,*], Eric C. Parent [2], Veronica Vleck [3] and Michael D. Kennedy [1]

1. Athlete Health Lab, Faculty of Kinesiology, Sport, & Recreation, University of Alberta, Edmonton, AB T6G 2H9, Canada; kennedy@ualberta.ca
2. Department of Physical Therapy, Faculty of Rehabilitation Medicine, University of Alberta, Edmonton, AB T6G 2G4, Canada; eparent@ualberta.ca
3. CIPER, Faculdade de Motricidade Humana, Universidade de Lisboa, 1499-002 Cruz Quebrada-Dafundo, Lisboa, Portugal; vvleck@fmh.ulisboa.pt
* Correspondence: falkneto@ualberta.ca

Citation: Falk Neto, J.H.; Parent, E.C.; Vleck, V.; Kennedy, M.D. The Training Characteristics of Recreational-Level Triathletes: Influence on Fatigue and Health. *Sports* 2021, *9*, 94. https://doi.org/10.3390/sports9070094

Academic Editor: Nicolas Babault

Received: 9 April 2021
Accepted: 18 June 2021
Published: 25 June 2021

Publisher's Note: MDPI stays neutral with regard to jurisdictional claims in published maps and institutional affiliations.

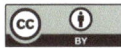

Copyright: © 2021 by the authors. Licensee MDPI, Basel, Switzerland. This article is an open access article distributed under the terms and conditions of the Creative Commons Attribution (CC BY) license (https://creativecommons.org/licenses/by/4.0/).

Abstract: Little is known about how recreational triathletes prepare for an Olympic distance event. The aim of this study was to identify the training characteristics of recreational-level triathletes within the competition period and assess how their preparation for a triathlon influences their health and their levels of fatigue. During the 6 weeks prior to, and the 2 weeks after, an Olympic distance triathlon, nine recreational athletes (five males, four females) completed a daily training log. Participants answered the Daily Analysis of Life Demands Questionnaire (DALDA), the Training Distress Scale (TDS) and the Alberta Swim Fatigue and Health Questionnaire weekly. The Recovery-Stress Questionnaire (REST-Q) was completed at the beginning of the study, on the day before the competition, and at the end of week 8. Training loads were calculated using session-based rating of perceived exertion (sRPE). The data from every week of training was compared to week 1 to determine how athletes' training and health changed throughout the study. No changes in training loads, duration or training intensity distribution were seen in the weeks leading up to the competition. Training duration was significantly reduced in week 6 ($p = 0.041$, d = 1.58, 95% CI = 6.9, 421.9), while the number of sessions was reduced in week 6 (Z = 2.32, $p = 0.02$, ES = 0.88) and week 7 (Z = 2.31, $p = 0.02$, ES = 0.87). Training was characterized by large weekly variations in training loads and a high training intensity. No significant changes were seen in the DALDA, TDS or REST-Q questionnaire scores throughout the 8 weeks. Despite large spikes in training load and a high overall training intensity, these recreational-level triathletes were able to maintain their health in the 6 weeks of training prior to an Olympic distance triathlon.

Keywords: training loads; monitoring; illness; recovery; triathlon

1. Introduction

Triathlon is a unique sport that requires athletes to excel in swimming, cycling and running over a variety of distances. Amateur triathletes make up the majority of participants [1]. Success in the sport requires that triathletes possess above average aerobic power and muscular endurance, along with well-developed anaerobic capacities for surges in pace and for the final moments of the race [2–4]. To be able to prepare for the demands of the sport while mastering the three disciplines, and depending on race distance [2,5–8], age-group triathletes have been reported to train between 8 and 16 h per week.

To maintain this training volume, triathletes may continue to train even when injured, by increasing their training load in another exercise mode to that in which the injury was sustained [4,9,10]. This approach to management of training loads and shifting of training to other modes when injured may expose recreational level triathletes to higher levels of risk for sustaining negative, training related, health outcomes [11]. The intensity at which the training sessions are performed may also be an issue [12]. According to previous research, recreational endurance athletes often perform easy sessions at a pace that is considered too hard [13], whilst not pushing hard enough on the intense training days. This can lead to a program with a higher overall intensity. This itself is linked to delayed recovery following training [14], a greater potential for the occurrence of non-functional overreaching [2,13] and potentially a higher likelihood of the occurrence of injuries [4,15]. Too much intense training can also be detrimental to performance. In endurance sports, a polarized approach, with a focus on training at lower intensities (below the lactate threshold), and with few key sessions at higher intensities, is likely the most effective way to elicit performance improvements [16,17].

The training frequency that is involved in preparation for triathlon competition, and possible associated difficulty in balancing their training and other life commitments, may also lead recreational-level triathletes to experience high levels of stress [18]. General life stress can negatively influence athletes' health status [19], blunt the adaptive response to endurance or resistance training programs [20,21] and moderate the relationship between fatigue and recovery [22]. The monitoring of amateur triathletes' training loads and well-being, to help balance their training and life stress and to improve the chances of early detection of negative health and performance outcomes, is therefore important [23].

Training loads can be monitored with different methods that are related to changes in performance, health and fatigue [3,15,24]. The session rating of perceived exertion (sRPE) is accepted as a valid measure of training load. It may be predictive of illnesses when a spike in training load occurs [24]. Monitoring fatigue levels throughout a training program, however, can be a challenging task. Even though many physiological measures have been investigated, most show little validity or practical application [3,15]. In this context, subjective measures (such as questionnaire-based surveys of mood and perceived stress,) have proven as or more effective than objective measures (such as blood markers and heart rate responses) [15,23,25,26].

Even though far more recreational level age-groupers prepare for the (1.5 km swim, 40 km bike, 10 km run) Olympic distance (OD) competition than do so for the (3.9 km swim, 180 km bike, 42.2 km run) Ironman distance (IR) [1], little is known about their training practices and associated health status. Only one detailed longitudinal prospective investigation of training, maladaptation and training status markers in OD athletes appears to exist [27]. Vleck monitored 51 British National Squad OD specialists over a seven month lead up to the World OD Championships (weeks 20–23 of which included their World Championship qualifying and National Championship OD races). As her 1996 study predated the inception of draft legal racing for Elites, Vleck's subjects were preparing for competition over what is nowadays the amateur OD triathlon format. However, their OD performance times over the study period (of 1:57:04 ± 0:19:55 hh:mm:ss for males and 2:10:30 ± 0:16:41 hh:mm:ss for females), would, even now, place them at the top level of such competition As such, they would be categorized as "well trained." We are only aware of one (6 month) prospective longitudinal investigation of training volume and intensity distribution, in the lead up to competition, of recreational level triathletes [2]. The study of Neal et al. [2], however, involved IR distance athletes. The only, albeit retrospective, comparison of training in IR vs. OD athletes that exists [4] and that used the same methods of data collection for both groups, suggests them to differ in training practice. To date, no prospective longitudinal study of training and maladaptation in recreational level OD triathletes has been published in the academic literature.

The purpose of this study, therefore, was to monitor the training characteristics of recreational-level triathletes in the lead up to an OD triathlon competition and assess how the participants' training influenced measures of health and fatigue. As the phenomenon has been reported with other endurance sports athletes [13], it was hypothesized that recreational triathletes would spend a disproportionate amount of their training time at higher exercise intensities. This would lead the participants to report high levels of fatigue, stress and negative health symptoms on a weekly basis.

2. Materials and Methods

The study was approved by a local Research Ethics Board (Pro00082267). Participants were informed of the risks and benefits of the study prior to signing an informed consent document. Recruitment occurred online via social media and the website of the following events: World Triathlon Series (WTS) Edmonton, WTS Montreal and the Vancouver Triathlon. All the events occurred between July and September of 2018.

2.1. Subjects

The participants were required to have 3 or more years of experience training for and competing in Olympic distance events. In this case, 11 participants (6 males, 5 females), with ages varying between 30 and 47 years old (39.2 ± 5.8, mean ± SD) volunteered for the study and competed in one of the aforementioned events. All the participants were classed as recreational athletes as they were competing in the amateur ("age-group") category, were not part of a regional or national development center and trained and competed in their leisure time [7,8]. None reported training as their main occupation. The Olympic distance race times of our subjects were slower than those of well-trained male age-groupers who had similar triathlon training experience [28]. This confirms the recreational nature of the participants in the current study.

2.2. Measurements

The participants agreed to record their training programs within the 6 weeks leading up to an Olympic distance triathlon that was the key event of their season- and over the 2 weeks that followed the event. A questionnaire was used to cover participants' experience in the sport (i.e., their years of training and competition), and how long they had been training or competing in swimming, cycling and running. Information on the participants' best performance in prior Olympic distance events, the age at which they started training and competing in triathlon, and their past training practice (e.g., their hours of training per week, training frequency and longest session in each exercise mode) was also collected. Lastly, the participants were asked about how many triathlons (over any distance) they had competed in within the current and past years.

2.2.1. Training Monitoring

Training was monitored via a customized online training log that was developed for this study. The participants were instructed to maintain their regular training programs while tracking every session. The training log required participants to report their session goal, activity type (e.g., tempo run, intervals), exercise mode and session rating of perceived exertion (sRPE) [24]. The study participants were also asked to report on other types of sessions that they performed (other modes of endurance training, such as rowing or resistance training sessions, for example) and describe what they were.

2.2.2. Training Load Calculations

External training loads were calculated as the total duration of each session (in minutes) across each week, and separated by mode of training (swimming, cycling, running). The participants' internal loads were calculated using the session rating of perceived exertion method (sRPE) that was developed by Foster [24], with the duration of each session multiplied by the rate of perceived exertion (1–10) that was assigned by the athlete to that session. Training monotony, an index of training variability defined as the daily mean load divided by the standard deviation of the load calculated over a week, was determined for each week [24]. Training strain (the product of training load and monotony) was also calculated weekly [24].

2.2.3. Training Intensity Distribution (TID)

The TID of the athletes was calculated based on the sRPE that was reported for each session. This method was chosen as the researchers did not have data on the participants' maximal heart rates, and it allowed for an easier collection of the intensity of the swimming sessions. Nevertheless, there is evidence to support the use of sRPE for assessing training intensity distribution in endurance athletes [16]. Sessions with a RPE of 4 or lower were considered as zone 1, a RPE of 5 or 6 were considered to equate to zone 2 and a RPE of 7 and above was considered as zone 3 [16]. The duration of each session was then assigned to its respective intensity zone (1, 2 or 3) so that the total amount of time within each zone could be calculated for each mode of exercise (swimming, cycling and running).

2.2.4. Self-Reported Measures of Health, Fatigue and Illness

At the end of each training week, participants were sent three questionnaires: the Daily Analysis of Life Demands (DALDA), the Training Distress Questionnaire and the Alberta Swim Fatigue and Health Questionnaire (details of which are provided below), via a digital link. The athletes were instructed to return the completed forms to the researchers within 24 h of receipt.

The DALDA was formulated on the basis of multiple tests for response consistency that were conducted in swimmers [26]. The reliability criterion was a stress or source item being responded to in the exact same manner on four of five occasions, each 14 days apart, by at least 80% of athletes. If this was not the case, the item was deleted. After this initial evaluation, 9 questions to assess general stress levels and their source (part A) and another 25 questions aimed at determining symptoms of health and fatigue (part B), remained in the questionnaire. Completion of the DALDA involves the athlete rating himself/herself as being either "worse than normal", "normal" or "better than normal" on each variable. As they can be representative of an increased level of (negative) stress [5,26], changes in the numbers of "worse than normal" scores are used to monitor athlete's health. The DALDA can be repeatedly administered during a training period [26] and is sensitive to changes in training loads. In triathletes undergoing a period of intensified training, the questionnaire was considered a practical test to monitor changes in recovery and health [5].

The Training Distress Scale Questionnaire (TDS) [25] both quantifies the psychobiological response to training and helps identify athletes who are at risk of training-induced distress. The TDS was developed from the seven items of the Profile of Mood States (POMS) [29] that Raglin and Morgan [25] considered to be the best identifiers of an athlete in distress. The questionnaire was initially validated in swimmers, across seven time points of their season. It was found to have a mean successful prediction rate of 69.1% ($p < 0.05$). The scale was later both cross-validated and found to be equally effective at identifying athletes in distress, in track and field athletes [25]. The TDS consists of 7 items to which participants rate their mood responses using a 5-point Likert scale (that ranges from "0—not at all" to "4—extremely"). Lower overall scores are taken to mean that the athlete is displaying a better mood state.

Lastly, the Alberta Swim Fatigue and Health questionnaire (ASFH) [30] was used to determine health and fatigue status, as well as general attributes that are associated with good health, on a weekly basis. The ASFH has previously been used to detect changes in respiratory symptoms with manipulations in training load [30], whilst also being used to assess changes in health and fatigue in varsity athletes. The questionnaire collects information about the athletes' overall wellbeing and health, in addition to their respiratory symptoms. Aches and soreness were identified as either a headache or general body ache (that was not specific), joint ache or pain, or muscle soreness, which was separated by body segments (e.g., lower back, shoulders, quadriceps, calves, etc.). A niggle was defined as a nagging pain that still allowed participants to train, although it could force participants to modify their training. If participants had to modify their training, the extent to which it was modified was also reported (i.e., no modification, to a minor extent, to a moderate extent, to a major extent, cannot participate at all).

At study baseline, 48 h prior to the OD race and 2 weeks post-event, the athletes also completed the Recovery Stress Questionnaire for Athletes (REST-Q). The REST-Q, which was initially validated in rowers [31], measures both the frequency of current stress and the frequency of recovery associated activities. It consists of 77 items (19 scales with four items each, plus a warm-up item), each with values ranging from 0 (never) to 6 (always), indicating how often the athlete has participated in activities over the past 3 days and nights [31]. Each of the scales has been rated as both reliable (with Cronbach's α for each scale ranges of between 0.68 and 0.89), and to possess good test-retest reliability [31]. For the purposes of this study, total stress was calculated as the sum of the 10 stress subscales, while total recovery was calculated as the sum of the 9 recovery subscales. The athletes' recovery-stress balance was calculated as the total stress score minus the total recovery score [6]. High scores in stress-associated scales reflect intense subjective strain, while high scores in the recovery associated scales reflect adequate recovery [6,31].

Saw et al. [23] and others [3,5,6,30] have demonstrated that such questionnaires can accurately reflect acute and chronic changes in well-being in response to alterations in training loads and are likely associated with changes in objective measures of training, health and fatigue. Previous studies in well-trained, but not elite, triathletes have also identified that questionnaires such as the DALDA and the REST-Q might play an important role in detecting alterations in levels of fatigue during a period of intensified training [5,6].

2.3. Data Analysis

Statistical analysis was performed using IBM SPSS® Statistics v.24 (IBM, Armonk, New York, NY, USA), with the significance level set at $p \leq 0.05$. Data distribution was checked with the Shapiro-Wilk test. A repeated-measures analysis of variance (ANOVA) was used to compare changes between week 1 and every subsequent week to analyze how training changed over time relative to baseline. Health and fatigue symptoms during the 8 weeks of the study were also compared to week 1. Partial eta square effect sizes are reported (η^2) and interpreted as small (0.01), medium (0.06) and large (0.14). When a main effect of time was found, post-hoc comparisons were performed using the Bonferroni correction, with Cohen's d calculated to report effect sizes (d) of pairwise comparisons between weeks (0–0.2 = trivial, 0.2–0.6 = small, 0.6–1.2 = moderate, 1.2–2.0 = large and >2 = very large) [32]. To control for alpha level inflation, only pairwise comparisons between week 1 and every subsequent week were performed. When Mauchly's test was significant, a Greenhouse-Geiser adjustment was used to determine the significance level of the test. If the assumption of normality was violated, Friedman's Test was utilized to assess the main effect of time, with Kendall's W used to report effect sizes (W). When the main effect of time was significant, the Wilcoxon-Signed Rank test was used to determine differences between weeks, with effect sizes (ES) calculated for each comparison ($r = Z/\sqrt{N}$) and interpreted as 0.10–small, 0.30–moderate, and 0.50–large effect [33]. Correlation analyses between weekly training characteristics (training loads, monotony and strain, and training time in zones 2 and 3) and both the "worse than normal" scores on the DALDA questionnaire and the scores on the TDS were performed using Spearman's Rank Test.

3. Results

The data of two individuals (one male and one female) were excluded from analysis, as a result of failure to complete the training log or to maintain a training routine. The final study subject number was nine, therefore. The characteristics of the study participants are presented in Table 1.

Table 1. Participants' self-reported training characteristics.

Characteristics	Mean (Range)
Age when started triathlon training (years)	33.6 (19–42)
Experience of training and competing in triathlon (years)	4.5 (3–12)
Swimming Experience (years)	6.5 (3–15)
Cycling Experience (years)	7.0 (3–15)
Running Experience (years)	14.2 (3–30)
Number of triathlons performed last season (any distance)	3.7 (2–5)
Training volume in the previous year (hours) [#]	341 ± 185 (150–674)
Number of triathlon specific sessions per week in the past year (overall and per mode) [#]	7.3 ± 1.5 (5.0–9.0)
Swimming [#]	2.2 ± 1.0 (1.0–4.0)
Cycling	3.0 (2.0–3.5)
Running [#]	2.7 ± 0.6 (2.0–4.0)
Training volume per week in the past year (hh:mm:ss)	
Overall	08:48:00 (3:30:00–13:30:00)
Swimming	2:24:00 (00:30:00–05:00:00)
Cycling	03:48:00 (01:12:00–06:00:00)
Running	02:24:00 (01:00:00–06:00:00)
Longest session (hh:mm:ss) in the past year	
Swimming	01:16:36 (00:50:21–02:00:00)
Cycling	03:18:24 (01:30:00–07:00:00)
Running	01:52:20 (01:00:00–03:00:00)
Average finishing time for Olympic Distance triathlon in week 6 (range) (hh:mm:ss)	02:39:06 (02:25:00–02:51:45)
Males	2:36:00 (2:17:12–2:58:00)
Females	2:40:48 (2:30:30–2:46:00)

[#] Data presented as mean ± standard deviation.

Two athletes won their age-group category, and one did not finish the race due to injury. Given their age and/or the number of finishers in each of their respective age-groups, we were able to confirm that the athletes in our study would not be classified as "fast, well-trained age-group Olympic distance triathlete" (s) [28]. Rather, this study deals with recreational level age-group triathletes. According to the training history questionnaire, the participants had an average of 5 years of experience in triathlon and a greater training history in one of the disciplines, with running being the most common. The athletes reported performing more cycling and running sessions in a week than swimming sessions. The number of cycling and running sessions that were accomplished in a week were similar.

3.1. Training Characteristics

The training characteristics of the participants is presented in Table 2.

3.1.1. Training Duration (Min) and Time Spent within Each Training Zone

Total training duration changed significantly over the 8 weeks ($F(7, 56) = 4.126$, $p = 0.014$, $\eta^2 = 0.340$). When compared to week 1, total training volume was significantly lower in week 6 ($p = 0.041$, 95% CI = 6.93, 421.95, d =1.58, 414.08 ± 170.5 vs. 199.6 ± 97.6 min). Over the 8 weeks of training, no significant changes were seen in the overall time spent in zone 1 ($F(7, 56) = 1.225$, $p = 0.305$, $\eta^2 = 0.133$) or zone 2 ($\chi^2 (7) = 9.00$, $p = 0.252$, W = 0.143). However, a significant difference for time spent in zone 3 was found ($\chi^2 (7) = 22.56$, $p = 0.002$, W = 0.358). Compared to week 1, the time spent in zone 3 was significantly shorter in week 6 ($Z = 2.52$, $p = 0.012$, ES = 0.95, median = 78 vs. 0 min), week 7 ($Z = 2.10$, $p = 0.036$, ES = 0.79, median = 78 vs. 0 min) and week 8 ($Z = 1.960$, $p = 0.050$, ES = 0.74, median = 78 vs. 40 min).

Table 2. Training characteristics of recreational-level triathletes for 8 weeks (data presented as median, 25th percentile, 75th percentile).

Variable	Week 1	Week 2	Week 3	Week 4	Week 5	Week 6	Week 7	Week 8	p-Value	Effect Size
Training Loads sRPE (A.U) [#]	2292.4 ± 1058.5	1911.2 ± 915.4	2429.7 ± 729.1	2166.7 ± 866.4	1949.9 ± 864.1	2129.6 ± 465.5	968.4 ± 577.3	1665.8 ± 621.3	<0.001	$\eta^2 = 0.447$
Training Duration (hh:mm:ss)	07:43:48 (03:54:12, 09:05:05)	06:52:48 (04:40:12, 08:46:30)	06:49:00 (05:56:36, 08:42:42)	06:37:48 (03:28:12, 07:53:24)	04:54:00 (03:51:36, 07:59:24)	02:58:48 (02:01:12, 04:15:00) [a]	02:39:36 (01:55:12, 06:04:12)	04:56:24 (02:03:36, 07:037:48)	0.014	$\eta^2 = 0.340$
Time in Zone 1 (hh:mm:ss)	02:53:24 (01:45:00, 04:36:00)	02:55:12 (01:27:00, 05:06:00)	02:00:00 (00:00:00, 03:34:12)	02:45:36 (01:05:24, 04:27:00)	01:54:36 (00:34:00, 03:42:00)	02:00:00 (01:02:30, 02:34:48)	02:33:00 (00:45:12, 05:23:24)	02:18:00 (00:37:30, 04:39:00)	0.305	$\eta^2 = 0.133$
Time in Zone 2 (hh:mm:ss)	00:39:00 (00:00:00, 02:24:06)	01:37:12 (00:37:18, 03:46:30)	02:03:00 (00:28:30, 03:00:06)	00:40:00 (00:00:00, 03:01:30)	01:00:00 (00:00:00, 02:09:00)	01:07:00 (00:00:00, 02:34:48)	00:00:00 (00:00:00, 00:43:42)	01:15:00 (00:38:30, 03:31:48)	0.252	W = 0.143
Time in Zone 3 (hh:mm:ss)	01:18:00 (00:46:00, 03:00:00)	00:28:00 (00:00:00, 01:42:00)	03:42:36 (00:55:00, 04:28:48)	01:36:00 (00:00:00, 03:24:00)	01:26:00 (00:35:30, 04:09:00)	00:00:00 (00:00:00, 00:55:52) [a]	00:00:00 (00:00:00, 00:40:30) [a]	00:40:00 (00:06:00, 01:09:00) [a]	0.002	W = 0.358
Training Monotony (A.U)	1.0 (0.9, 1.3)	1.2 (0.8, 1.3)	0.7 (0.6, 1.5)	1.1 (0.8, 1.4)	0.9 (0.8, 1.4)	0.6 (0.6, 0.8) [a]	0.7 (0.6, 1.3)	0.9 (0.8, 1.2)	0.008	W = 0.303
Training Strain (A.U)	2322.1 (1585.5, 2910.4)	2206.0 (1214.8, 3376.8)	1930.9 (1338.1, 3871.0)	2908.6 (1210.6, 3790.4)	1800.9 (1253.1, 3144.3)	1403.8 (1070.5, 1716.3) [a]	601.1 (363.7, 1927.6)	1545.8 (1147.1, 2592.2)	0.024	W = 0.256
Number of Sessions per week	9.0 (5.5, 10.5)	7.0 (6.5, 8.0)	8.0 (6.0, 9.5)	7.0 (6.0, 9.0)	6.0 (5.0, 8.0)	6.0 (4.0, 6.5) [a]	5.0 (4.0, 8.0) [a]	7.0 (6.0, 8.5)	0.007	W = 0.308
Swimming sessions per week	2.0 (1.0, 3.0)	2.0 (1.0, 3.0)	3.0 (2.0, 3.0)	1.0 (1.0, 3.0)	2.0 (1.0, 3.0)	2.0 (1.0, 2.5)	1.0 (1.0, 2.5)	2.0 (0.0, 3.0)	0.553	W = 0.093
Cycling sessions per week	2.0 (1.5, 3.5)	3.0 (2.0, 3.0)	3.0 (2.0, 3.0)	2.0 (2.0, 3.0)	3.0 (1.0, 4.0)	2.0 (1.0, 3.0)	1.0 (1.0, 2.5)	1.0 (0.0, 3.5)	0.180	W = 0.161
Running sessions per week	3.0 (2.0, 3.5)	2.0 (1.5, 3.0)	2.0 (1.0, 3.0)	2.0 (0.0, 3.5)	2.0 (0.5, 3.0)	2.0 (0.5, 2.0)	1.0 (0.0, 2.0) [a]	3.0 (2.0, 3.0)	0.019	W = 0.267
Number of other sessions per week	1.0 (0.0, 2.0)	0.0 (0.0, 1.0)	0.0 (0.0, 1.0)	1.0 (0.0, 1.0)	0.0 (0.0, 1.5)	0.0 (0.0, 0.5)	1.0 (0.0, 1.5)	0.0 (0.0, 3.0)	0.142	W = 0.173

[a] denotes a significant difference from week 1 ($p < 0.05$); [#] data presented as mean ± standard deviation; A.U (arbitrary units).

3.1.2. Total Time Spent Swimming, Cycling and Running and Time Spent in Zones 1, 2 and 3 for Each Mode

No significant differences across the 8 weeks were found for total swimming time (χ^2 (7) = 10.29, p = 0.173, W = 0.163). Total cycling time (F(7, 56) = 2.483, p = 0.027, η^2 = 0.237) was significantly changed across the 8 weeks, but no differences in relation to week 1 were found. Total running time differed across the 8 weeks (χ^2 (7) = 16.39, p = 0.022, W = 0.260), with running time in week 6 (Z = 2.54, p = 0.011, ES = 0.96, median = 27 vs. 105 min) and week 7 (Z = 2.07, p = 0.038, ES = 0.78, median = 31 vs. 105 min) being lower when compared to week 1. No differences were found for time spent in zones 1 or 2 for swimming, cycling or running. Time spent in zone 3 was significantly different across weeks for swimming (χ^2 (7) = 16.21, p = 0.023, W = 0.257) and cycling (χ^2 (7) = 23.33, p = 0.001, W = 0.370). However, post-hoc comparison only showed a significant difference between week 1 and week 6 for cycling in zone 3 (Z = 2.023, p = 0.043, ES = 0.76, median = 25 vs. 0 min). For running, time spent in zone 3 was significantly different across the 8 weeks (χ^2 (7) = 19.52, p = 0.007, W = 0.310), with week 6 (Z = 2.36, p = 0.018, ES = 0.89, median = 0 vs. 53 min) and week 7 (Z = 2.36, p = 0.018, ES = 0.89, median = 0 vs. 53 min) presenting a significantly lower duration at this intensity compared to week 1.

3.1.3. Number of Sessions per Week

There was a significant difference in the number of sessions performed each week (χ^2 (7) = 19.04, p = 0.007, W = 0.308). When compared to week 1, participants maintained their training frequency until week 6, when frequency was reduced (Z = 2.32, p = 0.02, ES = 0.88, median = 6.0 vs. 9.0). Training frequency was also reduced the week after the competition, with week 7 being significantly different than week 1 (Z = 2.31, p = 0.02, ES = 0.87, median = 5.0 vs. 9.0).

There was no difference in the number of swimming (χ^2 (7) = 5.88, p = 0.553, W = 0.09) and cycling sessions (χ^2 (7) = 10.16, p = 0.180, W = 0.16) that were performed over the 8 weeks. However, the number of running sessions changed significantly (χ^2 (7) = 16.82, p = 0.019, W = 0.26), with a higher number of sessions on week 1 when compared to week 7 (Z = 1.98, p = 0.048, ES = 0.75, median = 3.0 vs. 1.0 sessions). The number of other types of sessions performed throughout the 8 weeks did not change (χ^2 (7) = 10.92, p = 0.142, W = 0.17). Of the other sessions performed, only 1 participant performed some form of cross training, with the rowing and paddling sessions included in the training load calculations. Resistance training and yoga were the only other types of session that were performed and were not included in the training load calculations.

3.2. Training Load, Training Monotony and Training Strain

Whilst training loads changed significantly over time (F(7, 56) = 3.971, p = 0.001, η^2 = 0.332), no differences were found between week 1 and the other weeks of training. The average training load of the event was 1371.2 ± 248.2 A.U. To assess if the overall load was reduced in the week of the event, the training load for week 6 was calculated with and without the load from the event. Removing the competition load from the training load calculations for week 6 did not lead to a significant difference between week 1 and week 6. Training monotony changed significantly during the 8 weeks (χ^2 (7) = 19.07, p = 0.008, W = 0.30), with a significantly lower value for week 6 when compared to week 1 (Z = 2.54, p = 0.011, ES = 0.96, median = 1.0 vs. 0.6). Similarly, significant differences over the 8 weeks were reported for training strain (χ^2 (7) = 16.11, p = 0.024, W = 0.25), with pairwise comparisons showing a higher training strain during week 1 when compared to week 6 (Z = 2.42, p = 0.015, ES = 0.91, median = 2322.1 vs. 1403.8).

3.3. Self-Reported Measures of Health, Fatigue and Stress

No significant changes were reported for the DALDA questionnaire (χ^2 (7) = 12.54, p = 0.084, W = 0.224) and the Training Distress Scale (χ^2 (7) = 9.01, p = 0.252, W = 0.16) throughout the 8 weeks. For the REST-Q, no significant differences were found among responses at baseline, 48 h prior to the event, or two weeks after it (F(2, 14) = 0.803, p = 0.46, η^2 = 0.103).

For the Alberta Swim Fatigue and Health Questionnaire, weeks 6 and 7 presented some of the lowest reports of negative health symptoms (i.e., cold, flu, upset stomach, not feeling good overall), muscular aches and soreness and niggles. Symptoms were reported every week by at least 40% of participants, and every week at least 2 participants reported that they had to modify their training (Table 3).

Table 3. Descriptive athletes' health status data according to the Alberta Swim Fatigue and Health Questionnaire (n = 9).

	Week 1	Week 2	Week 3	Week 4	Week 5	Week 6	Week 7	Week 8
Number of athletes who reported aches and soreness	6	7	5	9	7	5	9	6
Number of athletes who reported niggles	8	7	7	7	6	5	7	6
Number of athletes who modified training	3	5	2	5	3	3	2	3

Correlation Analysis between Training Loads and Questionnaire Responses

No significant correlations were observed between training loads, monotony or strain and participants' responses to the DALDA or Training Distress questionnaire. Similarly, no significant correlation was found between the time spent in either zone 2 or zone 3 and the scores on each questionnaire.

4. Discussion

This study examined the training characteristics of recreational-level triathletes in the 6 weeks leading up to an Olympic distance triathlon and the 2 weeks after the event. The participants in this study had a training frequency that ranged between 5 and 9 sessions per week. The weekly training duration averaged 6.2 h per week from weeks 1 to 5, with weeks 7 and 8 showing a decrease in training duration. Not considering the athletes' Olympic distance triathlon, week 6 saw a significant reduction in training duration when compared to week 1, with athletes averaging just under 3 h of training. These training volumes are below what has been reported for 16 well-trained, but not elite triathletes, who had a minimum weekly training volume of 10 h [6]. Compared to athletes training for longer distance triathlons, the average weekly training volume was also lower, as previous research has identified that recreational-level Ironman triathletes train on average 14.1 h per week [7,8]. While these differences can be expected given the duration of the events (Ironman vs. Olympic distance), it must be acknowledged that the difference can be in part explained by the fact that data collected prospectively, such as in this study, can differ from retrospective data, as in the above-mentioned study. Nevertheless, training volume in this group of recreational triathletes was still larger than single mode recreational endurance athletes, such as half-marathon and marathon runners [7,34], and cyclists with similar years of experience as the athletes in this study [35].

Despite the importance of monitoring and reporting training volume, training loads are more relevant as these can determine if an athlete is adapting to the training program, assess fatigue and recovery status, and minimize the risks of non-functional overreaching, injury and illness [15]. The average load (Figure 1) in the weeks prior to the competition (2150.01 A. U., from weeks 1 to 5) is slightly higher than the average of 2000 A.U [6] reported by a group of well-trained male triathletes completing a four-week progressive, self-prescribed loading regime. While similar, the higher loads in the present study were achieved despite a lower average weekly training volume, indicating that weekly sessions were perceived to be performed at a higher intensity in this group of athletes. In addition, some of the reported loads in the current study were surprisingly high. For example, Coutts et al. [6] put a group of participants through a 4-week period of training overload designed to lead to overreaching. Weekly training loads started at upwards of 3000 A.U, a value that was reached by 5 of the 9 participants in this study at least once during the 8 weeks. One participant in this study also had a weekly load greater than what was reported by Coutts et al. [6] during their second week of overload (3.884 A.U vs. 3.809 A.U).

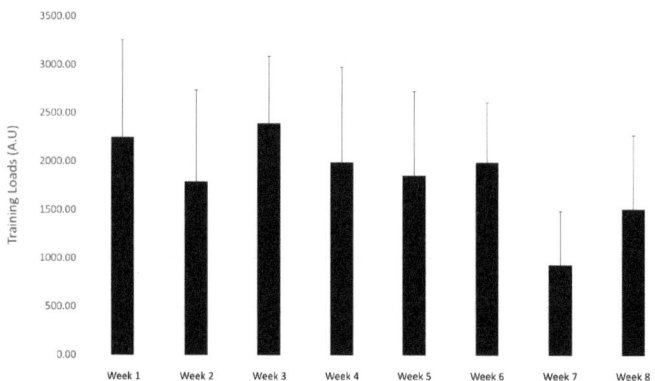

Figure 1. Average training loads (A.U) throughout the 8 weeks of training.

The training loads of the participants in this study were characterized by a high degree of variability throughout the eight weeks, with no discernible pattern in the five weeks leading up to the event. For the whole group, loads were reduced by 17% from week 1 to week 2 (2292.4 vs. 1911.2 A.U), only to increase by 27% (1911.2 vs. 2429.7) in week 3. While loads were reduced by an average of 10% in weeks 4 and 5 (Figure 1), an analysis of individual numbers confirms that large spikes in loads between weeks were frequent (Supplementary Material). Indeed, all participants doubled their loads from the previous week at least once throughout the study. As an example, one participant had a reduction in load of 33% in week 3 compared to week 2 (1064.2 A.U and 1603.4 A.U, respectively), followed by an increase of 122% in week 4 (2362.3 A.U), and a reduction of 60% in week 5 (948 A.U). These large variations in training loads can be detrimental to athletes' health. An association between training loads and injuries has been established, with large spikes in loads linked to an increased chance of injury, with the risk potentially remaining elevated for many weeks [36]. These spikes in load could also be related to an increased incidence of banal infections, a potential early sign of non-functional overreaching [24].

Similar to what occurred with training loads, no pattern was seen in the changes in training intensity distribution throughout the weeks of training (Figure 2). A high variability in the percentage of time spent in each training zone throughout the training program was also found. The only difference in TID found throughout the study was in the amount of training that was performed in Zone 3. Due to the competition, the athletes spent a greater amount of time in this intensity zone during week 6, and subsequently reduced the amount of time training in this zone in the two weeks after the competition. In addition, the athletes' training intensity over the 8 weeks confirmed our initial hypothesis, with participants' training intensity distribution favoring higher intensity sessions. Particularly, athletes spent an average of 47% of their training time in zone 1, with more than half of training spent in zones 2 and 3 (25% and 28%, respectively). When the time spent in zones 2 and 3 is considered together, only 2 out of the 8 weeks had a greater amount of time in zone 1 than in zones 2 and 3.

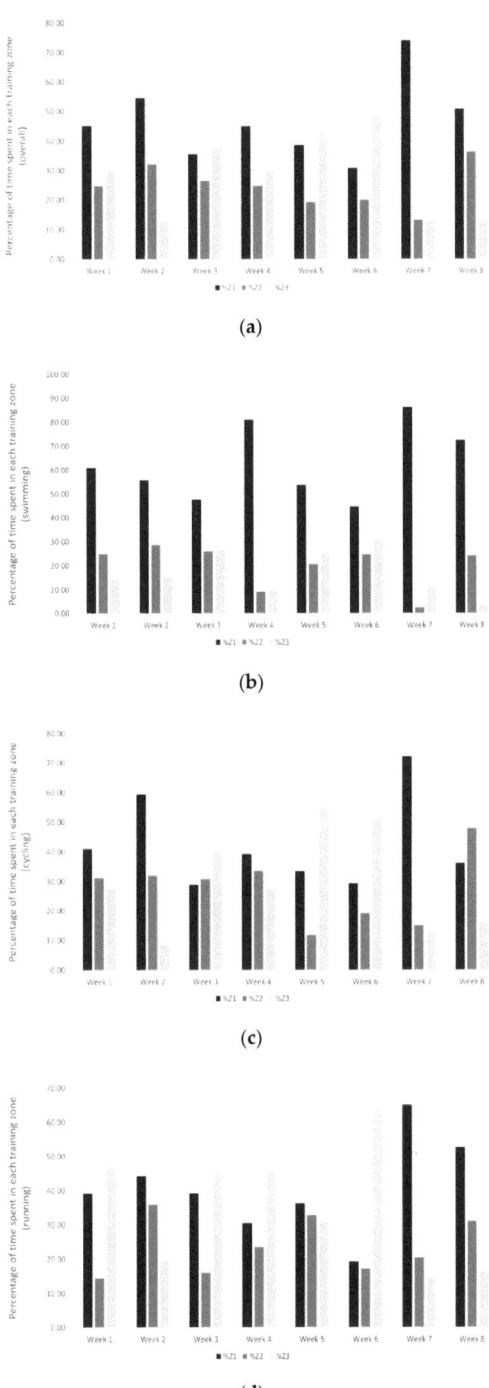

Figure 2. Training intensity distribution based on 3-zone model across the 8 weeks of training. (**a**) overall, (**b**) swimming, (**c**) cycling, (**d**) running. %Z1 = percent of time spent in zone 1, %Z2 = percent of time spent in zone 2, %Z3 = percent of time spent in zone 3.

The athletes' TID varied for each discipline, with swimming having a higher percentage of training time in zone 1 when compared to cycling and running. As many overuse injuries in triathlon are associated with cycling and running, particularly with the performance of intense sessions [4], the high volume of training in zones 2 and 3 in these disciplines could be cause for concern. For example, over the 8 weeks of training, the time spent in zone 3 during cycling was higher than that in zone 1 in weeks 3 and 5. Similar results were seen in the TID in running, where the amount of time spent in zone 3 was higher than that in zone 1 in 3 of the 5 weeks prior to the competition.

This high volume of training spent at higher intensities can be detrimental to athletes' performance. Improvements in endurance performance have been shown to be inversely related to the time spent at threshold intensities [2,17], with previous research showing that adaptations to training are related to the time spent in zone 1 (below the first ventilatory threshold) [37]. In addition, too much training time in zone 2 (between the first and second ventilatory thresholds) is also linked to symptoms of non-functional overreaching and a higher incidence of injuries [3,4,13]. Furthermore, Seiler et al. [14] demonstrated that training above the first ventilatory threshold (VT1), which demarcates the upper range of zone 1, can significantly delay recovery. This is particularly troubling for sports where training frequency can be high, such as triathlon, since it is possible that athletes would not be fully recovered prior to the following session.

Nevertheless, despite the large spikes in training loads between weeks and a training intensity distribution that favored higher intensities, contrary to our hypothesis, there were no significant changes in the athletes' fatigue and recovery status based on the questionnaires that were used. Only two injuries were reported, with one being due to a fall from the bike. However, high scores in the questionnaires, indicating a lack of recovery or presence of negative health symptoms were seen even in weeks with lower training loads. As recreational athletes struggle to maintain a balance between training and their regular life commitments [18], it is possible that general stress has an even greater impact on these athletes' self-reported measures of fatigue, illness and health. Otter et al. [22] reported that in a group of female endurance athletes (including five triathletes), recovery was hindered throughout the year of training in moments when general stress was higher. Further evidence also exists to support the notion that amateur triathletes have more difficulty in dealing with stress than those at the elite level [38], and other studies [20,21] have shown that for the general population, a cautious approach would be advisable when engaging in strenuous exercise if under chronic stress.

Even though these athletes were apparently healthy according to standard measures of fatigue, recovery and health (the DALDA, the TDS and the REST-Q), signs and symptoms associated with excessive training and not enough recovery were evident. Particularly, muscle soreness, aches and niggles were reported in the Alberta Swim Fatigue and Health Questionnaire every week by at least 40% of the athletes, with 20% of them having to modify their training on a weekly basis. This modification to training is similar to what has been previously reported in the literature, with athletes often increasing the load in another discipline when necessary [3]. While further research is needed to understand these athletes' approach to training, it is possible that the need to modify their training and the participants' approach to managing their complaints of muscle soreness, niggles and aches could help in explaining the high variations in weekly training loads.

In summary, the results of this study show that the participants incurred no significant changes in their health status in the 6 weeks prior to, or within two weeks after, competing in an OD triathlon. This situation occurred in spite of the athletes not having appeared to follow what is currently considered to be the ideal training practice for training for endurance events. Certainly, recreational triathletes should attempt to minimize large variations in training loads (as were reported for this group)-as such variations may have negative consequences for health and performance [2,6,24]. Age-group triathletes may also benefit from performing a higher proportion of their training at lower intensities (i.e., zone 1 in a 3-zone model), whilst limiting the volume of training that is accomplished above the first ventilatory threshold. In this group [2], performance improvements have been associated with a higher training volume in zone 1 and a reduced volume of training in zone 2. Doing high volumes of intense training sessions may also augment the risk of the athlete sustaining overuse injuries [4,15]. We recognize that working with a coach might lead to a reduction, on the part of the athlete, in the incidence of such training errors. We acknowledge, however, that such errors may persist even when the athlete's sessions are prescribed by a coach, if he/she performs the training at a different intensity than that which has been advocated [13].

Whilst this exploratory investigation has brought important information for coaches and athletes to light, the results should be interpreted with caution. For example, the small number of participants may partly explain why symptoms of fatigue were identified by the Alberta Swim Fatigue Health Questionnaire, but not by the other self-reported measures of health and fatigue that were implemented with them. Even though the nine athletes in question all exhibited similar training patterns (i.e., large variations in training loads and high volume of training being performed in intensity zones 2 and 3), the sample size of this study also precludes the drawing of definitive conclusions from it about recreational level triathletes as a whole. Previous research has also suggested that subjective measures of training maladaptation can be associated with, and, ideally, should be monitored alongside, objective measures [23]. Longer prospective longitudinal studies, that involve more participants; and that assess both subjective and objective measures of health, fatigue and performance, are needed if we are to better understand the inter-relationships between training characteristics and health in recreational triathletes.

5. Conclusions

The cohort of age-group triathletes in this study presented a random pattern of training throughout the 6 weeks prior to the competition, with large variations in training loads between weeks, along with several sessions performed at higher intensities (zones 2 and 3). Such approach to training could lead to a greater incidence of injuries, lack of recovery and reduced performance [2,4,14,24]. Nevertheless, no changes in the participants' fatigue and recovery status were found with the DALDA and TDS questionnaires. Still, this information was captured by the Alberta Swim Fatigue and Health Questionnaire. It is possible that training for a competitive event for some of the recreational athletes in this group was a balancing act between the hours of training and general life. This corroborates a recent study in which recreational endurance athletes, particularly triathletes, reported their struggle to find the time to train [18] and how they felt the need to push beyond their comfort levels to stimulate the desired adaptations. While such behaviors could help explain the results seen in this study, further research should assess the training characteristics of recreational athletes and seek to both understand the reasons behind their training patterns, and how such training patterns impact the athletes' health and performance.

Supplementary Materials: The following are available online at https://www.mdpi.com/article/10.3390/sports9070094/s1, Figures S1–S9: Individual Training Loads for each participant.

Author Contributions: Conceptualization, J.H.F.N. and M.D.K.; methodology, J.H.F.N. and M.D.K.; formal analysis, J.H.F.N., M.D.K., V.V. and E.C.P.; investigation, J.H.F.N., V.V. and M.D.K.; data curation, J.H.F.N. and E.C.P.; writing—original draft preparation, J.H.F.N.; writing—review and editing, J.H.F.N., M.D.K., V.V. and E.C.P.; supervision, M.D.K. and E.C.P. All authors have read and agreed to the published version of the manuscript.

Funding: This research was funded by "The University of Alberta President's Council for the Creative Performing Arts Human Performance Fund", grant number RG264 and "The APC was funded by The University of Alberta President's Council for the Creative Performing Arts Human Performance Fund". V.V. acknowledges the support of the Fundação para a Ciência e a Tecnologia—as expressed by Grant UIDB/00447/2020 to CIPER—Centro Interdisciplinar para o Estudo da Performance Humana (unit 447).

Institutional Review Board Statement: The study was conducted according to the guidelines of the Declaration of Helsinki, and approved by the Research Ethics Committee of the University of Alberta (Pro00082267, 29 May 2018).

Informed Consent Statement: Informed consent was obtained from all subjects involved in the study.

Data Availability Statement: The data presented in this study are available on request from the corresponding author. The data are not publicly available due to privacy reasons.

Acknowledgments: The authors would like to thank the athletes for their participation in this study. We would also thank the WTS Edmonton committee (Sheila O'Kelly, Stephen Boudreau, Kelly Livingstone) and Trevor Soll for their assistance.

Conflicts of Interest: The authors have no conflict of interest to declare.

References

1. Rios, L. *USA Triathlon Membership Survey*; USA Triathlon: Colorado Springs, CO, USA, 2016.
2. Neal, C.M.; Hunter, A.M.; Galloway, S.D. A 6-month analysis of training-intensity distribution and physiological adaptation in Ironman triathletes. *J. Sports Sci.* **2011**, *29*, 1515–1523. [CrossRef]
3. Vleck, V.; Millet, G.P.; Alves, F.B. The impact of triathlon training and racing on athletes' general health. *Sports Med.* **2014**, *44*, 1659–1692. [CrossRef]
4. Vleck, V.E.; Bentley, D.J.; Millet, G.P.; Cochrane, T. Triathlon event distance specialization: Training and injury effects. *J. Strength Cond. Res.* **2010**, *24*, 30–36. [CrossRef]
5. Coutts, A.J.; Slattery, K.M.; Wallace, L.K. Practical tests for monitoring performance, fatigue and recovery in triathletes. *J. Sci. Med. Sport* **2007**, *10*, 372–381. [CrossRef]
6. Coutts, A.J.; Wallace, L.K.; Slattery, K.M. Monitoring changes in performance, physiology, biochemistry, and psychology during overreaching and recovery in triathletes. *Int. J. Sports Med.* **2007**, *28*, 125–134. [CrossRef] [PubMed]
7. Rüst, C.A.; Knechtle, B.; Knechtle, P.; Rosemann, T. A comparison of anthropometric and training characteristics between recreational female marathoners and recreational female Ironman triathletes. *Chin. J. Physiol.* **2013**, *56*, 1–10. [CrossRef]
8. Rust, C.A.; Knechtle, B.; Knechtle, P.; Wirth, A.; Rosemann, T. A comparison of anthropometric and training characteristics among recreational male Ironman triathletes and ultra-endurance cyclists. *Chin. J. Physiol.* **2012**, *55*, 114–124. [CrossRef]
9. Vleck, V. *Epidemiology of Injury in Olympic Sports*; Caine, D.J., Harmer, P.A., Schiff, M.A., Eds.; Wiley-Blackwell: Chichester, UK, 2010.
10. Vleck, V.; Hoeden, D. Epidemiological aspects of illness and injury. In *Triathlon Medicine*; Springer Nature: Basel, Switzerland, 2019; pp. 19–41.
11. Korkia, P.K.; Tunstall-Pedoe, D.S.; Maffulli, N. An epidemiological investigation of training and injury patterns in British triathletes. *Brit. J. Sport Med.* **1994**, *28*, 191–196. [CrossRef]
12. Vleck, V. The changing relationship between multidisciplinary (triathlon) exercise and health across the lifespan. In *Research on Human Kinetics-Multidisciplinary Perspectives*; Alves, F.R.O., Pereira, L.M., Araujo, D., Eds.; Lisbon University Press: Lisbon, Portugal, 2018; pp. 185–198.
13. Foster, C.; Esten, P.L.; Brice, G.; Porcari, J.P. Differences in perceptions of training by coaches and athletes. *S. Afr. J. Sports Med.* **2001**, *8*, 3–7.
14. Seiler, S.; Haugen, O.; Kuffel, E. Autonomic recovery after exercise in trained athletes: Intensity and duration effects. *Med. Sci. Sports Exerc.* **2007**, *39*, 1366–1373. [CrossRef]
15. Halson, S.L. Monitoring training load to understand fatigue in athletes. *Sports Med.* **2014**, *44* (Suppl. 2), S139–S147. [CrossRef]
16. Hydren, J.R.; Cohen, B.S. Current Scientific Evidence for a Polarized Cardiovascular Endurance Training Model. *J. Strength Cond. Res.* **2015**, *29*, 3523–3530. [CrossRef]
17. Stöggl, T.L.; Sperlich, B. The training intensity distribution among well-trained and elite endurance athletes. *Front. Physiol.* **2015**, *6*, 295. [CrossRef] [PubMed]
18. McCormick, A.; Meijen, C.; Marcora, S. Psychological demands experienced by recreational endurance athletes. *Int. J. Sport Exerc. Psychol.* **2018**, *16*, 415–430. [CrossRef]
19. Pearce, P.Z. A practical approach to the overtraining syndrome. *Curr. Sports Med. Rep.* **2002**, *1*, 179–183. [CrossRef] [PubMed]
20. Ruuska, P.S.; Hautala, A.J.; Kiviniemi, A.M.; Makikallio, T.H.; Tulppo, M.P. Self-rated mental stress and exercise training response in healthy subjects. *Front. Physiol.* **2012**, *3*, 51. [CrossRef] [PubMed]
21. Stults-Kolehmainen, M.A.; Sinha, R. The effects of stress on physical activity and exercise. *Sports Med.* **2014**, *44*, 81–121. [CrossRef] [PubMed]
22. Otter, R.T.; Brink, M.S.; van der Does, H.T.; Lemmink, K.A. Monitoring Perceived Stress and Recovery in Relation to Cycling Performance in Female Athletes. *Int. J. Sports Med.* **2016**, *37*, 12–18. [CrossRef]
23. Saw, A.E.; Main, L.C.; Gastin, P.B. Monitoring the athlete training response: Subjective self-reported measures trump commonly used objective measures: A systematic review. *Brit. J. Sport Med.* **2016**, *50*, 281–291. [CrossRef]
24. Foster, C. Monitoring training in athletes with reference to overtraining syndrome. *Med. Sci. Sports Exerc.* **1998**, *30*, 1164–1168. [CrossRef]

25. Raglin, J.S.; Morgan, W.P. Development of a scale for use in monitoring training-induced distress in athletes. *Int. J. Sports Med.* **1994**, *15*, 84–88. [CrossRef]
26. Rushall, B.S. A tool for measuring stress tolerance in elite athletes. *J. Appl. Sport Psychol.* **1990**, *2*, 51–66. [CrossRef]
27. Vleck, V. *Triathlete Training and Injury Analysis—An Investigation in British National Squad and Age-Group Triathlete*; VDM Verlag Publishers: Saarbrücken, Germany, 2010; pp. 98–153.
28. Aoyagi, A.; Ishikura, K.; Nabekura, Y. Exercise Intensity during Olympic-Distance Triathlon in Well-Trained Age-Group Athletes: An Observational Study. *Sports* **2021**, *9*, 18. [CrossRef]
29. McNair, D.M.; Lorr, M.; Droppleman, L.F. *Profile of Mood States (POMS)–Revised Manual*; Education and Industrial Testing Service: San Diego, CA, USA, 1991.
30. Davies, R.D.; Parent, E.C.; Steinback, C.D.; Kennedy, M.D. The Effect of Different Training Loads on the Lung Health of Competitive Youth Swimmers. *Int. J. Exerc. Sci.* **2018**, *11*, 999–1018.
31. Kellmann, M.; Günther, K.D. Changes in stress and recovery in elite rowers during preparation for the Olympic Games. *Med. Sci. Sports Exerc.* **2000**, *32*, 676–683. [CrossRef]
32. Hopkins, W.G.; Marshall, S.W.; Batterham, A.M.; Hanin, J. Progressive statistics for studies in sports medicine and exercise science. *Med. Sci. Sports Exerc.* **2009**, *41*, 3–13. [CrossRef]
33. Tomczak, M.; Tomczak, E.W.A. The need to report effect size estimates revisited. An overview of some recommended measures of effect size. *Trends Sport Sci.* **2014**, *21*, 19–25.
34. Leyk, D.; Erley, O.; Gorges, W.; Ridder, D.; Ruther, T.; Wunderlich, M.; Sievert, A.; Essfeld, D.; Piekarski, C.; Erren, T. Performance, Training and Lifestyle Parameters of Marathon Runners Aged 20–80 Years: Results of the PACE-study. *Int. J. Sports Med.* **2009**, *30*, 360–365. [CrossRef]
35. Schultz, S.J.; Gordon, S.J. Recreational cyclists: The relationship between low back pain and training characteristics. *Int. J. Exerc. Sci.* **2010**, *3*, 79–85.
36. Drew, M.K.; Cook, J.; Finch, C.F. Sports-related workload and injury risk: Simply knowing the risks will not prevent injuries: Narrative review. *Br. J. Sports Med.* **2016**, *50*, 1306–1308. [CrossRef]
37. Muñoz, I.; Cejuela, R.; Seiler, S.; Larumbe, E.; Esteve-Lanao, J. Training-Intensity Distribution During an Ironman Season: Relationship With Competition Performance. *Int. J. Sports Physiol. Perf.* **2014**, *9*, 332–339. [CrossRef]
38. Olmedilla, A.; Torres-Luque, G.; García-Mas, A.; Rubio, V.J.; Ducoing, E.; Ortega, E. Psychological Profiling of Triathlon and Road Cycling Athletes. *Front. Psychol.* **2018**, *9*, 825. [CrossRef]

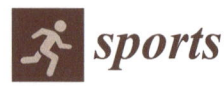

Article

Exercise Intensity during Olympic-Distance Triathlon in Well-Trained Age-Group Athletes: An Observational Study

Atsushi Aoyagi [1], Keisuke Ishikura [2] and Yoshiharu Nabekura [3,*]

[1] Graduate School of Comprehensive Human Sciences, University of Tsukuba, 1-1-1 Tennodai, Tsukuba, Ibaraki 305-8574, Japan; atsushi.aoyagi.1992@gmail.com
[2] Faculty of Management, Josai University, 1-1 Keyakidai, Sakado, Saitama 350-0295, Japan; ishikura@josai.ac.jp
[3] Faculty of Health and Sport Sciences, University of Tsukuba, 1-1-1 Tennodai, Tsukuba, Ibaraki 305-8574, Japan
* Correspondence: nabekura.yoshihar.fm@u.tsukuba.ac.jp

Abstract: The aim of this study was to examine the exercise intensity during the swimming, cycling, and running legs of nondraft legal, Olympic-distance triathlons in well-trained, age-group triathletes. Seventeen male triathletes completed incremental swimming, cycling, and running tests to exhaustion. Heart rate (HR) and workload corresponding to aerobic and anaerobic thresholds, maximal workloads, and maximal HR (HR_{max}) in each exercise mode were analyzed. HR and workload were monitored throughout the race. The intensity distributions in three HR zones for each discipline and five workload zones in cycling and running were quantified. The subjects were then assigned to a fast or slow group based on the total race time (range, 2 h 07 min–2 h 41 min). The mean percentages of HR_{max} in the swimming, cycling, and running legs were 89.8% ± 3.7%, 91.1% ± 4.4%, and 90.7% ± 5.1%, respectively, for all participants. The mean percentage of HR_{max} and intensity distributions during the swimming and cycling legs were similar between groups. In the running leg, the faster group spent relatively more time above HR at anaerobic threshold (AnT) and between workload at AnT and maximal workload. In conclusion, well-trained male triathletes performed at very high intensity throughout a nondraft legal, Olympic-distance triathlon race, and sustaining higher intensity during running might play a role in the success of these athletes.

Keywords: multisport; endurance performance; intensity profile; swimming; cycling; running; heart rate; aerobic threshold; anaerobic threshold; workload

Citation: Aoyagi, A.; Ishikura, K.; Nabekura, Y. Exercise Intensity during Olympic-Distance Triathlon in Well-Trained Age-Group Athletes: An Observational Study. *Sports* 2021, *9*, 18. https://doi.org/10.3390/sports9020018

Received: 20 December 2020
Accepted: 18 January 2021
Published: 21 January 2021

Publisher's Note: MDPI stays neutral with regard to jurisdictional claims in published maps and institutional affiliations.

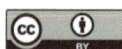

Copyright: © 2021 by the authors. Licensee MDPI, Basel, Switzerland. This article is an open access article distributed under the terms and conditions of the Creative Commons Attribution (CC BY) license (https://creativecommons.org/licenses/by/4.0/).

1. Introduction

Triathlon is a multidisciplinary endurance sport consisting of swimming, cycling, and running over a variety of distances [1]. The most common distances include the sprint (25.75 km, ~1 h), half-Ironman (113 km, ~4–5 h), and Ironman (226 km, ~8–17 h), and the most popular is the so-called Olympic distance (OD), consisting of standard distances for swimming (1.5 km), cycling (40 km), and running (10 km), for a total of 51.5 km. Scientific interest in the triathlon has significantly increased since the introduction of the 51.5-km race in the 2000 Summer Olympics, held in Sydney [2]. The total competition time of the OD race ranged from about 1 h 50 min to 2 h 40 min, with swimming accounting for 16%–19% (20–30 min), cycling of about 50%–55% (60–80 min), and running around 29%–31% (30–50 min) [3,4].

It is necessary to discern the physiological response and requirements during competition to optimize training and recovery, and to identify factors associated with performance. The efficient transition between two sequential legs of the triathlon has received considerable attention, e.g., the swim–cycle [5,6] and cycle–run [7,8] transitions have been well studied. Additionally, previous studies have assessed the acute consequences induced by the OD race, which include muscle [9,10] and intestinal damage [9], muscle fatigue [10], dehydration (>2%–4% body mass due to high sweat rates and high core temperatures, i.e., >39 °C) [11,12], systemic inflammation [13], transient immune suppression [14], reduced pulmonary diffusing capacity [15], and decreased aerobic exercise capacity [16,17].

Although a large number of studies have investigated the physiological responses and acute consequences of multidisciplinary and endurance sporting events, relatively few have addressed the sustained exercise intensity encountered during an actual OD race. Oxygen consumption ($\dot{V}O_2$) and blood lactate concentration (BLa) are two of the main parameters used to quantify exercise intensity [18]. However, it is difficult to measure these variables during actual competition. Over the past two decades, heart rate (HR), as a marker of internal load, has been used to estimate exercise intensity [19,20], by relating individual competition HR values measured in the field with those obtained in a laboratory incremental test [20–22]. In addition, the combination of internal load (HR) and external load (workload, i.e., speed and power output (PO)) can provide important information about the physiological demands during endurance events [19]. Thus, knowledge of exercise intensity profiles based on internal and external loads can facilitate greater comprehension of the physiological demands of the OD triathlon.

Studies investigating exercise intensity during an actual OD race are sparse. According to Bernard et al. [21], the mean relative HR and workload of elite triathletes during cycling in OD race were 91% ± 4% of the maximal heart rate (HR_{max}) and 60% ± 8% of the maximal aerobic power (MAP), although these measurements were not reported during the swimming and running legs. A study conducted by Le Meur et al. [22] of the mean relative HR and workload during an OD race in relation to the individual metabolic capacities of elite triathletes assessed at each exercise mode (i.e., swimming, cycling, and running) reported 91%–92% of HR_{max} for swimming, 90%–91% of HR_{max} and 61.4%–63.4% of MAP for cycling, and 93%–94% of HR_{max} for running. However, the cohorts of these studies [21,22] were limited to elite triathletes. While elite triathletes compete in draft legal cycling, in which a competitor is permitted to draft within a sheltered position behind another, nonelite or age-group triathletes usually compete in nondraft legal racing. Drafting directly affects exercise intensity by reducing $\dot{V}O_2$ (−14%) and HR (−7%), as compared to nondraft cycling with the same external load (speed) by triathletes [23]. Hence, it is necessary to distinguish between draft legal and nondraft legal races. To the best of our knowledge, only two studies have reported the exercise intensity sustained during actual nondraft legal OD races [24,25]. However, these were limited by reporting the absolute values of both HR (bpm) and workload (swimming speed, km·h^{-1}; cycling PO, W; and running speed, km·h^{-1}) [24] or the relative HR, but not workload, during cycling and running (not swimming), similar to an OD race (swimming:, 1.0 km; cycling, 30 km; and running, 8 km) [25]. Therefore, no study to date has investigated the relative exercise intensity sustained and the distribution of intensity during the entire duration of an actual nondraft legal OD race.

Furthermore, in other endurance events, there is an obvious tendency toward reduced relative intensity in relation to increased race duration. In ultra-endurance events of more than 8 h, such as the Ironman triathlon [26] and the 65-km run of a mountain ultra-marathon [27], the relative intensity during competition was lower than the ventilatory threshold (VT) and 80% of the HR_{max}. Hence, these intensities have been proposed as an "ultra-endurance threshold" [6]. In the 42-km marathon (~2.5–5 h), the mean relative HR is reportedly around 80%–90% of HR_{max} [28,29], which is similar to the HR at VT [30]. During a shorter event, such as a 5–10 km running (~15–55 min), the mean HR values are reportedly higher (~90–96% of HR_{max}) [28]. On the other hand, the relative intensity that can be sustained during an endurance race may also be related to differences in performance levels [31,32]. Thus, even among triathletes, the relative intensity during an OD triathlon could also differ, depending on the exercise duration and/or performance level.

Therefore, the aim of this study was (i) to estimate, using competition HR and workload data, the relative exercise intensity in all three disciplines during a nondraft legal OD race in well-trained, age-group triathletes, and (ii) to compare the estimated intensity of fast and slow triathletes. We hypothesized that triathletes would maintain a high level of intensity throughout the race, and that faster triathletes could perform the race at higher relative intensity than slower triathletes.

2. Materials and Methods

2.1. Study Design

This study was conducted in two phases consisting of laboratory tests and during-race monitoring. The laboratory tests included an incremental swimming test, an incremental cycling test, and an incremental treadmill running test, which were performed randomly and separated by a minimum of 2 days and maximum of 20 days. Competition measurements of each participant were conducted during the OD race with a nondraft legal cycling leg and were timed as close as possible to all laboratory tests (mean ± standard deviation, 45 ± 26 days).

2.2. Subjects

The study cohort consisted of 17 well-trained, age-group male triathletes (Table 1) who met the following inclusion criteria: (1) regular training of at least five sessions per week for a triathlon competition; (2) not suffering from any present injury, which could have possibly hampered their performance, and nonsmokers; and (3) a minimum of one year of experience competing in triathlons. The median time for completion of the OD race based on pooled data was 2:16:13 h:min:s. The subjects were split into two groups according to the total time of the OD race. Participants with times not less than 2:16:13 were assigned to the faster group and those with times greater than 2:16:13 was assigned to the slower group. The study protocol was approved by the Ethics Committee of the University of Tsukuba (project identification code: Tai 30–24) and conducted in accordance with the ethical principles for medical research involving human subjects as described in the Declaration of Helsinki. All subjects provided written informed consents to participate in the study.

Table 1. Characteristics and Olympic-distance race times of the faster and slower groups.

	All (N = 17)	Faster (n = 9)	Slower (n = 8)
Subject characteristics			
Age (yr)	23.1 ± 6.7	24.3 ± 8.4	21.6 ± 4.2
Height (cm)	173.8 ± 5.9	174.2 ± 5.2	173.4 ± 7.0
Mass (kg)	65.1 ± 5.5	64.9 ± 6.1	65.3 ± 5.2
Body Fat (%)	10.3 ± 1.7	9.8 ± 1.4	10.9 ± 1.9
BMI	21.5 ± 1.1	21.4 ± 1.5	21.7 ± 0.3
Triathlon experience (yr)	4.1 ± 6.1	5.4 ± 8.1	2.6 ± 2.4
Olympic-distance race times			
Swimming (h:min:s)	0:26:28 ± 0:04:01	0:23:34 ± 0:01:49	0:29:45 ± 0:03:10 **
Cycling (h:min:s)	1:10:33 ± 0:02:53	1:08:54 ± 0:02:19	1:12:25 ± 0:02:19 *
Running (h:min:s)	0:42:49 ± 0:04:39	0:39:57 ± 0:02:14	0:46:02 ± 0:04:37 **
Total (h:min:s)	2:19:50 ± 0:09:38	2:12:24 ± 0:02:54	2:28:12 ± 0:07:11 **

Values are means ± SD. N, number of subjects; BMI, body mass index. The nonparametric Mann–Whitney U test was used to detect statistically significant differences between the groups. * $p < 0.05$; ** $p < 0.01$.

2.3. Laboratory Tests

The subjects were instructed to refrain from consuming caffeine and alcohol and from heavy training on the day before the tests, as well as to consume a light meal at least 3 h before each laboratory test. During the 3-h period preceding the tests, only ad libitum water ingestion was permitted. During all laboratory tests, HR was collected via a HR monitor (HRM-Tri; Garmin Ltd., Olathe, KS, USA) across the chest with sampling at 1 Hz. Body mass was measured with a body fat monitor scale (TBF-102; Tanita, Tokyo, Japan) before the cycling and running tests.

2.3.1. Incremental Swimming Test

The subjects completed a two-part test consisting of a submaximal intermittent test and a maximal incremental test that were performed in a swimming flume at a constant water temperature of 25.8 ± 0.8 °C. The subjects wore their own technical trisuits, standard swimming caps, and goggles throughout the incremental swimming test. The submaximal intermittent test was performed first. The swimming speed of the submaximal intermittent test was individualized according to the average swimming speed of the most recent 1500-m time trial (S_{1500}) of each triathlete. The speed for the initial stage was 70% of S_{1500} and increased by 5% at each subsequent stage for a total five to seven stages, each consisting of 4 min of exercise and 2 min of rest. Before the test and after each stage, blood samples were obtained from the fingertip and the BLa was measured with a lactate analyzer (Lactate Pro 2; Arkray, Inc., Kyoto, Japan). The submaximal intermittent test was concluded when the BLa exceeded 4.0 mmol·L^{-1} or the rate of perceived exertion was ≥15. Following a 5-min recovery period after the submaximal intermittent test, the maximal incremental test was performed. The initial speed was set at that of the next to last stage of the submaximal intermittent test and then was increased by 0.03 m·s^{-1} every minute until volitional exhaustion, which was defined as the point at which the subject could no longer swim at the required speed.

2.3.2. Incremental Cycling Test

The maximal incremental test was performed on an electronically braked, indoor cycle trainer (CompuTrainer Pro; RacerMate Inc., Seattle, WA, USA), which allowed the subjects to use their own bicycles, at a constant room temperature of 25.2 ± 1.2 °C, relative humidity of 40.4% ± 8.3%, and barometric pressure of 755.4 ± 3.5 mmHg with an electric fan ensuring air circulation around the participant. The maximal incremental test was performed following a 5-min warm-up period (100 W) and a 5-min recovery period. The initial workload was set at 100 W and then increased by 20 W·min^{-1} and cadence was maintained at 80 or 90 rpm in accordance with race cadence of the individual until volitional exhaustion, which was defined as <75 or 85 rpm (i.e., a decrease of 5 rpm as compared with the cadence of the sustained during test) continuously for 5 s. To determine the PO during the test, which was used for analysis, the bicycles were fitted with calibrated power measuring pedals (Garmin Ltd.) at a sampling rate of 1 Hz.

2.3.3. Incremental Treadmill Running Test

The maximal incremental test was performed on a motorized treadmill (ORK-7000; Ohtake-Root Kogyo Co., Ltd., Iwate, Japan) at a grade of 1% to accurately reflect the energetic cost of outdoor running [33] following a 5-min warm-up period (9.0 km·h^{-1}) and a 5-min recovery period. The experimental environmental conditions were similar to those of the incremental cycling test. The initial speed was set at 9.0 km·h^{-1} and then increased by 0.6 km·h^{-1} every minute until volitional exhaustion, which was defined as the inability of the subject to continue running at the required speed. The treadmill belt speed, which was used for analysis, was measured with a hand-held tachometer (EE-1B; Nidec-Shimpo Corporation, Kyoto, Japan).

2.4. Gas Analysis

During the incremental cycling and treadmill running tests, $\dot{V}O_2$, carbon dioxide production ($\dot{V}CO_2$), minute ventilation ($\dot{V}_E$), ventilatory equivalent of oxygen ($\dot{V}_E/\dot{V}O_2$) and carbon dioxide ($\dot{V}_E/\dot{V}CO_2$), end-tidal partial pressure of oxygen ($P_{ET}O_2$) and carbon dioxide ($P_{ET}CO_2$), and respiratory exchange ratio (RER) were measured on a breath-by-breath basis using a computerized standard open circuit technique with a metabolic gas analyzer (AE-310s; Minato Medical Science Co., Ltd., Osaka, Japan).

Before both tests, the metabolic system was calibrated using known gas concentrations and a 2-L syringe in accordance with the manufacturer's instructions. Maximal $\dot{V}O_2$

($\dot{V}O_{2\,max}$), which was defined as the highest 1-min rolling average (20-s × 3), was attained when at least two of the following four criteria were met: (1) a leveling-off of $\dot{V}O_2$ despite an increase in PO or running speed, (2) peak RER $\geq$ 1.10, (3) peak HR $\geq$ 90% of age-predicted values, and (4) perceived exertion score at the end of the tests of $\geq$19. The gross efficiency during cycling was calculated as described in a previous study [34]. The running economy was expressed as the O_2 cost (ml·kg^{-1}·km^{-1}) and was calculated based on the last 1-min $\dot{V}O_2$ while running for 5 min (9.0 km·h^{-1}) [35].

2.5. Determination of Aerobic and Anaerobic Thresholds, and Maximal Workload

The predicted swimming speed and HR at both the lactate threshold (LT) and the onset of blood lactate accumulation (OBLA) of 4 mmol·L^{-1} were calculated using validated software (Lactate-E [36], version 2.0, National University of Galway, Galway, Ireland) based on the BLa, swimming speed, and HR collected during the incremental swimming test.

VT during cycling and running was determined using the criteria of an increase in both $\dot{V}_E/\dot{V}O_2$ and $P_{ET}O_2$ with no increase in $\dot{V}_E/\dot{V}CO_2$, whereas the respiratory compensation point (RCP) was determined using the criteria of an increase in both $\dot{V}_E/\dot{V}O_2$ and $\dot{V}_E/\dot{V}CO_2$, and a decrease in $P_{ET}CO_2$ [37,38]. Two independent observers determined the VT and RCP for cycling and running. Any disagreement was mediated by the opinion of a third investigator [39].

Based on previous studies [40,41], the LT obtained from the swimming test and the VT obtained from the cycling and the treadmill running tests were defined as the "aerobic threshold" (AeT), while the OBLA of 4 mmol·L^{-1} obtained from the swimming test and the RCP obtained from cycling and running test were defined as the "anaerobic threshold" (AnT).

Maximal swimming speed (SS$_{max}$) and maximal running speed (RS$_{max}$) were determined by the last stage of the maximal incremental test. When the subject was unable to complete 1 min at the current workload, the maximal workload was determined by adding a fraction of the final workload to the workload of the immediately preceding 1 min [42]. Maximal PO (PO$_{max}$) was determined as the highest 20-s rolling average attained during the incremental cycling test. These three variables were collectively referred to as the "maximal workload".

2.6. Competition Measurements

The OD races were nonunified between each individual because of the difficulty of securing a sufficient sample size among the participants of the same race. The distance of each OD race was the same and consisted of swimming for 1.5 km, cycling for 40 km, and running for 10 km. During all races, the subjects wore a HR monitor (HRM-Tri) across the chest with sampling at 1 Hz. Also, the subjects wore waterproofed portable global navigation satellite system (GNSS) units (ForeAthlete 920XT; Garmin Ltd., Olathe, KS, USA) on the wrist with sampling at 1 Hz to determine the speed throughout the race. To determine cycling PO during the race, the bicycles were fitted with calibrated power measuring pedals (Garmin Ltd.) set at a sampling rate of 1 Hz. Following completion of each race, performance times were obtained from official websites of the event. Air temperature, relative humidity, wind speed, and barometric pressure were obtained from the local meteorological agency within 1 h of the start of the race. Water temperature was measured with a water temperature gauge (CTH-1365; Custom Corporation, Tokyo, Japan) before the start of the race. Cumulated positive elevation during cycling and running was obtained from the GNSS units. The elevation to distance ratio was calculated by dividing the cumulated positive elevation by 40 (km, for cycling) or 10 (km, for running).

2.7. Exercise Intensity Zone Settings

Based on the HR measurements, the total time of each leg of the OD race was divided into three intensity zones based on the results of the laboratory tests in the corresponding exercise mode. The percentage of time spent in each zone was calculated as follows: less than AeT ($HR_{zone}1$), between AeT and AnT ($HR_{zone}2$), more than AnT ($HR_{zone}3$) [43,44]. Similar analysis of the PO measurements in the cycling leg [22,45] was also conducted: below 10% of PO_{max} ($PO_{zone}1$), between 10% of PO_{max} and AeT ($PO_{zone}2$), between AeT and AnT ($PO_{zone}3$), between AnT and PO_{max} ($PO_{zone}4$), and above PO_{max} ($PO_{zone}5$). In addition, using the average running speed (RS) at each 100 m in the running leg, an analysis similar to that for PO distribution was conducted based on the incremental running test results, rather than the incremental cycling test results.

2.8. Data Analysis

HR, PO, and speed obtained from the GNSS units were recorded with the GNSS units (Garmin Ltd.). The obtained data were exported to third party, open-source analysis software (Golden Cheetah, version 3.4, http://www.goldencheetah.org/), and further analysis was performed using Microsoft Excel software (version 2019, Microsoft Corporation, Redmond, WA, USA). Expired gas data were averaged across 20-s intervals using internal gas analysis software (version 3STG, AT Windows; Minato Medical Science Co., Ltd., Osaka, Japan), and exported to a.csv file. Further analysis was performed using Microsoft Excel 2019 software.

2.9. Statistical Analysis

All results are presented as the mean ± standard deviation unless otherwise indicated. Normal distribution of the data was tested using the Kolmogorov–Smirnov test. The nonparametric Mann–Whitney U test was used to detect statistically significant differences between groups. The effect size (ES) was evaluated as r (with 0.1 considered to be a small, 0.3 a medium, and 0.5 a large effect [46]). All statistical analyses were conducted using IBM SPSS Statistics version 26 (IBM Japan, Tokyo, Japan). A probability (p) value of ≤ 0.05 was considered statistically significant.

3. Results

The competition measurement data of the OD race were corrected from 10 races conducted in 2018 or 2019. The environmental conditions during the OD races are shown in Table 2. There were no significant differences observed between the two groups (all, $p \geq 0.16$; ES = 0.04–0.35). During the swimming leg of the race, most of the subjects wore their own wetsuits, with the exception one subject in each group who exercised in nonwetsuits.

The results of the three incremental tests of each exercise mode are summarized in Table 3. The faster group ($n = 9$) was superior to the slower group ($n = 8$) in speed at AeT and AnT and SS_{max} for the swimming test ($p < 0.01$, respectively, ES = 0.68–0.76), and PO at AeT ($p = 0.04$, ES = 0.51), PO_{max} ($p = 0.03$, ES = 0.53), and $\dot{V}O_{2\,max}$ (L·min^{-1} and ml·kg^{-1}·min^{-1}, $p = 0.01$ and < 0.01, respectively, ES = 0.61, 0.72, respectively) for the cycling test. However, there were no significant differences in the treadmill running test results between groups (all, $p \geq 0.14$; ES = 0.00–0.36).

3.1. Laboratory Tests

The subjects were instructed to refrain from consuming caffeine and alcohol and from heavy training on the day before the tests, as well as to consume a light meal at least 3 h before each laboratory test. During the 3-h period preceding the tests, only ad libitum water ingestion was permitted. During all laboratory tests, HR was collected via a HR monitor (HRM-Tri; Garmin Ltd., Olathe, KS, USA) across the chest with sampling at 1 Hz. Body mass was measured with a body fat monitor scale (TBF-102; Tanita, Tokyo, Japan) before the cycling and running tests.

Table 2. Environmental conditions during the Olympic-distance race of the faster and slower groups.

	All (N = 17)	Faster (n = 9)	Slower (n = 8)
Overall			
Air temperature (°C)	21.6 ± 3.7	20.9 ± 3.6	22.3 ± 3.9
Relative humidity (%)	64.3 ± 17.0	58.6 ± 15.2	70.0 ± 17.7
Wind speed (m·s^{-1})	3.5 ± 1.0	3.4 ± 0.9	3.6 ± 1.1
Barometric pressure (mmHg)	759.1 ± 7.1	760.8 ± 6.1	757.4 ± 8.1
Swimming			
Water temperature (°C)	20.3 ± 3.3	21.3 ± 3.1	20.1 ± 3.7
Cycling			
Cumulated positive elevation (m)	173.7 ± 115.6	147.8 ± 134.2	202.8 ± 90.3
Elevation to distance ratio (m·km^{-1})	4.3 ± 2.9	3.7 ± 3.4	5.1 ± 2.3
Running			
Cumulated positive elevation (m)	37.7 ± 31.3	28.7 ± 20.6	47.8 ± 39.2
Elevation to distance ratio (m·km^{-1})	3.8 ± 3.1	2.9 ± 2.1	4.8 ± 3.9

Values are means ± SD. N, number of subjects. No significant differences were observed between the groups ($p < 0.05$).

Table 3. Laboratory measurements of swimming, cycle ergometry, and treadmill running of the faster and slower groups.

	All (N = 17)	Faster (n = 9)	Slower (n = 8)
Swimming			
Speed at AeT (m·s^{-1})	0.88 ± 0.14	0.98 ± 0.10	0.78 ± 0.10 **
Speed at AnT (m·s^{-1})	0.93 ± 0.13	1.02 ± 0.10	0.84 ± 0.09 **
SS$_{max}$ (m·s^{-1})	1.07 ± 0.13	1.16 ± 0.09	0.96 ± 0.08 **
HR at AeT (bpm)	138 ± 17	142 ± 15	135 ± 19
HR at AnT (bpm)	150 ± 13	149 ± 10	151 ± 18
HR$_{max}$ (bpm)	185 ± 9	186 ± 9	182 ± 10
%HR$_{max}$ at AeT (%)	74.8 ± 6.7	76.0 ± 6.8	73.6 ± 6.7
%HR$_{max}$ at AnT (%)	81.2 ± 6.0	80.0 ± 4.8	82.5 ± 7.2
Cycling			
PO at AeT (W)	190 ± 32	203 ± 28	176 ± 33 *
PO at AnT (W)	252 ± 33	263 ± 32	239 ± 31
PO$_{max}$ (W)	343 ± 34	359 ± 34	325 ± 24 *
HR at AeT (bpm)	136 ± 15	140 ± 16	132 ± 14
HR at AnT (bpm)	156 ± 13	158 ± 16	154 ± 10
HR$_{max}$ (bpm)	183 ± 8	183 ± 9	182 ± 7
%HR$_{max}$ at AeT (%)	74.7 ± 6.5	76.6 ± 6.3	72.6 ± 6.5
%HR$_{max}$ at AnT (%)	85.6 ± 5.0	86.5 ± 6.2	84.6 ± 3.4
$\dot{V}O_{2\,max}$ (L·min^{-1})	3.8 ± 0.4	4.0 ± 0.3	3.6 ± 0.3 *
$\dot{V}O_{2\,max}$ (ml·kg^{-1}·min^{-1})	58.7 ± 5.9	62.4 ± 4.7	54.5 ± 3.9 **
% $\dot{V}O_{2\,max}$ at AeT (%)	63.7 ± 7.9	64.7 ± 5.5	62.6 ± 10.2
% $\dot{V}O_{2\,max}$ at AnT (%)	80.8 ± 6.2	81.2 ± 7.5	80.3 ± 4.8
GE (%)	21.3 ± 1.4	21.3 ± 1.2	21.3 ± 1.6

Table 3. Cont.

	All (N = 17)	Faster (n = 9)	Slower (n = 8)
Running			
Speed at AeT (km·h^{-1})	12.2 ± 1.2	12.6 ± 1.0	11.9 ± 1.3
Speed at AnT (km·h^{-1})	14.5 ± 1.5	14.9 ± 0.9	14.1 ± 2.0
RS$_{max}$ (km·h^{-1})	17.5 ± 1.0	17.8 ± 0.7	17.1 ± 1.2
HR at AeT (bpm)	154 ± 10	153 ± 13	155 ± 8
HR at AnT (bpm)	171 ± 13	171 ± 13	172 ± 12
HR$_{max}$ (bpm)	192 ± 9	190 ± 9	194 ± 9
%HR$_{max}$ at AeT (%)	80.1 ± 4.0	80.3 ± 4.6	79.8 ± 3.5
%HR$_{max}$ at AnT (%)	89.1 ± 4.4	89.6 ± 3.9	88.5 ± 5.1
$\dot{V}O_{2\,max}$ (L·min^{-1})	3.9 ± 0.4	4.0 ± 0.4	3.8 ± 0.4
$\dot{V}O_{2\,max}$ (ml·kg^{-1}·min^{-1})	60.4 ± 4.4	62.2 ± 2.8	58.5 ± 5.3
% $\dot{V}O_{2\,max}$ at AeT (%)	72.2 ± 6.1	71.8 ± 5.5	72.8 ± 7.0
% $\dot{V}O_{2\,max}$ at AnT (%)	86.9 ± 6.2	86.2 ± 3.9	87.6 ± 8.3
Running economy (ml·kg^{-1}·km^{-1})	217 ± 14	217 ± 9	216 ± 18

Values are means ± SD. N, number of subjects; AeT, aerobic threshold; AnT, anaerobic threshold; SS$_{max}$, Maximal swimming speed; HR, heart rate; HR$_{max}$, maximal heart rate; PO, power output; PO$_{max}$, Maximal power output, $\dot{V}O_{2\,max}$, maximal oxygen uptake; GE, gross efficiency; RS$_{max}$, Maximal running speed. * $p < 0.05$; ** $p < 0.01$. See text for explanations of AnT and AeT in each exercise mode.

3.2. Exercise Intensity of Each Leg

The mean exercise intensity of each leg of the OD race is shown in Table 4. The overall mean absolute workload was 1.03 ± 0.18 m·s^{-1} for swimming, 209.6 ± 24.3 W for cycling, and 14.1 ± 1.4 km·h^{-1} for running. The absolute workload was greater in the faster group than the slower group for swimming (1.14 ± 0.18 vs. 0.92 ± 0.09 m·s^{-1}, respectively, $p < 0.01$, ES = 0.68) and running (14.9 ± 0.8 vs. 13.2 ± 1.4 km·h^{-1}, respectively, $p = 0.02$, ES = 0.58). The absolute workload for cycling was also greater in the faster group than the slower group, although the difference was not significant ($p = 0.06$, ES = 0.47). The mean relative HR of all participants was 89.8% ± 3.7% of HR$_{max}$ for swimming, 91.1% ± 4.4% of HR$_{max}$ for cycling, and 90.7% ± 5.1% of HR$_{max}$ for running. There were no differences in mean relative HR between groups for swimming and cycling ($p = 0.25$ and 0.07, respectively, ES = 0.28, 0.44, respectively). However, the relative HR for running of the faster group was greater than that of the slower group ($p < 0.01$, ES = 0.65). The relative workloads and absolute HR values of each leg are shown in Table 4.

The absolute workloads and relative HR values (i.e., % of HR$_{max}$) of each leg during the OD race of all participants are shown in Figure 1. The average AeT, AnT, and maximal values of each laboratory test of each leg are shown for visual reference. The mean workload value shifted above workload at AnT in swimming, between workload at AeT and AnT in cycling, and slightly below workload at AnT, with the exception of the beginning and end of the leg, in running. The mean relative HR value remained above HR at AnT throughout the race.

3.3. Exercise Intensity Distribution during the Race

During the swimming, cycling, and running legs of the OD race, the HR distribution of all participants was 1.5% ± 2.3%, 2.8% ± 8.0%, and 4.1% ± 10.6% in HR$_{zone}$1, 6.6% ± 15.0%, 18.4% ± 24.0%, and 39.9% ± 38.5% in HR$_{zone}$2, and 91.9% ± 16.3%, 78.8% ± 28.1%, and 56.0% ± 42.1% in HR$_{zone}$3, respectively. There were no significant differences in HR distribution between groups in the swimming and cycling legs (all, $p \geq 0.20$; ES = 0.14–0.32; Figure 2). In running, however, the slower group had a higher percentage in HR$_{zone}$2

(65.4% ± 35.0% vs. 17.3% ± 25.9%, p = 0.02, ES = 0.58) and a lower percentage in $HR_{zone}3$ (26.2% ± 36.4% vs. 82.4% ± 26.6%, p = 0.01, ES = 0.60) as compared to the faster group (Figure 2).

The PO distribution of all participants was 5.8% ± 3.2% in $PO_{zone}1$, 30.0% ± 18.1% in $PO_{zone}2$, 36.3% ± 17.2% in $PO_{zone}3$, 22.8% ± 11.1% in $PO_{zone}4$, and 5.1% ± 2.8% in $PO_{zone}5$, respectively. There were no significant differences in PO distribution between the two groups (all, $p \geq 0.14$; ES = 0.09–0.35; Figure 3A). The RS distribution of all participants was 0.0% ± 0.0% in $RS_{zone}1$, 8.7% ± 12.5% in $RS_{zone}2$, 52.1% ± 28.9% in $RS_{zone}3$, 38.8% ± 31.0% in $RS_{zone}4$, and 0.5% ± 0.7% in $RS_{zone}5$, respectively. As compared to the slower group, the faster group had a higher percentage only in $RS_{zone}4$ (53.8% ± 31.7% vs. 21.9% ± 20.6%, p = 0.04, ES = 0.50) (Figure 3B).

Table 4. Mean absolute HR, mean relative HR, mean absolute workload, and mean relative workload of the faster (n = 9) and slower (n = 8) groups.

	Group	Swimming	Cycling	Running
Absolute workload [a]	All (N = 17)	1.03 ± 0.18	210 ± 24	14.1 ± 1.4
	Faster (n = 9)	1.14 ± 0.18	221 ± 26	14.9 ± 0.8
	Slower (n = 8)	0.92 ± 0.09 **	197 ± 15	13.2 ± 1.4 *
Relative workload (%maximal workload)	All (N = 17)	96.6 ± 8.8	61.3 ± 5.2	80.5 ± 4.9
	Faster (n = 9)	97.8 ± 10.0	61.5 ± 5.5	83.4 ± 2.9
	Slower (n = 8)	95.2 ± 7.7	61.0 ± 5.2	77.2 ± 4.5 *
Absolute HR (bpm)	All (N = 17)	166 ± 12	166 ± 9	174 ± 9
	Faster (n = 9)	170 ± 13	170 ± 7	179 ± 7
	Slower (n = 8)	162 ± 11	162 ± 8	169 ± 9 *
Relative HR (%HR_{max})	All (N = 17)	89.8 ± 3.7	91.1 ± 4.4	90.7 ± 5.1
	Faster (n = 9)	90.9 ± 3.1	93.1 ± 4.3	94.0 ± 2.2
	Slower (n = 8)	88.6 ± 4.1	89.0 ± 3.7	87.0 ± 5.1 **

Values are means ± SD. N, number of subjects; HR, heart rate; HR_{max}, maximal heart rate. * $p < 0.05$; ** $p < 0.01$.
[a] Swimming, speed (m·s^{-1}); Cycling, power output (W); Running, speed (km·h^{-1}).

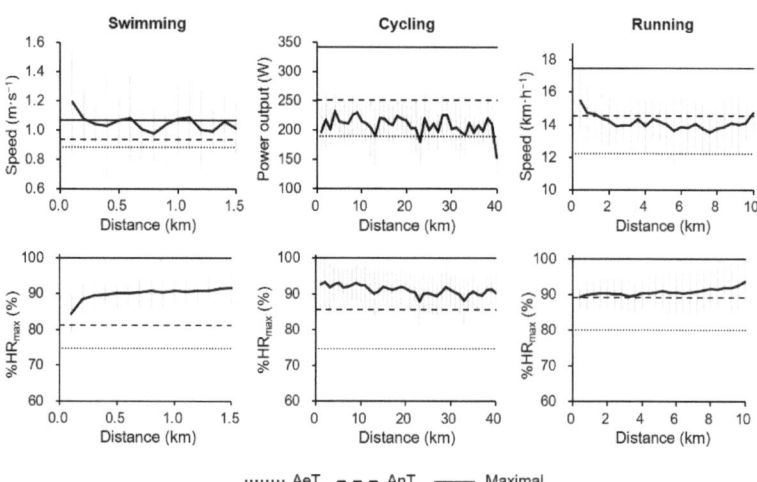

Figure 1. Profile of the percentage of maximal heart rate (%HR_{max}) and absolute workload (swimming speed, cycling power output, and running speed) in each leg during Olympic-distance races (N = 17). **Upper figures**: mean %HR_{max} at AeT (dotted line), %HR_{max} at AnT (dashed line), and HR_{max} (solid line). **Lower figures**: mean workload at AeT (dotted line), workload at AnT (dashed line), and maximal workload (solid line). See text for explanations of AeT, AnT, and maximal workload in each exercise mode.

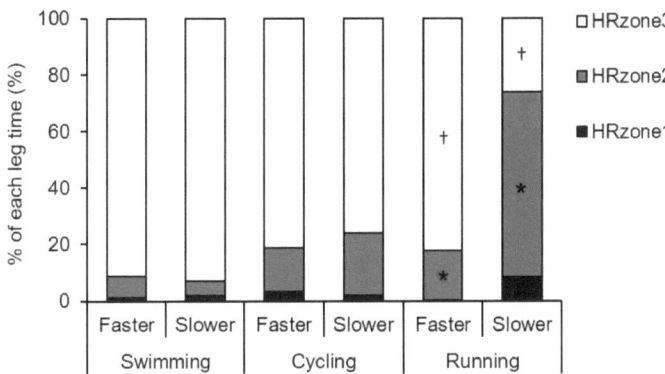

Figure 2. Time percentage in three intensity zones based on heart rate (HR) in each leg during Olympic-distance races in the faster ($n = 9$) and slower ($n = 8$) groups. * $p < 0.05$ in HR$_{zone}$2 in running leg. † $p < 0.05$ in HR$_{zone}$3 in running leg. Standard deviations have been eliminated to improve clarity. See text for explanations of HR$_{zone}$1, 2, and 3.

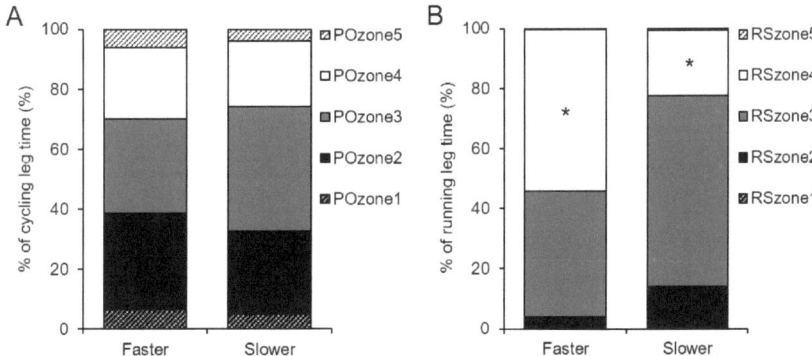

Figure 3. Time percentage in five intensity zones based on power output (PO, **A**) in the cycling leg and running speed (RS, **B**) in the running leg during Olympic-distance races in the faster ($n = 9$) and slower ($n = 8$) groups. No significant differences were observed between the groups in each PO$_{zone}$ in the cycling leg ($p > 0.05$). * $p < 0.05$ in RS$_{zone}$4 in the running leg. Standard deviations have been eliminated to improve clarity. See text for explanations of each PO$_{zone}$ and RS$_{zone}$.

4. Discussion

To the best of our knowledge, this study is the first to evaluate the relative exercise intensity of well-trained, age-group male triathletes at two performance levels according to the principle of test specificity in all disciplines during a nondraft legal OD race. The main findings of this study were as follows: (1) Well-trained, age-group male triathletes who completed the nondraft legal OD at a mean time (h:min:s) of 2:19:50 ± 0:09:38 (range, 2:07:16–2:41:07) demonstrated a high percentage of HR$_{max}$ (87% of HR$_{max}$~) throughout all three legs; (2) Faster triathletes had shorter times in all three legs with higher absolute workloads, but differences in relative intensity and intensity distribution were observed only in the running leg, as faster triathletes sustained higher intensity than slower triathletes.

4.1. Laboratory Tests and OD Triathlon Performance

The total performance times of the OD race in this study were close to those obtained in other studies with similar well-trained triathletes [47], but shorter than a study of recreational triathletes [48]. It is well known that successful endurance athletes are characterized by high levels of maximal ($\dot{V}O_{2\,max}$ and maximal workload) and submaximal (aerobic/anaerobic threshold and economy/efficiency) measures [49,50]. In the present study, the times to complete the swimming (−20.8%) and cycling (−4.9%) legs in an actual OD race were significantly shorter for the faster group in association with superior maximal and submaximal measures in the incremental swimming and cycling tests, as compared with the slower group. However, the time to complete the running leg was significantly shorter for the faster group (−13.2%), while there was no significant difference in any parameters in the incremental running test between the groups. These results suggest that the differences in swimming and cycling performance between the two groups were highly dependent on aerobic capacities, as assessed by specific incremental tests for each of the exercise modes. However, the difference in running performance between the two groups may have been due to factors other than aerobic capacities, as assessed by the incremental treadmill running test in this study. A review article [7] pointed out that the relationship between aerobic capacity measured separately in each leg and triathlon performance was not as high as in the respective single sports. A possible explanation for this finding may be that prior exercise affected the strength of the correlation between physiological variables specific to one discipline and performance in it under conditions characteristic of a triathlon competition [7,51].

4.2. Exercise Intensity during the Race

In the swimming leg, the mean relative intensities and the distribution of HR within the three intensity zones were similar between groups (Figure 2, Table 4). The mean relative HR of all participants was 89.8% of HR_{max}, which is comparable to previous reports of elite triathletes (91%–92% of HR_{max}) [22]. Surprisingly, the same level of relative HR (91.5% of HR_{max}) was reported in the Ironman swimming leg (3.8 km, ~1 h) [52]. Although there is an obvious tendency toward reduced relative intensity with relation to increased race duration [20,28], this relationship may not necessarily be linear in triathlon swimming. Wu et al. [24] compared absolute exercise intensities across the three triathlon races (sprint, Olympic, and half-Ironman distance) performed by the same triathletes and found no differences in mean speed across the races despite differences in swimming duration (range, approximately 0:11:00–0:30:00 h:min:s). Therefore, relative intensity is considered comparable across the three triathlon races. Taken together, there might be little difference in relative intensities during the swimming leg at different performance levels and different race durations (~1 h). However, it is unclear whether about 90% of HR_{max} is the upper limit of sustainable intensity during triathlon swimming or if intensity is controlled based on anticipation of the longer duration of exercise following the swimming leg.

A visual inspection of the relative HR profile (Figure 1) suggests that the HR remained above HR at AnT throughout the swimming leg, as most of the leg was performed in $HR_{zone}3$ (more than AnT), and the time spent in $HR_{zone}1$ (less than AeT) was negligible (Figure 2), because $HR_{zone}1$ was held only during the initial phase of the start of the race, when the triathletes began accelerating from the starting line. This is in agreement with a previous study demonstrating the HR distribution during 10-km cross-country skiing [19], during which the exercise duration (mean race time, 0:25:47 h:min:s) was comparable to the swimming leg in the present study (mean swimming time, 0:26:28 h:min:s).

Despite the stability of relative HR, large fluctuations above the AnT line were observed in the relative workload (Figure 1), which could be due to the influence of environmental factors. In open water swimming, the water conditions and tides can considerably affect absolute swimming speed and, therefore, relative swimming speed, even if the same relative HR is maintained.

In the cycling leg, all of the indicators of relative intensity were similar between groups (Figures 2 and 3A, and Table 4). The mean relative HR of all participants was 91.1% of HR_{max}. This value was nearly equal to those reported for elite triathletes during draft legal races (90%–92% of HR_{max}) [21,22] and clearly higher than those reported for ironman triathletes (83% of peak HR) [26]. This value was slightly lower than the those reported for nonelite triathletes with comparable $\dot{V}O_{2\,max}$ as the subjects in the present study (60.6 vs. 58.7 mL·kg^{-1}·min^{-1}, respectively) during nondraft legal short-course races (94.1% HR$_{max}$) [25], which may be partly due to some difference in the race distance of the cycling leg accompanied by differences in exercise duration between studies; i.e., the race distance and exercise duration were 30 km and 50.09 min in the previous study [25] and 40 km and 70.55 min in this study.

The mean relative workload in the cycling leg of all participants was 61.3% of PO$_{max}$, which was nearly equal to that of elite triathletes during the draft legal race (60%–63% of PO$_{max}$) [21,22]. However, some differences in the PO distribution evaluated with the same methodology were observed between the draft legal race in a previous study [22] and the nondraft legal race in the present study. In the former study [22], more time was spent in PO$_{zone}$1 (below 10% of PO$_{max}$) and PO$_{zone}$5 (above PO$_{max}$), with a comparatively shorter time in PO$_{zone}$3 (between the PO at AeT and AnT) and PO$_{zone}$4 (between the PO at AnT and PO$_{max}$) in the present study. This discrepancy may be related to drafting, group riding dynamics, and the course profile. Elite triathletes often compete in criterium or circuit courses with frequent technical corners requiring repeated accelerations and decelerations with rotating the position within the same pack. Meanwhile, cycling during nondraft legal events is more similar to that of an individual time trial, as reflected by the stability of PO during flat cycling [53]. Therefore, the difference in the PO distribution may be related to the application rule of drafting and/or the course profile, even though the mean relative PO was similar in both races.

As shown by the relative HR profile in Figure 1, the HR remained above HR at AnT throughout the cycling leg. However, the PO profile (Figure 1) suggests that the PO shifted between PO at AeT and AnT throughout the leg. This discordance might be suggestive of the residual effect of prior swimming and the subsequent physiological responses that differ from performing an isolated exercise, especially in the initial phase [54]. Another explanation might be cardiovascular drift, which is primarily characterized by a progressive decrease in stroke volume and a progressive increase in HR to maintain cardiac output during prolonged exercise [55]. The hyperthermia and dehydration that occur concomitantly with long-duration exercise influence the magnitude of cardiovascular drift in a graded fashion [56]. Glycogen depletion caused by prolonged exercise also affects the workload–HR relationship [57]. Therefore, HR during an OD race may overestimate the PO [58]. Even in the running leg, the relative HR level was higher than the relative workload level.

In the running leg, there were clear differences in relative intensity between the faster and slower groups. The mean relative HR was definitely higher in the faster group than the slower group (94.0% vs. 87.0% of HR$_{max}$) and slightly higher than the recreational triathletes (92.3% HR$_{max}$) [25], but on a comparable level for elite triathletes (93%–94% of HR$_{max}$) [22]. Additionally, the faster group spent more time in the high-intensity zones (i.e., larger values of HR$_{zone}$3 and RS$_{zone}$4) as compared to the slower group. The relative workload was also higher in the faster group than the slower group (83.4% vs. 77.2% of RS$_{max}$). Therefore, our hypothesis is supported only in the running leg.

It is interesting to note that clear differences in relative intensity between the two groups were observed only in the running leg in this study. In terms of the pacing strategy, it has been demonstrated that the slower, less experienced athletes tended to pace at too high an intensity at the beginning of the race, leading to a continuous decrease in exercise intensity for the remaining duration [32]. However, in the swimming and cycling legs in this study, there were no differences in any indicator of relative intensity or triathlon experience between the two groups. Thus, the effect of the height and distribution of relative intensity until the completion of the cycling leg may have had only a minor impact on the difference in relative intensity during the running leg between the two groups. On the other hand, before the start of the running leg, the slower group was exposed a longer duration of relative intensity (~10 min) at a level comparable to that of the faster group. This difference might have induced greater physiological and metabolic disruptions in the slower group, resulting in premature fatigue and impaired workload in the running leg.

Millet and Vleck [7] stated that the first transition (i.e., swim–cycle transition) is regarded as having a negligible effect on overall performance during the nondraft legal OD race. Meanwhile, a number of studies reported the effects of prior exercise on subsequent running [7,8,59–61] and the cycle–run transition is traditionally considered to be more important on performance during an OD race [7,8]. Prior cycling induces physiological/cardiorespiratory and biomechanical changes during subsequent running [8]. Several studies have reported that such changes (usually negative effects) might be related to the performance level of triathletes [62–66]. For example, Boussana et al. [62] observed significantly higher ventilatory responses and significantly greater decreases in respiratory muscle strength and endurance in competition triathletes than in the elite group in running following cycling performed at similar relative intensities, despite similar $\dot{V}O_{2\ max}$ and VT [62]. Therefore, in this study, the negative effects of prior exercise on physiological and biomechanical responses during subsequent running might have been larger in the slower group than the faster group, which could be related to the difference in relative intensity between the groups during the running leg. Further studies are required to specifically analyze the mechanisms underlying the difference in relative intensity induced by prior exercise.

From the point of view of exercise intensity throughout the OD race, relative HR remained above HR at AnT until the end of the cycling leg and remained at or above HR at AnT in the running leg in both groups. These values were higher than those previously reported for ultra-endurance events (race durations >8 h) [26,27] and a 42-km marathon (~2.5–5 h), during which intensity was approximated as AeT [30]. A possible explanation for the higher intensity during the OD race as compared to marathon—both with similar estimated energy expenditures (2000–2546 kcal) [67]—may lie in the degree of muscle fatigue derived from peripheral factors. Although the causes of muscle fatigue are complex and not completely understood, exercise-induced muscle damage is a primary cause of muscle fatigue during endurance sports [68]. While no direct comparison is available, expression levels of markers of muscle damage, such as creatine kinase and lactate dehydrogenase, are higher after marathon running [68] than after an OD triathlon [10]. Additionally, a reduction in the height of countermovement jump, which is also higher after a marathon [10,68], suggesting that exercise-induced fatigue of lower extremity muscles is greater while competing in a marathon as compared to an OD triathlon. Swimming and cycling are considered to produce minor damage to the involved muscles, while running—a weight-bearing exercise that includes concentric and eccentric contractions of the leg muscles—may produce more pronounced muscle damage while competing in a 42-km marathon. Another possible explanation could be related to the degree of glycogen depletion, as proposed in a previous report [69]. Glycogen depletion is also related to muscle fatigue during prolonged exercise [70]. Differences in muscle activities among the three exercise modes might be related to higher glycogen reserves in active muscles in each discipline of a triathlon as compared to strictly running in a marathon. However, further investigations are needed to elucidate the specific physiological responses during a triathlon.

4.3. Limitations

There were several methodological limitations to this study that should be acknowledged. First, the competition measurements were carried out in several separate OD races. This disparity may have added some bias to the analysis of the present study. However, there were no significant differences in environmental conditions or course profiles between the two groups (Table 2), and thus, the effects of these disparities were considered minor. Moreover, differences in the swimming conditions between the laboratory tests (i.e., flume swimming) and competition measurements (i.e., open water swimming) could affect the analysis of this study. Also, the air temperature in the laboratory tests (around 25 °C) was higher than that in the OD races (around 21.6 °C). Cardiovascular drift can occur in temperate conditions and greater effects are seen in high heat conditions [71], so the difference mentioned above could impact the $\dot{V}O_2$ or BLa vs. HR relationships. However, an electric fan provided airflow, and overall room ventilation was maintained throughout each test, which minimizes the possibility of a cardiovascular drift. Furthermore, each incremental test was performed at 45 ± 26 days from the competition measurements of the OD race in this study, while most previous similar studies performed incremental tests within 2 to 4 weeks before the OD race [21,22,25,72]. The individual training programs and different season calendars among our subjects made it difficult to arrive at a unified schedule in this study. Although the maximal and submaximal measures of triathletes are reportedly stable throughout the pre-competition to competitive period [73], future research examining exercise intensity during OD triathlon should attempt to use unified race conditions and schedules.

5. Conclusions

Mean exercise intensity during a nondraft legal OD triathlon was above 87% of HR_{max} derived from each exercise mode throughout all three legs in well-trained, age-group male triathletes. The majority of the swimming and cycling legs was spent at an intensity more than HR at AnT, while the exercise intensity during the running leg differed among individuals. The time to complete the whole OD race showed that the intensity of the faster triathletes was higher than that of the slower triathletes. The results of the present study suggest that sustaining higher intensity during the running leg might be important for success in nondraft legal OD triathlon races. These results may be beneficial for athletes, coaches, and researchers in the sense that they describe the characteristic performance profiles of the multisport nature of triathlon events. As such, the present research may give rise to better plan training and racing strategies.

Author Contributions: Conceptualization, A.A., K.I. and Y.N.; Data curation, A.A.; Formal analysis, A.A.; Funding acquisition, Y.N.; Investigation, A.A.; Methodology, A.A. and K.I.; Project administration, Y.N.; Resources, A.A., K.I. and Y.N.; Supervision, K.I. and Y.N.; Visualization, A.A.; Writing–original draft, A.A.; Writing–review & editing, A.A., K.I. and Y.N. All authors have read and agreed to the published version of the manuscript.

Funding: This research was supported in part by a grant from Advanced Research Initiative for Human High Performance (ARIHHP), University of Tsukuba.

Institutional Review Board Statement: The study was conducted according to the guidelines of the Declaration of Helsinki, and approved by the Ethics Committee of the University of Tsukuba (project identification code: Tai 30–24).

Informed Consent Statement: Informed consent was obtained from all subjects involved in the study.

Data Availability Statement: The data presented in this study are available on request from the corresponding author.

Acknowledgments: We would like to thank all participants for dedicating their time and effort toward this study. We would also like to thank the members of our laboratory for their support in performing this project.

Conflicts of Interest: The authors declare no conflict of interest.

References

1. Wu, S.S.; Peiffer, J.J.; Brisswalter, J.; Nosaka, K.; Abbiss, C.R. Factors influencing pacing in triathlon. *Open Access J. Sports Med.* **2014**, *5*, 223–234. [CrossRef] [PubMed]
2. Millet, G.P.; Bentley, D.J.; Vleck, V.E. The relationships between science and sport: Application in triathlon. *Int. J. Sports Physiol. Perform.* **2007**, *2*, 315–322. [CrossRef] [PubMed]
3. Revelles, A.B.F.; Granizo, I.R.; Sánchez, M.C.; Ruz, R.P. Men's triathlon correlation between stages and final result in the London 2012 Olympic Games. *J. Hum. Sport Exerc.* **2018**, *2*, 514–528.

4. Wu, S.S.X.; Peiffer, J.P.; Brisswalter, J.; Lau, W.Y.; Nosaka, K.; Abbiss, C.R. Influence of race distance and biological sex on age-related declines in triathlon performance: Part A. *J. Sci. Cycl.* **2014**, *3*, 42–48.
5. Bentley, D.; Libicz, S.; Jougla, A.; Coste, O.; Manetta, J.; Chamari, K.; Millet, G. The effects of exercise intensity or drafting during swimming on subsequent cycling performance in triathletes. *J. Sci. Med. Sport* **2007**, *10*, 234–243. [CrossRef]
6. Laursen, P.B.; Rhodes, E.C. Factors affecting performance in an ultraendurance triathlon. *Sports Med.* **2001**, *31*, 195–209. [CrossRef]
7. Millet, G.P.; Vleck, V.E. Physiological and biomechanical adaptations to the cycle to run transition in Olympic triathlon: Review and practical recommendations for training. *Br. J. Sports Med.* **2000**, *34*, 384–390. [CrossRef]
8. Walsh, J.A. The Rise of Elite Short-course triathlon re-emphasises the necessity to transition efficiently from cycling to running. *Sports* **2019**, *7*, 99. [CrossRef]
9. Tota, Ł.; Piotrowska, A.; Pałka, T.; Morawska, M.; Mikuľáková, W.; Mucha, D.; Żmuda-Pałka, M.; Pilch, W. Muscle and intestinal damage in triathletes. *PLoS ONE* **2019**, *14*, e0210651. [CrossRef]
10. Olcina, G.; Timón, R.; Brazo-Sayavera, J.; Martínez-Guardado, I.; Marcos-Serrano, M.; Crespo, C. Changes in physiological and performance variables in non-professional triathletes after taking part in an Olympic distance triathlon. *Res. Sports Med.* **2018**, *26*, 323–331. [CrossRef]
11. Logan-Sprenger, H.M. Fluid balance and thermoregulatory responses of competitive triathletes. *J. Therm. Biol.* **2019**, *79*, 69–72. [CrossRef]
12. Millard-Stafford, M.; Sparling, P.B.; Rosskopf, L.B.; Hinson, B.T.; DiCarlo, L.J. Carbohydrate-electrolyte replacement during a simulated triathlon in the heat. *Med. Sci. Sports Exerc.* **1990**, *22*, 621–628. [CrossRef] [PubMed]
13. Lopes, R.F.; Osiecki, R.; Rama, L.M.P. Biochemical markers during and after an Olympic triathlon race. *J. Exerc. Physiol. Online* **2011**, *14*, 87–96.
14. Park, C.H.; Kim, T.U.; Park, T.G.; Kwak, Y.S. Changes of immunological markers in elite and amateur triathletes. *Int. SportMed J.* **2008**, *9*, 116–130.
15. Caillaud, C.; Serre-Cousiné, O.; Anselme, F.; Capdevilla, X.; Préfaut, C. Computerized tomography and pulmonary diffusing capacity in highly trained athletes after performing a triathlon. *J. Appl. Physiol.* **1995**, *79*, 1226–1232. [CrossRef]
16. Le Gallais, D.; Hayot, M.; Hue, O.; Wouassi, D.; Boussana, A.; Ramonatxo, M.; Préfaut, C. Metabolic and cardioventilatory responses during a graded exercise test before and 24 h after a triathlon. *Eur. J. Appl. Physiol. Occup. Physiol.* **1999**, *79*, 176–181. [CrossRef]
17. Sultana, F.; Abbiss, C.R.; Louis, J.; Bernard, T.; Hausswirth, C.; Brisswalter, J. Age-related changes in cardio-respiratory responses and muscular performance following an Olympic triathlon in well-trained triathletes. *Eur. J. Appl. Physiol.* **2012**, *112*, 1549–1556. [CrossRef]
18. Hopkins, W.G. Quantification of training in competitive sports. *Sports Med.* **1991**, *12*, 161–183. [CrossRef]
19. Formenti, D.; Rossi, A.; Calogiuri, G.; Thomassen, T.O.; Scurati, R.; Weydahl, A. Exercise intensity and pacing strategy of cross-country skiers during a 10 km skating simulated race. *Res. Sports Med.* **2015**, *23*, 126–139. [CrossRef]
20. Padilla, S.; Mujika, I.; Orbañanos, J.; Angulo, F. Exercise intensity during competition time trials in professional road cycling. *Med. Sci. Sports Exerc.* **2000**, *32*, 850–856. [CrossRef]
21. Bernard, T.; Hausswirth, C.; Le Meur, Y.; Bignet, F.; Dorel, S.; Brisswalter, J. Distribution of power output during the cycling stage of a Triathlon World Cup. *Med. Sci. Sports Exerc.* **2009**, *41*, 1296–1302. [CrossRef] [PubMed]
22. Le Meur, Y.; Hausswirth, C.; Dorel, S.; Bignet, F.; Brisswalter, J.; Bernard, T. Influence of gender on pacing adopted by elite triathletes during a competition. *Eur. J. Appl. Physiol.* **2009**, *106*, 535–545. [CrossRef] [PubMed]
23. Hausswirth, C.; Lehénaff, D.; Dréano, P.; Savonen, K. Effects of cycling alone or in a sheltered position on subsequent running performance during a triathlon. *Med. Sci. Sports Exerc.* **1999**, *31*, 599–604. [CrossRef]
24. Wu, S.S.; Peiffer, J.J.; Brisswalter, J.; Nosaka, K.; Lau, W.Y.; Abbiss, C.R. Pacing strategies during the swim, cycle and run disciplines of sprint, Olympic and half-Ironman triathlons. *Eur. J. Appl. Physiol.* **2015**, *115*, 1147–1154. [CrossRef] [PubMed]
25. Zhou, S.; Robson, S.J.; King, M.J.; Davie, A.J. Correlations between short-course triathlon performance and physiological variables determined in laboratory cycle and treadmill tests. *J. Sports Med. Phys. Fitness* **1997**, *37*, 122–130.
26. Laursen, P.B.; Knez, W.L.; Shing, C.M.; Langill, R.H.; Rhodes, E.C.; Jenkins, D.G. Relationship between laboratory-measured variables and heart rate during an ultra-endurance triathlon. *J. Sports Sci.* **2005**, *23*, 1111–1120. [CrossRef]
27. Fornasiero, A.; Savoldelli, A.; Fruet, D.; Boccia, G.; Pellegrini, B.; Schena, F. Physiological intensity profile, exercise load and performance predictors of a 65-km mountain ultra-marathon. *J. Sports Sci.* **2018**, *36*, 1287–1295. [CrossRef]
28. Esteve-Lanao, J.; Lucia, A.; Dekoning, J.J.; Foster, C. How do humans control physiological strain during strenuous endurance exercise? *PLoS ONE* **2008**, *3*, e2943. [CrossRef]
29. Billat, V.L.; Petot, H.; Landrain, M.; Meilland, R.; Koralsztein, J.P.; Mille-Hamard, L. Cardiac output and performance during a marathon race in middle-aged recreational runners. *Sci. World J.* **2012**, *2012*, 810859. [CrossRef]
30. Shimazu, W.; Takayama, F.; Tanji, F.; Nabekura, Y. Relationship between cardiovascular drift and performance in marathon running. *Int. J. Sport Health Sci.* **2020**, 202036. [CrossRef]
31. Lima-Silva, A.E.; Bertuzzi, R.C.; Pires, F.O.; Barros, R.V.; Gagliardi, J.F.; Hammond, J.; Kiss, M.A.; Bishop, D.J. Effect of performance level on pacing strategy during a 10-km running race. *Eur. J. Appl. Physiol.* **2010**, *108*, 1045–1053. [CrossRef] [PubMed]
32. Stöggl, T.L.; Hertlein, M.; Brunauer, R.; Welde, B.; Andersson, E.P.; Swarén, M. Pacing, exercise intensity, and technique by performance level in long-distance cross-country skiing. *Front. Physiol.* **2020**, *11*, 17. [CrossRef]

33. Jones, A.M.; Doust, J.H. A 1% treadmill grade most accurately reflects the energetic cost of outdoor running. *J. Sports Sci.* **1996**, *14*, 321–327. [CrossRef] [PubMed]
34. Moseley, L.; Jeukendrup, A.E. The reliability of cycling efficiency. *Med. Sci. Sports Exerc.* **2001**, *33*, 621–627. [CrossRef] [PubMed]
35. Takayama, F.; Aoyagi, A.; Takahashi, K.; Nabekura, Y. Relationship between oxygen cost and C-reactive protein response to marathon running in college recreational runners. *Open Access J. Sports Med.* **2018**, *9*, 261–268. [CrossRef] [PubMed]
36. Newell, J.; Higgins, D.; Madden, N.; Cruickshank, J.; Einbeck, J.; McMillan, K.; McDonald, R. Software for calculating blood lactate endurance markers. *J. Sports Sci.* **2007**, *25*, 1403–1409. [CrossRef]
37. Buchfuhrer, M.J.; Hansen, J.E.; Robinson, T.E.; Sue, D.Y.; Wasserman, K.; Whipp, B.J. Optimizing the exercise protocol for cardiopulmonary assessment. *J. Appl. Physiol. Respir. Environ. Exerc. Physiol.* **1983**, *55*, 1558–1564. [CrossRef]
38. Pallares, J.G.; Moran-Navarro, R.; Ortega, J.F.; Fernandez-Elias, V.E.; Mora-Rodriguez, R. Validity and reliability of ventilatory and blood lactate thresholds in well-trained cyclists. *PLoS ONE* **2016**, *11*, e0163389. [CrossRef]
39. Esteve-Lanao, J.; San Juan, A.; Earnest, C.P.; Foster, C.; Lucia, A. How do endurance runners actually train? Relationship with competition performance. *Med. Sci. Sports Exerc.* **2005**, *37*, 496–504. [CrossRef]
40. Binder, R.K.; Wonisch, M.; Corra, U.; Cohen-Solal, A.; Vanhees, L.; Saner, H.; Schmid, J.-P. Methodological approach to the first and second lactate threshold in incremental cardiopulmonary exercise testing. *Eur. J. Cardiovasc. Prev. Rehabil.* **2008**, *15*, 726–734. [CrossRef]
41. Cejuela-Anta, R.; Esteve-Lanao, J. Training load quantification in triathlon. *J. Hum. Sport Exerc.* **2011**. [CrossRef]
42. Kuipers, H.; Verstappen, F.T.; Keizer, H.A.; Geurten, P.; van Kranenburg, G. Variability of aerobic performance in the laboratory and its physiologic correlates. *Int. J. Sports Med.* **1985**, *6*, 197–201. [CrossRef]
43. Esteve-Lanao, J.; Foster, C.; Seiler, S.; Lucia, A. Impact of training intensity distribution on performance in endurance athletes. *J. Strength Cond. Res.* **2007**, *21*, 943–949. [CrossRef] [PubMed]
44. Seiler, S.; Tønnessen, E. Intervals, thresholds, and long slow distance: The role of intensity and duration in endurance training. *Sportscience* **2009**, *13*, 32–53.
45. Granier, C.; Abbiss, C.R.; Aubry, A.; Vauchez, Y.; Dorel, S.; Hausswirth, C.; Le Meur, Y. Power output and pacing during international cross-country mountain bike cycling. *Int. J. Sports Physiol. Perform.* **2018**, *13*, 1243–1249. [CrossRef]
46. Fritz, C.O.; Morris, P.E.; Richler, J.J. Effect size estimates: Current use, calculations, and interpretation. *J. Exp. Psychol. Gen.* **2012**, *141*, 2. [CrossRef]
47. Hausswirth, C.; Bigard, A.X.; Guezennec, C.Y. Relationships between running mechanics and energy cost of running at the end of a triathlon and a marathon. *Int. J. Sports Med.* **1997**, *18*, 330–339. [CrossRef]
48. Butts, N.K.; Henry, B.A.; McLean, D. Correlations between VO2 max and performance times of recreational triathletes. *J. Sports Med. Phys. Fitness* **1991**, *31*, 339–344.
49. Suriano, R.; Bishop, D. Physiological attributes of triathletes. *J. Sci. Med. Sport* **2010**, *13*, 340–347. [CrossRef]
50. Millet, G.P.; Vleck, V.E.; Bentley, D.J. Physiological requirements in triathlon. *J. Hum. Sport Exerc.* **2011**, *6*, 184–204. [CrossRef]
51. Aoyagi, A.; Ishikura, K.; Shirai, Y.; Nabekura, Y. The relationship between running performance in the Olympic-distance triathlon and aerobic physiological variables, focusing on the three factors of the classic model. *Japan J. Phys. Educ. Health Sport Sci.* **2020**, *65*, 815–830. (In Japanese) [CrossRef]
52. Barrero, A.; Chaverri, D.; Erola, P.; Iglesias, X.; Rodríguez, F.A. Intensity profile during an ultra-endurance triathlon in relation to testing and performance. *Int. J. Sports Med.* **2014**, *35*, 1170–1178. [CrossRef] [PubMed]
53. Abbiss, C.R.; Quod, M.J.; Martin, D.T.; Netto, K.J.; Nosaka, K.; Lee, H.; Surriano, R.; Bishop, D.; Laursen, P.B. Dynamic pacing strategies during the cycle phase of an Ironman triathlon. *Med. Sci. Sports Exerc.* **2006**, *38*, 726–734. [CrossRef] [PubMed]
54. Delextrat, A.; Brisswalter, J.; Hausswirth, C.; Bernard, T.; Vallier, J.M. Does prior 1500-m swimming affect cycling energy expenditure in well-trained triathletes? *Can. J. Appl. Physiol.* **2005**, *30*, 392–403. [CrossRef]
55. Coyle, E.F. Cardiovascular drift during prolonged exercise and the effects of dehydration. *Int. J. Sports Med.* **1998**, *19* (Suppl. 2), S121–S124. [CrossRef]
56. Ganio, M.S.; Wingo, J.E.; Carrolll, C.E.; Thomas, M.K.; Cureton, K.J. Fluid ingestion attenuates the decline in VO2peak associated with cardiovascular drift. *Med. Sci. Sports Exerc.* **2006**, *38*, 901–909. [CrossRef]
57. Hargreaves, M.; Dillo, P.; Angus, D.; Febbraio, M. Effect of fluid ingestion on muscle metabolism during prolonged exercise. *J. Appl. Physiol.* **1996**, *80*, 363–366. [CrossRef]
58. O'Toole, M.; Douglas, P.; Hiller, W. Lactate, oxygen uptake, and cycling performance in triathletes. *Int. J. Sports Med.* **1989**, *10*, 413–418. [CrossRef]
59. Etxebarria, N.; Hunt, J.; Ingham, S.; Ferguson, R. Physiological assessment of isolated running does not directly replicate running capacity after triathlon-specific cycling. *J. Sports Sci.* **2014**, *32*, 229–238. [CrossRef]
60. Berry, N.T.; Wideman, L.; Shields, E.W.; Battaglini, C.L. The Effects of a duathlon simulation on ventilatory threshold and running economy. *J. Sports Sci. Med.* **2016**, *15*, 247–253.
61. De Vito, G.; Bernardi, M.; Sproviero, E.; Figura, F. Decrease of endurance performance during Olympic triathlon. *Int. J. Sports Med.* **1995**, *16*, 24–28. [CrossRef] [PubMed]
62. Boussana, A.; Hue, O.; Matecki, S.; Galy, O.; Ramonatxo, M.; Varray, A.; Le Gallais, D. The effect of cycling followed by running on respiratory muscle performance in elite and competition triathletes. *Eur. J. Appl. Physiol.* **2002**, *87*, 441–447. [PubMed]

63. Hue, O.; Le Gallais, D.; Boussana, A.; Chollet, D.; Prefaut, C. Performance level and cardiopulmonary responses during a cycle-run trial. *Int. J. Sports Med.* **2000**, *21*, 250–255. [CrossRef] [PubMed]
64. Hue, O.; Galy, O.; Le Gallais, D.; Préfaut, C. Pulmonary responses during the cycle-run succession in elite and competitive triathletes. *Can. J. Appl. Physiol.* **2001**, *26*, 559–573. [CrossRef] [PubMed]
65. Millet, G.P.; Millet, G.Y.; Hofmann, M.D.; Candau, R.B. Alterations in running economy and mechanics after maximal cycling in triathletes: Influence of performance level. *Int. J. Sports Med.* **2000**, *21*, 127–132. [CrossRef] [PubMed]
66. Millet, G.; Millet, G.; Candau, R. Duration and seriousness of running mechanices alterations after maximal cycling in triathlets: Influence of the performance level. *J. Sports Med. Phys. Fitness* **2001**, *41*, 147. [PubMed]
67. Kreider, R.B. Physiological considerations of ultraendurance performance. *Int. J. Sport Nutr. Exerc. Metab.* **1991**, *1*, 3–27. [CrossRef]
68. Del Coso, J.; Fernández de Velasco, D.; Fernández, D.; Abián-Vicen, J.; Salinero, J.J.; González-Millán, C.; Areces, F.; Ruiz, D.; Gallo, C.; Calleja-González, J.; et al. Running pace decrease during a marathon is positively related to blood markers of muscle damage. *PLoS ONE* **2013**, *8*, e57602. [CrossRef]
69. Hausswirth, C.; Bigard, A.X.; Berthelot, M.; Thomaïdis, M.; Guezennec, C.Y. Variability in energy cost of running at the end of a triathlon and a marathon. *Int. J. Sports Med.* **1996**, *17*, 572–579. [CrossRef]
70. Hermansen, L.; Hultman, E.; Saltin, B. Muscle glycogen during prolonged severe exercise. *Acta Physiol. Scand.* **1967**, *71*, 129–139. [CrossRef]
71. Wingo, J.E. Exercise intensity prescription during heat stress: A brief review. *Scand. J. Med. Sci. Sports* **2015**, *25* (Suppl. 1), 90–95. [CrossRef]
72. Hue, O.; Galy, O.; Le Gallais, D. Exercise intensity during repeated days of racing in professional triathletes. *Appl. Physiol. Nutr. Metab.* **2006**, *31*, 250–256. [CrossRef] [PubMed]
73. Galy, O.; Manetta, J.; Coste, O.; Maimoun, L.; Chamari, K.; Hue, O. Maximal oxygen uptake and power of lower limbs during a competitive season in triathletes. *Scand. J. Med. Sci. Sports* **2003**, *13*, 185–193. [CrossRef] [PubMed]

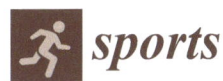

Article

The Prevalence of Legal Performance-Enhancing Substance Use and Potential Cognitive and or Physical Doping in German Recreational Triathletes, Assessed via the Randomised Response Technique

Sebastian Seifarth [1,2], Pavel Dietz [3], Alexander C. Disch [1], Martin Engelhardt [4] and Stefan Zwingenberger [1,*]

1. Department of Sports Medicine at the University Center for Orthopedics and Traumatology, University Medicine Carl Gustav Carus, Technical University Dresden, 01307 Dresden, Germany; Sebsei93@aol.de (S.S.); Alexander.Disch@uniklinikum-dresden.de (A.C.D.)
2. Bundeswehr Hospital Ulm, 89081 Ulm, Germany
3. Institute of Occupational, Social and Environmental Medicine, University Medical Centre of the University of Mainz, Mainz, Germany, 55131 Mainz, Germany; pdietz@uni-mainz.de
4. Department of Orthopedics, Trauma and Hand Surgery, Klinikum Osnabrück, 49076 Osnabrück, Germany; Martin.Engelhardt@klinikum-os.de
* Correspondence: Stefan.Zwingenberger@uniklinikum-dresden.de; Tel.: +49-172-790-8318

Received: 28 July 2019; Accepted: 21 November 2019; Published: 26 November 2019

Abstract: This study investigated the use of performance-enhancing substances in recreational triathletes who were competing in German races at distances ranging from super-sprint to long-distance, as per the International Triathlon Union. The use of legal drugs and over-the-counter supplements over the previous year, painkillers over the previous 3 months, and the potential three-month prevalence of physical doping and or cognitive doping in this group were assessed via an anonymous questionnaire. The Randomised Response Technique (RRT) was implemented for sensitive questions regarding "prescription drugs [. . .] for the purpose of performance enhancement [. . .] only available at a pharmacy or on the black market". The survey did not directly state the word "doping," but included examples of substances that could later be classed as physical and or cognitive doping. The subjects were not required to detail what they were taking. Overall, 1953 completed questionnaires were received from 3134 registered starters at six regional events—themselves involving 17 separate races—in 2017. Of the respondents, 31.8% and 11.3% admitted to the use of dietary supplements, and of painkillers during the previous three months, respectively. Potential physical doping and cognitive doping over the preceding year were reported by 7.0% (Confidence Interval CI: 4.2–9.8) and 9.4% (CI: 6.6–12.3) of triathletes. Gender, age, experience in endurance sports, and number of weekly triathlon training hours were linked to potential physical or cognitive doping. Given the potentially relevant side effects of painkiller use and physical and or cognitive doping, we recommend that educational and preventative measures for them be implemented within amateur triathlons.

Keywords: doping; painkillers; triathlon; recreational athletes; risk factors; RRT

1. Introduction

The World Anti-Doping Agency (WADA) declares doping as fundamentally contrary to the spirit of sport [1], and this is the moral basis for them producing an annual list of banned substances. These substances can be divided in two groups according to their mode of action. Physical doping agents (e.g., sympathomimetics, anabolic steroids, or erythropoietin) have a direct effect on physical aspects of the body. In contrast, cognitive doping agents (which include stimulants such as amphetamines, methylphenidate, and antidepressants) target the central nervous system. All such substances often have multiple unexpected side effects. Even over-the-counter painkillers can provoke life-threatening risks such as hyponatraemia, uncontrolled haemorrhage, and myocardial or renal infarction [2,3]. Often these side effects are unknown or simply ignored [4]. To protect the athlete's health, it is important to avoid the non-therapeutic use of multiple substances.

Investigations into state-sponsored doping in Russia and into positive doping cases at the World Athletics Championships have recently highlighted that doping is a major problem in elite sports [5–7]. Given the high extent of substance abuse amongst elite athletes, it is likely that a substantial number of recreational athletes behave in the same way [8–10].

As in all endurance sports, a considerable amount of doping cases are reported in triathlons [11–13]. However, triathletes are a diverse population, with some athletes competing in a total race distance of less than 15 km, whilst others race over more than 220 km [14]. Although the latter so-called "long-distance" group only represents approximately one-tenth of all recreational triathletes [15], it is the only triathlete group thus far within which the prevalence of doping has been examined [4,11,12,16]. When such athletes were asked whether they had used banned substances over the previous 12 months, the doping prevalence was found to exceed 10% [11,12,16]. Yet the real number of substance abusers remains an estimated value. Even doping controls underestimate the actual number of abuse by a factor of 8 [17]. This, to our knowledge, is the first study to investigate the doping behaviour of recreational triathletes racing over a wide range of distances (from super-sprint up to long-distance) as per the official International Triathlon Union (ITU).

2. Materials and Methods

2.1. Sample, Ethics, Races, Procedure

Ethical approval to perform this study was obtained from the local University Ethical Committee (document number: EK 74022017). Triathletes were surveyed at six different triathlon events in central Germany in 2017. The race distances that were involved ranged from super-sprint to long-distance triathlons (Table 1).

Table 1. The official International Triathlon Union (ITU) distances are presented, with the associated competition distances of swimming, cycling, and running [14] as well as the event locations, where athletes of the corresponding distances were interviewed. Race location: Gera (G), Jena (J), Koberbach (K), Leipzig (L), Moritzburg (M), Nordhausen (N).

Official Distance	Swim (km)	Bike (km)	Run (km)	Race Location
Super-sprint	0.4	10	2.5	G, K, J
Sprint	0.75	20	5	G, M, K, J, L, N
Olympic	1.5	40	10	G, M, K, L, N
Half-distance	1.9	90	21	M, N
Long-distance	3.9	180	42.2	M

The paper-based questionnaire was distributed from the race registration offices on the day before and on the race day, at each event. A written explanation of the study was provided at the same locale. The athletes were informed within the aforesaid explanation that the act of submitting the questionnaire implied their informed consent to participate in the study. The athletes were requested to complete the survey prior to or directly after race registration. All the forms were in the German language. The questionnaires were handed to age-group starters for all the available race distances. For this reason, the dataset obtained is more representative of the average recreational athlete than that collected by previous studies, all of which were exclusive to long-distance athletes [11,12]. For the purposes of anonymity, all the completed forms were collected in a black box and no information about the name, birth date, the distance raced, nor the estimated finish time of the participant was requested. The term "doping" was circumvented in the questionnaire in order to reduce any problems with compliance that this might cause [11]. It was replaced by the German equivalent of "prescription drugs [...] with the goal of increasing (mental or physical) performance. Substances that can only be obtained from a pharmacy or on the black market". This indirect method of questioning was chosen because it typically yields higher prevalence rates for sensitive issues and thus a more valid picture of athletes' behaviour [12].

2.2. Questionnaire

At the beginning of the questionnaire, the athletes were informed both of the purpose of the survey and that participation was anonymous and voluntary. The Randomised Response Technique (RRT) was used to estimate the 12-month prevalence of prohibited substances [18]. The complete RRT question to assess the prevalence of physical doping is shown in Table 2. This assessment period was chosen, instead of life time prevalence, in order to obtain comparable data to those of previous studies. Some information was obtained via closed questions with respect to sex (male/female), A-level (i.e., possession of a German diploma that qualifies the holder for university admission, yes/no), training in a group (yes/no), ingestion of painkillers during training/competition (prophylactic/therapeutic/rest in case of pain/no pain), 12-month prevalence for the use of legal and freely available substances for physical (yes/no), and cognitive (yes/no) enhancement. The next set of questions related to biographical data (e.g., age, height, and weight) and training behaviour such as previous years of training in endurance sports, and number of weekly training hours in swimming/cycling/running. Finally, the athletes were asked which triathlon distances (out of super-sprint, sprint, Olympic-distance, half-distance, and long-distance) they had competed over within the past 12 months. The athletes were also asked to give details of painkiller intake and the underlying rationale for said intake. The athletes' motivation for supplementation was consequently divided into prophylactic vs. therapeutic and training vs. competition related use. In order to question the gateway hypothesis, the question about dietary supplements differentiated between the intake of physical (e.g., bronchodilator) or mental (e.g., concentration-enhancing) substances. The said hypothesis states that the usage of freely available substances may lead to the later abuse of prohibited substances for the purpose of performance enhancement [19].

Table 2. The Randomised Response Technique (RRT) procedure to assess for potential physical doping and cognitive doping.

Physical doping	Please consider a certain birthday (yours, your mother's, etc.). Is this birthday in the first third of a month (first to tenth day)? If yes, please proceed to Question A; if no, please proceed to Question B.
Question A	Is this birthday in the first half of the year (prior to the first of July)?
Question B	Have you taken substances to increase your physical performance within the past 12 months that are only available at a pharmacy, at the doctor's office, or on the black market (e.g., anabolic steroids, erythropoietin, stimulants, growth hormones)? Note that only you know which of the questions you will answer
	Yes　　　　　　　　　　　　　　No
Cognitive doping	Please consider a certain birthday (yours, your mother's, etc.). Is this birthday in the first third of a month (first to tenth day)? If yes, please proceed to Question A; if no, please proceed to Question B.
Question A	Is this birthday in the first half of the year (prior to the first of July)?
Question B	Have you taken substances to increase your mental performance in the past 12 months that are only available at a pharmacy, at the doctor's office, or on the black market (e.g., stimulants, cocaine, methylphenidate, antidepressants, beta-blockers, modafinil)? Note that only you know which of the questions you will answer
	Yes　　　　　　　　　　　　　　No

2.3. Randomised Response Technique (RRT)

RRTs are specifically developed to obtain more valid estimates when sensitive topics are studied, through their guarantee of a maximum amount of anonymity to the respondent [11,18,20]. In the present survey, a paper-and-pencil version of the unrelated question model (UQM) was used to estimate the potential prevalence of physical and cognitive doping ($\hat{\pi}_s$) [21]. The UQM as it was used for the present study has been explicitly described by previous articles [11,12,22]. An explicit example of its calculation is provided by Franke et al. [23]. Similarly to their study, we used a probability for receiving the sensitive question (p) of 245.25/365.25. Afterwards the participants who were randomised to the sensitive group were asked a sensitive question (Questions B, Table 2), whilst the others were asked a neutral question.

The probability for answering the neutral question with "yes" (π_n) was 181.25/365.25. With this model, even the interviewer is unable to know whether the interviewee has answered the sensitive question or not. Furthermore, the RRT can be used to assess separate doping-prevalence values for sub-categories (e.g., females vs. males, users vs. non-users of painkillers), if the number of participants for several groups is high enough. For the purposes of this study the term "potential doping" is used for those athletes who (after completion of the RRT) gave a positive answer to the sensitive question. This definition differs from the WADA definition of doping i.e., "doping is the occurrence of one or more of the anti-doping rule violations set forth in Article 2.1 through Article 2.10 of the Code" [24]. In order to minimise the time that was taken to complete the survey, and thereby maximise compliance, we did not ask the athletes to identify what substance(s) they were taking. Strictly speaking, therefore, our data relate to the potential prevalence, rather than the actual prevalence, of doping in German recreational triathletes. Our methodology, however, allows our results to be directly compared to those of the only previously published triathlete specific studies in this area [11,12].

2.4. Statistics

Descriptive data are presented as mean ± SD values for continuous scaled variables and as numbers and percentages for non-continuous scaled variables. They were obtained using SPSS software, version 22. Prevalence estimates ($\hat{\pi}_s$) for physical and cognitive doping are presented as percentages with 95% confidence intervals (CI) and standard error (SE), as obtained via MATLAB version R2015a. The continuous variables "age" and "years doing endurance sports" were dichotomized by median. The splitting enabled us to calculate separate prevalence estimates, for example for younger/older athletes. Post-hoc power analyses [25] were performed for all RRT calculations, in order to test whether the sample sizes were adequate.

3. Results

A total of 3134 recreational athletes, on the start lists for six different triathlon events, were surveyed. Overall, 1989 (63.5%) questionnaires were received from them (Tables 1 and 3). Of these, 1953 forms (98.2%) were sufficiently completed and evaluated. More than half of all the questionnaires ($n = 1046$; 53.6%) were collected at the Schlosstriathlon Moritzburg (sprint, Olympic, half-distance, and long-distance) event, and about one-fifth ($n = 419$; 21.5%) were obtained at the Leipzig (sprint and Olympic-distance) triathlon. The other races that were surveyed yielded smaller amounts of data: 170 forms at Powertriathlon Gera (8.7%, involving super-sprint, sprint, and Olympic-distance races); 127 forms at Koberbachtalsperre (6.5%, from super-sprint, sprint, and Olympic-distance triathlons); 106 forms at Paradiestriathlon Jena (5.4%, from super-sprint and sprint races); and 84 forms at ICAN Nordhausen (4.3%, for Olympic-distance and half-distance triathlons). Of the study participants, 76.4% ($n = 1491$) were male. The mean athlete age was 39.6 years. Subject and event characteristics are presented in Table 3.

Table 3. The distribution of athletes from the different locations, with biographical data, and training behaviour. Race location: Gera (G), Jena (J), Koberbach (K), Leipzig (L), Moritzburg (M), Nordhausen (N).

Race Athletes	$n = 3134$
Participants (Total)	$n = 1989$
Response Rate	63.5%
Location	
Moritzburg	53.6% ($n = 1046$)
Leipzig	21.5% ($n = 419$)
Gera	8.7% ($n = 170$)
Koberbach	6.5% ($n = 127$)
Jena	5.4% ($n = 106$)
Nordhausen	4.3% ($n = 84$)
Gender	76.4% male ($n = 1477$)
	23.6% female ($n = 456$)
Age in years, (mean; SD)	18–80 (39.6 ± 10.7)
Height cm, (mean; SD)	150–202 (177.9 ± 8.4)
Weight in kg, (mean; SD)	46–130 (78.7 ± 11.6)
BMI kg/m^2, (mean; SD)	Male 14.8–41.3 (24.0 ± 2.4)
	Female 14.7–34.6 (21.9 ± 2.4)
A-Level (German diploma, qualifies the holder for university admission)	69.2% yes ($n = 1351$)
	30.0% no ($n = 586$)
Years of triathlon-specific training, years (mean; SD)	0–50 (11.9 ± 9.7)
Hours swimming/week (mean; SD)	0–12 (1.56 ± 1.23)
Hours bike/week, (mean; SD)	0–20 (4.20 ± 3.00)
Hours running/week (mean; SD)	0–20 (2.79 ± 1.87)
Hours of training in total (mean; SD)	0–39 (8.56 ± 2.14)
distances	
No distance raced	14.8% ($n = 289$)
Super-sprint (race location G, J, K)	4.8% ($n = 94$)
Sprint (race location G, J, K, L, M, N)	51.2% ($n = 999$)
Olympic (race location G, K, L, M, N)	43.7% ($n = 853$)
Half-Distance (race location M, N)	24.1% ($n = 470$)
Long-Distance (race location M)	8.9% ($n = 173$)

3.1. Dietary Supplements and Painkillers

Of the study respondents, 31.8% declared that they had taken dietary supplements, 6.9% reported the use of cognitive enhancers and 9.7% stated that they had used physical enhancers. Intake of substances from both of the latter groups was reported by 14.2% of the athletes who took part in the study.

Painkiller use within the previous three months was reported by 11.3% of participants. We found slight differences between training and competition in the underlying rationale that was given for such intake. The prevalence of within competition painkiller use for therapeutic reasons (3.5%) was similar to that for prophylactic (3.6%) reasons. However, during training sessions more athletes used painkillers to treat their pain (4.7%), than to avoid it (2.0%). Furthermore, we identified that the intake of painkillers was associated with the use of just potential physical doping, or the use of potential physical and cognitive doping substances. More athletes used painkillers when they had raced an Olympic-distance triathlon. Additionally, we found that the use of painkillers is less likely amongst first-time starters. The use of legal and freely available substances by the study participants is summarised in Table 4.

Table 4. Twelve-month prevalence for the use of legal substances and 3-month prevalence for painkillers, divided into therapeutic and prophylactic use.

Physical Enhancement only	9.5% ($n = 186$)	
Cognitive enhancement only	6.8% ($n = 133$)	
Both	14.0% ($n = 274$)	
None	68.3% ($n = 1334$)	
Use of painkillers during the last 3 months	11.1% ($n = 218$)	
	Prophylactic use	Therapeutic use
During training	2.0% ($n = 39$)	4.7% ($n = 92$)
During competition	3.6% ($n = 70$)	3.5% ($n = 69$)

3.2. RRT Results for Physical and Cognitive Doping

The survey, which used the Unrelated Question Model (UQM), demonstrated an overall prevalence of potential physical doping in its respondents over the previous year of 7.0% (CI: 4.2–9.8). The following factors increased an athletes' prevalence for potential physical doping: more than 10 years of experience in doing endurance sports (9.4%), an age older than 39 years (9.8%), participation in an Olympic-distance event (9.3%), training more than 8 h per week (8.0%), and not training in a group (8.6%).

In comparison, the prevalence for potential cognitive doping was higher in those athletes who usually trained in a group (11.2%). Female athletes (13.2%) and athletes who did not race during the 12 months leading up to the study (15.0%) were also more willing to enhance their cognitive performance than were male or experienced athletes. The overall prevalence of potential cognitive doping was found to be 9.4% (CI: 6.6–12.3). There was an association between the intake of painkillers during the last three months and potential physical or cognitive doping. However, no significant correlation was detected between the use of dietary supplements and the use of prohibited substances. All associated influences, as well as the overall intake rate of performance-enhancing drugs, can be found in Tables 5 and 6 and Table S1. The overall hours of weekly training of the athletes was calculated as the summation of the weekly number of hours that they spent swimming, cycling, and running. Detailed statistical analyses are attached as supplementary data to this paper (Table S2).

Table 5. Influence of the longest distance raced on potential doping prevalence. The standard error (SE) is provided. Post-hoc power analyses (Power) were performed to verify the results.

Variable (Longest Distance Raced over Last 12 Months)			Doping Prevalence $\hat{\pi}_s$ in % (Positive Answers after RRT)	SE ($\hat{\pi}_s$)	Power
None	Physical doping	$n = 287$	2.7	0.034	0.22
	Cognitive doping	$n = 298$	15.2	0.038	1
Super-sprint or sprint	Physical doping	$n = 550$	6.9	0.026	0.88
	Cognitive doping	$n = 567$	11.4	0.027	1
Olympic distance	Physical doping	$n = 475$	9.3	0.029	0.96
	Cognitive doping	$n = 494$	9.8	0.028	0.98
Half-distance or long-distance	Physical doping	$n = 491$	7.6	0.028	0.9
	Cognitive doping	$n = 509$	3.5	0.026	0.42

Table 6. Factors associated with potential doping. The continuous scaled variables that are marked '#' were dichotomised by median, and post-hoc power analyses (Power) were performed.

Variable			Doping Prevalence $\hat{\pi}_s$ in % (Positive Answers after RRT)	SE ($\hat{\pi}_s$)	Power
Gender					
female	Physical doping	n = 419	5.6	0.029	0.66
	Cognitive doping	n = 437	13.2	0.031	1
male	Physical doping	n = 1381	7.5	0.016	1
	Cognitive doping	n = 1428	8.3	0.016	1
A-level (German diploma, qualifies the holder for university admission)					
yes	Physical doping	n = 1264	7.4	0.017	1
	Cognitive doping	n = 1306	12.0	0.018	1
no	Physical doping	n = 524	4.7	0.026	0.61
	Cognitive doping	n = 547	2.7	0.025	0.32
Years doing endurance sports #					
≤10 years	Physical doping	n = 963	6.3	0.019	0.96
	Cognitive doping	n = 1000	8.0	0.019	1
>10 years	Physical doping	n = 658	9.4	0.024	1
	Cognitive doping	n = 679	10.4	0.024	1
Training in a group					
yes	Physical doping	n = 907	5.4	0.02	0.89
	Cognitive doping	n = 936	11.2	0.021	1
no	Physical doping	n = 883	8.6	0.021	1
	Cognitive doping	n = 918	8.0	0.02	1
Age #					
≤39 years	Physical doping	n = 933	4.6	0.019	0.8
	Cognitive doping	n = 956	10.0	0.02	1
>39 years	Physical doping	n = 844	8.9	0.022	1
	Cognitive doping	n = 885	8.7	0.021	1
Competition performed within the last 12 months					
yes	Physical doping	n = 1523	7.8	0.016	1
	Cognitive doping	n = 1577	8.6	0.016	1
no	Physical doping	n = 280	2.8	0.034	0.22
	Cognitive doping	n = 284	15.0	0.039	1
Use of legal/freely available substances					
yes	Physical doping	n = 554	7.7	0.026	0.93
	Cognitive doping	n = 574	9.4	0.026	0.98
no	Physical doping	n = 1239	6.7	0.017	1
	Cognitive doping	n = 1284	9.4	0.017	1
Use of analgesics during the last three months					
yes	Physical doping	n = 198	11.8	0.045	0.88
	Cognitive doping	n = 209	13.5	0.056	0.84
no	Physical doping	n = 1605	6.4	0.015	1
	Cognitive doping	n = 1659	9.0	0.015	1
Overall hours of training per week #					
≤8 h	Physical doping	n = 995	8.0	0.02	1
	Cognitive doping	n = 1028	13.4	0.02	1
>8 h	Physical doping	n = 807	5.1	0.021	0.82
	Cognitive doping	n = 839	4.7	0.02	0.78

4. Discussion

Our study found that a significant proportion of recreational triathletes both used painkillers and potentially implemented physical and cognitive doping. Previous studies of long-distance triathletes have shown them to use substances such as anabolic steroid hormones, erythropoietin growth hormones, and amphetamines [11,17]. Such substance abuse is not only associated with triathlon. Numerous studies of professional athletic sports athletes in the late 1990s detected a prevalence of steroid abusers of 20% [9,26–28]. Recreational level athletes in sports such as football, athletics, tennis, handball, or gymnastics have also been reported to use physical doping [13]. Depending on the sport in question, lifetime doping prevalence values varied between 4% and 30% of athletes.

In triathlon, just two surveys in this field have been conducted to date [11,12,16]. Both examined 12-month prevalence as opposed to lifetime prevalence. They reported 10% to 18% of long-distance triathletes to have implemented potential physical doping over the year leading up to their being surveyed [11]. In our athletes, who were racing over more of the more commonly raced triathlon distances, overall potential prevalence, over an equivalent assessment period, was 7.0% for physical doping and 9.4% for cognitive doping. Our values were obtained from a questionnaire that was almost identical to that of Dietz et al. [11]. The only difference from the latter survey was the fact that, as they are legally available in some countries, we removed caffeine (pills) from the list of examples of potential cognitive doping that was provided within it. Instead, we listed caffeine as an example of an "legal and over-the-counter drug […] with the goal of increasing mental performance". This minor difference between the two questionnaires is unlikely to account for the differences in the results that were obtained from them. The lower prevalence of doping in recreational triathletes racing super-sprint as compared to long-distance triathlons that has been reported for long-distance triathletes (i.e., 13% cognitive; 15.1% physical doping) [11,12,16] may be related to the high proportion of athletes who were performing their first triathlon ($n = 289$) in our study.

We identified five key factors to be associated with potential physical or cognitive doping. Firstly, we found that athletes who were more than 39 years of age more often reported the use of physical enhancing drugs than did younger athletes. Dietz et al. did not detect age as a predictor for physical doping in recreational long-distance triathletes [11]. Secondly, we identified that proportionally more females than males used potential cognitive doping. This finding contradicts that of Dietz et al. They reported proportionally more male than female long-distance triathletes to utilise cognitive doping [11]. Thirdly, the athletes in our study who had over 10 years of competitive endurance sports experience more often used physical doping substances than those who had less. This finding agrees with that of Dietz et al. [11]. Fourthly, we found that athletes who spent more than 8 h training per week (with the population dichotomised by median) more often used physical doping than those who trained less than 8 h in total. This relationship between weekly training time and potential susceptibility to doping has not previously been either examined or reported. Lastly, we found that, of the athletes in our sample, the Olympic-distance triathletes presented the highest prevalence of use of prohibited substances for physical doping. This is also a novel finding. Additionally, we observed that novice athletes showed the lowest tendency to enhance their performance through (potential) physical doping, and that athletes who were racing over a longer distance exhibited a higher prevalence of potential physical doping. These were not unexpected findings. Long-distance athletes may be more predisposed to feeling that they require prohibited substances, as a consequence of both greater physiological demand and greater financial costs of competition being placed upon them as compared to short-distance athletes. In contrast, we found that athletes racing shorter distances, or even those who were racing their first triathlon, tended to use potential cognitive doping more often. This could theoretically be explained by novices possessing a higher level of race-associated excitement or anxiety than experienced athletes who are competing over longer distances.

It has been hypothesised that the likelihood of future doping may be increased when an athlete uses nutritional supplements or painkillers [29]. In order to test this so called "gateway hypothesis", we also asked our athletes whether they had used such substances. In total, 593 of our athletes (31.8%) declared the use of legal and freely available supplements to enhance their personal performance. Athletes who used nutritional supplements had a slightly higher prevalence for potential physical doping (7.7%) than athletes who had not used nutritional supplements (6.7%). The prevalence for potential cognitive doping among both populations was also the same (9.4%). However, as we were unable to detect a statistically significant association between nutritional supplementation and potential doping, our results cannot be said to support the gateway hypothesis.

In addition to the use of nutritional supplements, painkiller use is widespread amongst recreational athletes. Most common is the intake of non-steroidal anti-inflammatory drugs (NSAIDs) or other over-the-counter analgesics [3,9]. One study reported more than half of recreational marathon runners to admit to the intake of NSAIDs [2], (presumably or partly) as a means of pain avoidance [2–4,16,30]. A survey of participants in the IRONMAN®-Brazil suggested a similar prevalence value—up to 60%—for long-distance triathletes [4]. European investigations, however, have revealed remarkably lower prevalence values, at about one-third up to one-sixth of this (9.2%–20.4%) [11,16]. The 3-month prevalence for painkillers of our study was 11.2% and comparable to the results of previous European studies. Perhaps different attitudes towards the use of painkillers in general could be responsible for this extreme geographical variation in painkiller intake by triathletes.

Two of the advantages of this study are its relatively large sample size and the fact that we used the RRT to guarantee a higher level of anonymity to its respondents than might otherwise have been the case. Although failure on the part of athletes in a hurry to understand the RRT procedure could have had an impact on some answers, these factors are likely to have had an overall positive impact on the validity of our data. Nonetheless, it is important to note that, in accordance with the previous research in this field [11,12], we did not ask those of our study subjects who responded positively to the sensitive question to enumerate exactly what they were taking. Nor, so as to minimise the administration time and maximise compliance, were our study participants provided with a "self-check list" of the substances that fulfilled the WADA definition of doping at the time of survey administration. Being amateurs, our athletes were unlikely to already be well versed in the contents of the WADA list. Clearly there is a possible "trade-off" between the fact that administration of an optional survey of this type around the (compulsory) procedure of race registration could increase its subject pool, and the fact that athletes who are there may be "time-limited". In accordance with the work of Dietz et al. [11], we took "potential doping" to be synonymous with a positive answer to the sensitive questions of the RRT i.e., whether the athlete had taken "prescription drugs [. . .] with the goal of increasing (mental or physical) performance [. . .] that can only be obtained from a pharmacy or on the black market". We only appended examples of doping substances, as opposed to the full WADA list, to these sensitive questions. It is a potential limitation of our study that the fact that our prevalence values were obtained through the use of a simpler definition of doping [1] than that of WADA means that our data cannot be directly compared to any future data that are obtained in strict accordance with the WADA definition of doping.

That notwithstanding, our key findings that recreational triathletes racing over the most common triathlon distances use "prescription drugs [. . .] that can only be obtained from a pharmacy or on the black market with the goal of increasing (mental or physical) performance" as well as pain killers to improve their performance are important. This is despite the fact that (1) doping and medical abuse are not necessarily the same thing, (2) the use of prescribed drugs as ergogenic aids is not necessarily medical abuse, and (3) the use of prescribed drugs to enhance (sporting) performance does not necessarily constitute doping. Previous research has shown that intake of any of such substances comes with the possibility of life-threatening side effects. Our work demonstrates a need to improve awareness of the risks and to reduce the intake of such substances in recreational triathletes, through the implementation of targeted education prevention and programmes.

Supplementary Materials: The following are available online at http://www.mdpi.com/2075-4663/7/12/241/s1, Table S1: Influence of the longest distance raced on doping prevalence, Table S2: Factors associated with physical and cognitive doping.

Author Contributions: Conceptualisation, S.S., P.D. and S.Z.; methodology, S.S., P.D. and S.Z.; formal analysis, P.D.; investigation, S.S.; data curation, S.S.; writing—original draft preparation, S.S. and P.D.; writing—review and editing, P.D., A.C.D., M.E. and S.Z.; project administration, S.Z.

Funding: Open Access Funding by the Publication Fund of the TU Dresden.

Acknowledgments: This research was supported by the President of the Thüringer Triathlon Verband Jürgen Rockstroh, who provided orientation with regard to the selection of the right locations. We also thank the organisers of the triathlon competitions of Gera, Jena, Koberbachtalsperre, Nordhausen, Leipzig, and Moritzburg for their support. We would also like to show our gratitude to Jette Fietzek, Falk Haase, Estelle Heyne, David Hoffmann, Steffen Jabin, Maria Lehmann, Theodor Popp, Martin Serfling, and Madlen Schiewek for their assistance during the survey. Special thanks are given Susanne Zeeb for comments that greatly improved the manuscript. Further, we thank Anita Marquart and Thomas Dörfer for their help with the translation. We are grateful to Geoffrey Lee for rewriting the manuscript to optimise the English language. Finally, our special gratitude goes to Veronica Vleck for her invaluable help during rewriting and optimizing the manuscript.

Conflicts of Interest: The authors declare no conflict of interest.

References

1. World Anti-Doping Agency. Prohibited List 2018. 2017. Available online: https://www.wada-ama.org/en/media/news/2015-09/wada-publishes-2016-prohibited-list (accessed on 11 November 2019).
2. Almond, C.S.; Shin, A.Y.; Fortescue, E.B.; Mannix, R.C.; Wypij, D.; Binstadt, B.A.; Duncan, C.N.; Olson, D.P.; Salerno, A.E.; Newburger, J.W.; et al. Hyponatremia among runners in the Boston Marathon. *N. Engl. J. Med.* **2005**, *352*, 1550–1556. [CrossRef] [PubMed]
3. Kuster, M.; Renner, B.; Oppel, P.; Niederweis, U.; Brune, K. Consumption of analgesics before a marathon and the incidence of cardiovascular, gastrointestinal and renal problems: A cohort study. *BMJ Open* **2013**, *3*. [CrossRef] [PubMed]
4. Gorski, T.; Cadore, E.L.; Pinto, S.S.; da Silva, E.M.; Correa, C.S.; Beltrami, F.G.; Kruel, L.F. Use of NSAIDs in triathletes: Prevalence, level of awareness and reasons for use. *Br. J. Sports Med.* **2011**, *45*, 85–90. [CrossRef] [PubMed]
5. de Hon, O.; Kuipers, H.; van Bottenburg, M. Prevalence of Doping Use in Elite Sports: A Review of Numbers and Methods. *Sports Med.* **2015**, *45*, 57–69. [CrossRef] [PubMed]
6. McLaren, R.H. WADA Investigation of Sochi Allegations 2016. Available online: https://www.wada-ama.org/sites/default/files/resources/files/mclaren_report_part_ii_2.pdf (accessed on 16 July 2016).
7. Ulrich, R.; Pope, H.G., Jr.; Cleret, L.; Petroczi, A.; Nepusz, T.; Schaffer, J.; Kanayama, G.; Comstock, R.D.; Simon, P. Doping in Two Elite Athletics Competitions Assessed by Randomized-Response Surveys. *Sports Med.* **2018**, *48*, 211–219. [CrossRef]
8. Braun, H.; Koehler, K.; Geyer, H.; Kleiner, J.; Mester, J.; Schanzer, W. Dietary supplement use among elite young German athletes. *Int. J. Sport Nutr. Exerc. Metab.* **2009**, *19*, 97–109. [CrossRef]
9. Kläber, M. Fitness-Studios und ihre Dopingavantgarde Die Zeitschrift für Sport, Recht und Medizin. *Doping* **2011**, *2*, 164–170.
10. Wanjek, B.; Rosendahl, J.; Strauss, B.; Gabriel, H.H. Doping, drugs and drug abuse among adolescents in the State of Thuringia (Germany): Prevalence, knowledge and attitudes. *Int. J. Sports Med.* **2007**, *28*, 346–353. [CrossRef]
11. Dietz, P.; Ulrich, R.; Dalaker, R.; Striegel, H.; Franke, A.G.; Lieb, K.; Simon, P. Associations between physical and cognitive doping–a cross-sectional study in 2997 triathletes. *PLoS ONE* **2013**, *8*, e78702. [CrossRef]
12. Schroter, H.; Studzinski, B.; Dietz, P.; Ulrich, R.; Striegel, H.; Simon, P. A Comparison of the Cheater Detection and the Unrelated Question Models: A Randomized Response Survey on Physical and Cognitive Doping in Recreational Triathletes. *PLoS ONE* **2016**, *11*. [CrossRef]
13. Frenger, M.; Pitsch, W.; Emrich, E. Sport-Induced Substance Use-An. Empirical Study to the Extent within a German Sports Association. *PLoS ONE* **2016**, *11*. [CrossRef]
14. ITU. *ITU Competition Rules 2017*; ITU: Lausanne, Switzerland, 2016.
15. Zwingenberger, S.; Valladares, R.D.; Walther, A.; Beck, H.; Stiehler, M.; Kirschner, S.; Engelhardt, M.; Kasten, P. An epidemiological investigation of training and injury patterns in triathletes. *J. Sports Sci.* **2014**, *32*, 583–590. [CrossRef] [PubMed]
16. Dietz, P.; Dalaker, R.; Letzel, S.; Ulrich, R.; Simon, P. Analgesics use in competitive triathletes: Its relationship to doping and on predicting its usage. *J. Sports Sci.* **2016**, *34*, 1965–1969. [CrossRef] [PubMed]
17. Striegel, H.; Ulrich, R.; Simon, P. Randomized response estimates for doping and illicit drug use in elite athletes. *Drug Alcohol Depend.* **2010**, *106*, 230–232. [CrossRef] [PubMed]

18. Lensvelt-Mulders, G.J.L.M.; Hox, J.J.; van der Heijden, P.G.M.; Maas, C.J.M. Meta-Analysis of Randomized Response Research:Thirty-Five Years of Validation. *Sociol. Methods Res.* **2005**, *33*, 319–348. [CrossRef]
19. Kandel, D.; Kandel, E. The Gateway Hypothesis of substance abuse: Developmental, biological and societal perspectives. *Acta Paediatr.* **2015**, *104*, 130–137. [CrossRef]
20. Lensvelt-Mulders, G.J.L.M.; Hox, J.J.; van der Heijden, P.G.M. How to Improve the Efficiency of Randomised Response Designs. *Qual. Quant.* **2005**, *39*, 253–265. [CrossRef]
21. Greenberg, B.G.; Abul-Ela, A.-L.A.; Simmons, W.R.; Horvitz, D.G. The Unrelated Question Randomized Response Model.: Theoretical Framework. *J. Am. Stat. Assoc.* **1969**, *64*, 520–539. [CrossRef]
22. Dietz, P.; Striegel, H.; Franke, A.G.; Lieb, K.; Simon, P.; Ulrich, R. Randomized response estimates for the 12-month prevalence of cognitive-enhancing drug use in university students. *Pharmacotherapy* **2013**, *33*, 44–50. [CrossRef]
23. Franke, A.G.; Bagusat, C.; Dietz, P.; Hoffmann, I.; Simon, P.; Ulrich, R.; Lieb, K. Use of illicit and prescription drugs for cognitive or mood enhancement among surgeons. *BMC Med.* **2013**, *11*, 102. [CrossRef]
24. WADA. *WORLD ANTI-DOPING CODE 2015 - with Amendments 2019*; WADA: Montreal, QC, Canada, 2019; p. 156.
25. Ulrich, R.; Schroter, H.; Striegel, H.; Simon, P. Asking sensitive questions: A statistical power analysis of randomized response models. *Psychol. Methods* **2012**, *17*, 623–641. [CrossRef] [PubMed]
26. Striegel, H.; Simon, P.; Wurster, C.; Niess, A.M.; Ulrich, R. The use of nutritional supplements among master athletes. *Int. J. Sports Med.* **2006**, *27*, 236–241. [CrossRef] [PubMed]
27. Kujath, P.; Boss, C.; Wulff, P.; Bruch, H.-P. Medikamentenmißbrauch beim Freizeitsportler im Fitneßbereich, in Deutsches Ärzteblatt. *Dtsch. Arzteb.* **1998**, *95*, 953–957.
28. Löllgen, H. Doping und Medikamentenmißbrauch im Sport, in Deutsches Ärzteblatt. *Dtsch. Arzteb.* **1998**, *95*, 950–952.
29. Backhouse, S.H.; Whitaker, L.; Petroczi, A. Gateway to doping? Supplement use in the context of preferred competitive situations, doping attitude, beliefs, and norms. *Scand. J. Med. Sci. Sports* **2013**, *23*, 244–252. [PubMed]
30. Corrigan, B.; Kazlauskas, R. Medication use in athletes selected for doping control at the Sydney Olympics (2000). *Clin. J. Sport Med.* **2003**, *13*, 33–40. [CrossRef] [PubMed]

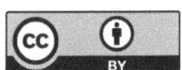

© 2019 by the authors. Licensee MDPI, Basel, Switzerland. This article is an open access article distributed under the terms and conditions of the Creative Commons Attribution (CC BY) license (http://creativecommons.org/licenses/by/4.0/).

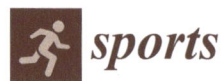

Article

Motivation Regulation among Black Women Triathletes

Candace S. Brown [1,2]

[1] Department of Public Health Sciences, University of North Carolina, Charlotte, NC 28223, USA; cbrow342@uncc.edu or candace.brown@duke.edu

[2] Motivated Cognition and Aging Brain Lab, Center for Cognitive Neuroscience, Duke University, Box 90999 Durham, NC 27708, USA

Received: 20 July 2019; Accepted: 5 September 2019; Published: 10 September 2019

Abstract: There is a paucity of information on motivation among U.S. minority triathletes. This study aimed to understand the extrinsic motivation and regulators of Black women triathletes using a modified version of the valid Motivations of Marathoners Scale and semi-structured interviews, for triathletes. The Self Determination Theory guided the dual method assessment of the extrinsic motivators and the regulators external, introjection, and integrated. Using MANOVA, data from (N = 121) triathletes were compared across participant categories of age, body mass index, and distance. Results showed a significant age difference with younger women displaying more motivation. Descriptive means indicated integration as the greatest regulator of motivation. The statements 'to compete with myself' and 'to be more fit,' had the highest means among the women. A sub-sample of 12 interviews were conducted revealing 16 extrinsic themes. Six were related to the regulator integration and two unexpectedly related to the regulator, identified. Integrated themes, including coping mechanisms, finishing course, improvement, accomplishment, and physical awareness were most represented. This research fills gaps of understanding extrinsic motivation and the regulators of a group not previously explored. Future research on motivation among triathletes may benefit knowing how motivations are regulated, as to promote personalized training and participation.

Keywords: motivation; triathletes; regulation; Black women

1. Introduction

Motivation is simply defined as the, "direction and intensity of one's effort," [1] (p. 51) and is self-initiated for direction and sustainability leading toward a goal. Preparation for sport participation is intentional. Therefore, the behavioral construct of motivation is principal to understanding why people choose to participate in sport [2].

Motivation to participate in sport and understanding cultural constructs have drawn from an array of theoretical perspectives from many disciplines. The Self Determination Theory (SDT) is a macro theory of human motivation that addresses issues such as self-regulation, psychological needs, life goals and aspirations, energy and vitality, and a host of other issues related to well-being and life domains [3]. It specifically determines how behavior describes both personal choice and outside influence, therefore, allowing for an examination of the differential effects of motivation that underlie the behavior of sport participation [3,4]. However, behavior is not always intrinsically motivated and certain external pressures (e.g., social) may motivate individuals to participate in sport even though it does not interest them.

A sub-theory of the SDT, the Organismic Integration Theory (OIT), explains the external contextual processes that serve as barriers or facilitators in behavior regulation [5]. A central assumption of the OIT is that extrinsic motivation can be measured by regulators of a continuum that range from external regulation to integrated regulation [5]. This continuum of motivational regulators stimulate behavior as athletes interact with their sport environment. The four associated regulators are described through associated processes of rewards or punishments (external), due to self-control (introjected), of personal importance (identified), and having self-awareness (integrated) [3].

Research on motivation and sport reports differences in motivation based on sport level; whereas, intercollegiate and elite athletes report higher levels of motivation compared to intramural athletes and non-elite athletes [6]. Specifically, understanding motivation in the sport of triathlon provides researchers access to an extreme sport where exercise regimens can be in excess of 20 h per week as it requires practice in the three separate sports of swimming, cycling, and running [7]. Studies on triathletes reporting differences by sex report women to have a higher fitness motivation, lower mean external regulation than men [2,8]. Motivation for initially pursuing the sport and remaining in the sport has been documented. Social reasons for participating have included a 'sense of belonging' [9] and physical health motivation has been related to increasing or maintaining fitness [10]. Additionally, researchers have also long considered psychological health of participation in triathlons with the literature demonstrating an increase of self-esteem, self-efficacy, and the suggested transformative effect participation has on body image [9].

Most studies on motivation among triathletes have been conducted primarily with White men and women, demonstrating a paucity in research on participants of minority status in the United States. Indeed, the number of Black people who participate in the sport is significantly lower than that of their White counterparts. Data from the 2016 survey conducted by USA Triathlon (USAT) indicated only 1% of members were Black triathletes [11]. In the same year, the Centers for Disease Control and Prevention estimated that only 44.4% of U.S. Black adults met the 2008 U.S. physical activity guidelines which were to engage in at least 150 min of weekly moderate intensity aerobic activity and to complete muscle strengthening activities that work all major muscle groups at least twice weekly [12]. Black women are a most sedentary group in the United States exercise, thus contributing to the high number of those diagnosed with death-causing conditions such as coronary heart disease and cancer [13,14].

However, Black women who participate in triathlons represent a group of successful exercisers with limited exposure in research. The only known study on Black women to participate in a minority-based triathlon program ($N = 25$) reported that the top motivational reason for participation was to improve their health and fitness (84%). Furthermore, while many of the participants (48%) reported they were motivated by the group to prepare for a triathlon, receiving encouragement from friends was one of the lowest responses for motivation, at 28 percent [15]. Therefore, the purpose of this study was to explore the extrinsic motivation and regulators of Black women who participate in triathlons to further develop an understanding of motivation among triathletes.

A measure used to understand varying motivation and underlying themes for participating in sporting events and activities is the Motivations for Marathoners Scale (MOMS). Developed by Masters, Ogles, and Jolton [16], the MOMS uses four motivational categories: physical health, social, achievement and psychological to assess motivation. Within these four categorical measures (Physical Health, Achievement, Psychological and Social) of the MOMS, there are nine scales (i.e., General Health Orientation, Weight Control, Affiliation, Recognition, Competition, Personal Goal Achievement, Psychological Coping, Self-Esteem, and Life Meaning). The MOMS has been used in several studies related to athletes who participate in sport disciplines related to triathlon. Male cyclists were more motivated by Competition, and female cyclists the scale Weight Concern, as reasons for cycling [17]. Participants of cause-related (to support charity) Aquabike (i.e., swim and cycle) and cycling only events were significantly more motivated by Personal Goal Achievement ($p < 0.001$) and Competition ($p < 0.001$) compared to those who participated in non-cause-related events [18]. Triathletes registered with Triathlon Australia indicated life meaning to be the only significant variable between the elite and non-elite triathletes, (F = 4.395, $p < 0.05$), whereas elite participants felt they had more life purpose for competing in triathlons [19]. Lovett utilized a modified version of the MOMS by adding words synonymous to represent the exercises completed by triathletes (e.g., swim, bike, and run) reporting that women have greater personal goal achievement and self-esteem scores than males [20].

While these studies yielded demographic differences in the motivation among majority triathletes, what remained unclear is whether there were similar motivations among triathletes that identify as Black. The MOMS only identifies how much motivation is determined by the scales. For example, enjoyment of participating in sports has been interpreted as intrinsic motivation and competition as an extrinsic motivation, interpreted [21,22]. This study purposed to explore the motivations of Black women triathletes and to identify the regulators associated with extrinsic motivations.

A proposed link between the SDT motivations, OIT regulators and a modified version of the MOMS, intended for use with triathletes and renamed the Motivations of Marathoners Scale for Triathletes (MOMS-T). The MOMS-T was constructed to explore the motivations and regulators of Black women (BW) triathletes. Not previously done with the MOMS, the working hypothesis of this study was formed from the scale descriptions of the MOMS and from the review of qualitative descriptions of extrinsic motivation from Lamont and Kennelly [10]. The exploratory SDT/OIT/MOMS-T model would provide an understanding of how the women perceived their regulation based on their narratives. The following questions drove the analysis of the interviews:

(1) Do narratives of Black women triathletes support the placement of the MOMS-T scales weight control and competition as external regulated?
(2) Do narratives of Black women triathletes support the placement of the MOMS-T scales recognition and self-esteem as introjection regulated?
(3) Do narratives of Black women triathletes support the placement of the MOMS-T scales health orientation, personal goals, and psychological coping as integration?

It was hypothesized that external regulation would be the measured sum of the scales weight control and competition. The sum of scales recognition and self-esteem was introjection. Integration regulation was measured as a sum of scales health orientation, personal goals, and psychological coping.

The objective of this exploratory study was to understand the regulations of the extrinsic motivations, among BW triathletes. This information may inform future research using the MOMS-T and the development of programming for women interested in increasing their physical activity, and possibly completing a triathlon.

2. Materials and Methods

A dual method of collecting both quantitative and qualitative data guided this study [2]. The quantitative goals of the study were to use the previously validated Motivations of Marathoners Scale for Triathletes (MOMS-T) to assess extrinsic motivation for triathlon participation among BW triathletes and identify whether rates of extrinsic regulators varied by age, body mass index (BMI), and triathlon distance. The quantitative approach was non-experimental with a correlational design that was used to administer a web-based survey. The primary qualitative goal was to gain a better descriptive understanding of the relationship between extrinsic motivation and the regulators. The qualitative approach was completed through semi-structured interviews with a subset of the BW triathletes who had recently completed the web-based survey. Intrinsic motivation and their regulators are not reported here because they are less likely to explain how controlled factors effect motivation. The results reported here are based on combined data of the extrinsic motivations of the sample.

2.1. Procedures

Following approval from the Virginia Commonwealth University (VCU) Institutional Review Board, BW triathletes were recruited for participation in the study. Inclusion criteria for participation included self-identifying as a Black woman, age $\geq$ 36 years, U.S. resident, and either completion of an individual triathlon between the years 2012 and 2014 or preparing for an individual triathlon in 2015. Potential participants were directed to a web link by VCU's secure web-based system (RedCap) that included informed consent forms, a demographic questionnaire, and the MOMS-T survey. Following consent and completion of all forms related to the quantitative phase of the study, the women were invited to participate in a semi-structured interview to further explore their motivations that were identified in the survey. Interviewed participants signed a separate consent form and agreed to the use of pseudonyms for confidentiality. Audio recording and field notes were used to keep an accurate account of the conversation between the interviewer and participants. In addition, field notes assisted in recording of follow-up questions, included descriptions of non-verbal communication, and reflected notes on the participants' experiences. The study survey and interviews were conducted for 12 weeks, from February to May 2015.

2.2. Population and Sampling

Multiple sampling strategies were used for this study. Snowball sampling was used to identify Black triathlete women for study participation. Early sampled participants ($N = 320$) were sent emails from the national triathlon organization, USA Triathlon (USAT). In addition, multiple triathlete social networks, including The Black Triathletes Association, Sisters Tri-ing, the International Association of Black Triathletes, Sole Tri-Sisters, and Realizing Your Potential Everyday, posted the study information on their Facebook© pages. Early participants were asked to identify other triathletes who met eligibility criteria to participate in the study. Many of the participants did this by 'tagging' other women on the Facebook© social media pages where the original study information had been posted.

Purposive stratified sampling was used to select interviewees. Selection was based on age, estimated BMI, and distance of most completed triathlons. Those who completed the survey first, and agreed to do the interview, were first considered for the interview. Projected quotas allowed for qualitative comparisons among 12 participants with nine varying attributes. Quotas were set to represent an equal number of participants from each stratification variable. To achieve further sample representativeness, participants were from different USAT regions and states. Those who completed the surveys first, were willing to be interviewed, and met the necessary criterion of the remaining projected quotas were contacted first for interviews. Potential interviewees were first emailed and follow-up conversations through either email or telephone followed to set up the interview.

2.3. Instruments in the Study

Three instruments were used for this study to quantitatively and qualitatively assess the triathletes. The descriptive demographic and triathlon participation information was assessed via the Motivation of Triathlon Participation Questionnaire. The MOMS-T characterized motivation for participation in triathlons and the Motivations of Marathoners Scale for Triathletes Interview Guide (MOTIG) inquired additional information related to the motivations in the MOMS-T [13].

The Motivations of Triathlon Participation Questionnaire comprised 16 items (open and closed) related to the demographics (e.g., educational status, relationship status), triathlon participation, and current training regimen. Age was separated into two categories with ages 36–49 representing middle age and those 50+ and older representing the older age group. Four BMI categories, including underweight, normal weight, overweight, and obese, were calculated from participant self-reports of weight and height [23]. The distances and number of triathlons completed were self-reported as either Sprint, Olympic, Half-Ironman, or Ironman [24].

The MOMS-T is a revised form of the valid and reliable Motivations of Marathoners Scale in which four of the 56 statements included the exercises 'cycling and swimming' to replace 'running' and the word 'triathlete(s)' replaced 'runner(s)' to assesses motivation to participate in triathlons [13,16]. A similar form for triathletes, previously validated, involves a 7-point Likert scale to assess the importance of participation, where the number 1 indicates that the statement is "not a reason" and the number 7 indicates the statement is a "very important" reason for participation [20]. The score on each MOMS-T scale is the mean of the survey items that compose that scale.

The previously published Motivations of Triathletes Interview Guide (MOTIG) is an exploratory instrument developed specifically to complement the questions in the MOMS-T survey [13]. Its purpose was to encourage an in-depth dialogue that would reveal the thoughts, attitudes, and opinions about motivation to participate in triathlons through a newly developed method of 'Survey Transformation'. In addition, the MOTIG inquired further to identify specific regulators of the extrinsic scales of the MOMS-T. The MOTIG facilitated discussion with participants by asking them to retrospectively consider personal perceptions from their recently completed MOMS-T survey. Corresponding statements from the MOMS-T were rewritten with an introductory clause related to the MOMS-T scale and followed by an item from the scale. For example, to transform the MOMS-T Psychological Coping scale, interviewees were prompted with the statement, "My motivation is connected to my coping ability so I am able ... ", and an item from the MOMS-T scale followed, 'To concentrate on my thoughts.' Two to three follow-up prompts to facilitate discussion were also used for each of the 27 open-ended MOTIG items. The semi-structured format allowed for flexibility and exploration of new concepts and themes.

2.4. Converging the SDT, OIT, and MOMS-T

Before the analysis, the conversion of SDT motivations, OIT regulators, and data from Lamont and Kennelly was used to propose which MOMS-T scales for participating in triathlons were extrinsic [10,21]. Key words describing the extrinsic motivation of this study were matched with the scales within the MOMS-T. Table 1 illustrates the process that led the creation of the extrinsic MOMS-T scales to the OIT-associated regulators. External regulation, considered to be the least self-determined form of motivation, would regulate the MOMS-T scales weight control and competition. Triathletes who engaged in the sport to avoid negative feelings or reprimand from others, were *introjection* regulated through the scales self-esteem, and recognition. Those with integrated regulation chose to participate in triathlons because they had fully developed their value systems. Those values were attached with personal goal achievement, health orientation, and psychological coping. The only regulator that was not included to have a link with the MOMS-T was *identified*. This regulator is theorized to represent participation in a sport, even if the activity is unattractive [25]. It was believed that the women who participated in a triathlon would disregard any notion of the activity being 'unattractive,' participate if it meant their personal goals would be met and would, therefore, already identify as a triathlete.

Table 1. Converging the Motivations of Marathoners Scale for Triathletes (MOMS-T) scales and Organismic Integration Theory (OIT) regulators.

MOMS-T Scale	MOMS-T Descriptions	SDT Keywords	OIT Regulator
General Health Orientation	Improve health, prolong life, stay physically active	Synthesis of goals	Integration
Weight Concern	Look leaner, control weight, reduce weight	External reward	External
Recognition	Earn respect, feel pride from others, earn recognition	Ego Involvement	Introjection
Competition	Compete with others, be faster than friends, placement achievement	External Rewards	External
Personal Goal Achievement	Improve speed, push myself, improve overall time	Synthesis	Integration
Psychological Coping	Be less anxious, distraction from worries, improve mood	Congruence	Integration
Self-Esteem	Improve self-esteem, improve confidence, sense of achievement	Self-esteem	Introjection

2.5. Statistical Analysis

The quantitative analytic plan was to use IBM SPSS Statistics (version 22) to assess participants' extrinsic motivation for participating in triathlons and to identify differences of the seven scales and three regulators. Mean values of the 7-point Likert-format scale were calculated from the extrinsic MOMS-T statements (General Health Orientation, Weight Control, Recognition, Competition, Personal Goal Achievement, Psychological Coping, and Self-Esteem). Next, a new dependent variable termed "extrinsic motivation" was calculated by aggregating each individual's mean scores across her/his responses to MOMS-T items on the extrinsic scales. MANOVA analysis would show the correlation between the dependent regulators (weight control and competition = external; recognition and self-esteem = introjection; health orientation, personal goals, and psychological coping = integration regulation) and variables age, BMI and distance.

The qualitative analysis descriptive comparisons of the most motivating and least motivating MOMS-T items for this study population were assessed. To accomplish this, thematic analysis of qualitative data was conducted to further explore the relationship between motivation and regulators identified in the MOMS-T survey by participants. The researcher based the interview questions in the questionnaire on the quantitative MOMS-T survey and developed three additional questions to understand how the women started in the sport and their plans for continuation of the sport. All participants chose pseudonyms to protect their identities. The audio recording was transcribed verbatim and the field notes were used as supplemental data. All collected data were entered into the qualitative data analysis program, Atlas ti.7 and quotations representing categories of extrinsic motivation, identified by phrases, sentences, or paragraphs, were assigned a label. The labels were then categorized and regrouped according to their similarities. Categories reflecting more than 70% of the interviews were identified as adequately saturated [26]. These categories were then collapsed into common definitions to help identify themes to explain the participants' motivational views. Member checking and peer review of the codes and themes were conducted to promote trustworthiness of the data.

3. Results

3.1. Quantitative Results

A total of 140 people responded to the survey with 121 meeting the inclusion criteria. Nineteen were excluded: (a) three for criteria exclusion (one under criterion age and two men); (b) nine for duplicate submission, and seven for incompletion). Two of the incomplete survey participants were contacted and encouraged to complete their surveys as they had, at least, completed the demographic portion of the survey. Table 2 displays the survey participant characteristics. Among 118 participants who provided their age, most were younger (76.9%). BMI calculations from self-reported height and weight data, indicated most of the triathletes were either normal or overweight (61.2%). The data from the one participant who was calculated to be underweight were collapsed into the normal weight category. More than 90% of participants had completed a triathlon in the past 3 years, and the 8.3% of participants who had not yet completed a triathlon expected to complete a triathlon by the end of 2015. The Sprint distance triathlon category was the most completed triathlon distance among participants (48.8%).

Table 2. Study participant characteristics.

Variable	Values	Mean	Number	Percentage
Age (years)	36–49	-	93	76.9%
	50+	45.6	25	20.7%
	Missing	-	3	2.5%
BMI	Normal	-	37	30.6%
	Overweight	-	37	30.6%
	Obese	-	31	25.6%
	Missing	-	16	13.2%
Distance completed	Not completed	-	10	8.3%
	Sprint	-	59	48.8%
	Olympic	-	15	12.4%
	Half-ironman	-	17	14.0%
	Ironman	-	17	14.0%
	Missing	-	3	2.5%

The descriptive statistics of the seven scales which included 43 (of the 56) survey items show the possible minimum and maximum numbers indicate that health orientation, personal goal achievement, and recognition had large ranges. Psychological coping and self-esteem, with higher min and max scores, also had large ranges. When compared to the other scales, weight control and competition had low ranges; both scales only had four values. While the range of these scales varied widely, participants were more closely aligned with health orientation, personal goal achievement, and recognition. The statistics are presented in Appendix A.

Means and standard deviations were calculated for the motivational statements and presented in Table 3. The highest rated extrinsic motivational statements were 'compete [with] self' (M = 6.1, SD = 1.1) within Personal Goal Achievement and '[to be] more fit,' within Health Orientation (M = 6.1, SD = 1.2). The lowest rated extrinsic motivational statements were 'beat new person' was (M = 2.0, SD = 1.5) for the scale Competition and 'compliments from others' (M = 2.2, SD = 1.5) for Recognition.

Table 3. Extrinsic Motivational Statements.

Scale	Highest Motivational Item	N	Mean	SD	Lowest Motivational Item	N	Mean	SD
Health Orientation	more_fit	119	6.059	1.188	reduce_heartattack	120	4.500	2.268
Weight Control	leaner_look	119	4.773	1.955	reduce_weight	119	4.176	2.154
Personal Goal Achievement	compete_self	119	6.160	1.112	beat_time	119	3.933	2.170
Competition	compete_others	120	3.242	1.932	beat_new_person	117	2.034	1.531
Recognition	famfriends_proud	118	2.754	1.719	compliments_othe	120	2.167	1.525
Psychological Coping	improve_mood	119	3.807	2.001	less_depressed	119	2.798	2.048
Self-Esteem	meaning_life	120	3.708	2.047	feel_whole	118	2.737	1.874

The descriptive statistics of the extrinsic regulation variables (aggregated by responses to the extrinsic scales) and categories of age, BMI, and distance indicated integration regulation was the highest, and external regulation was the lowest, in all categories. Older participants (50+) reported more integration regulation than the younger participants did, those with normal BMI strata reported less integration regulation compared to the participants who were obese (which was only slightly more than those who were overweight), and the triathletes who participated in Ironman distances displayed more integration regulation than that of the triathletes preferring the three shorter triathlon distances. The table is presented in Appendix B.

Results of MANOVA indicated a significant difference between the two age categories (Wilks' Λ = 0.068, $p > 0.05$). The mean for the younger women (36–49 years old) was higher than for the older women (50+ years old). Next, two-way MANOVA analysis indicated the dependent regulator variables External, Introjection, Integration and Intrinsic, (which is not reported here) were only correlated with age and distance (Wilks' Λ = 0.01, $p > 0.05$). The age and distance model of predicted means with confidence intervals, ndicated that the integration, was the regulator of motivation for this population.

3.2. Qualitative Results

Interview results are based on a purposive sample ($N = 12$) of participants' perceptions and interpretations as triathletes and as Black women. Eligibility for an interview was contingent on completing the demographics and MOMS-T survey. Of the 121 survey participants, 118 (97%) were eligible. Eleven face-to-face interviews were conducted in the U.S. states of North Carolina, Virginia, Georgia, Illinois, Michigan, Colorado and Massachusetts. These states represented the Mideast, Southeast, North Central, and Northeast USA Triathlon regions. One telephone interview was conducted with a participant from California, of the West region. Presented in Appendix C are the characteristics of the interview participants (using pseudonyms), including six participants in each age group (36–49; 50+), four Sprint, two Olympic, three Half-Ironman, and three Ironman finishers; and four of the participants had a normal BMI, five were overweight, and three were obese.

There were 508 quotations related to extrinsic motivation. These quotations were coded and were separated among the original seven extrinsic scales. As set in the proposal, the researcher identified categories that were adequately saturated, reflecting more that 70% quotations. The scales within the MOMS are not as easily defined into a regulated style simply based on the scale itself. Rather, the themes within the styles are what mitigate whether a scale is external, introjection, integration, or identification.

There were 16 total themes gleaned from the qualitative data. Eleven themes, including weight maintenance, physical attraction, competition, medals, confidence, fear, competition, coping mechanism, finishing course, improvement, accomplishment, and physical awareness were directly related to the extrinsic MOMS-T scales and regulators. The theme—depression—is also included as the saturation was close at 69%. Transition and inspiration were themes related to the not-previously included regulator, identification, and to the new proposed MOMS-T scale, Triathlete Lifestyle. Two themes, encouragement and family, are not presented in this manuscript because of their dual relationship with the intrinsic scale, Affiliation. Figure 1 represents the total of seven scales, four extrinsic regulators, and 14 themes from the qualitative data. This section presents an analysis of the interviews and is based on the generalization of what the researcher understood about participants' personal values and beliefs. The researcher examined whether the participant's views about the MOMS-T motivations were supported by the intended regulators.

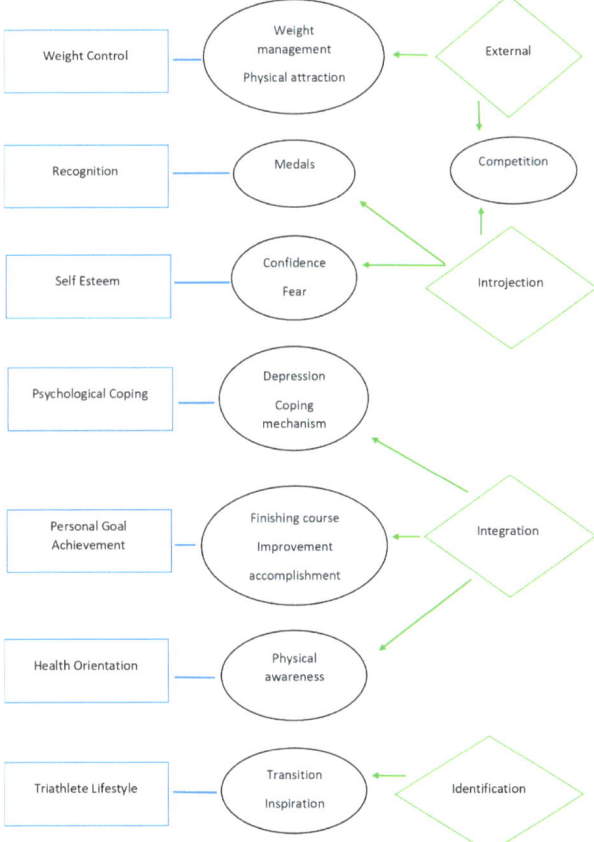

Figure 1. The relationship between the MOMS-T Scales, themes, and their OIT Regulators. On the **left** (blue rectangles) are the MOMS-T scales. In the **middle** (black circles), are the themes derived from the qualitative interviews. To the **right** (green diamonds), are the OIT extrinsic regulators.

External regulated. The SDT scales, weight control and competition, were initially thought to be external regulated. Signified by the themes, weight maintenance and physical attractiveness, women were either ordered by physicians or encouraged themselves to lose weight due to medical issues. The desired effect of weight loss was to have a more defined 'lean' look of one who is athletic. Being lean was perceived to be more physically attractive and was evaluated based on mirror appearance or achieving the status of a 'triathlete' (one who completed a triathlon).

Rado explained that being physically attractive is "[being] as fit as you're genetically able to be." Competition, however, presented factors of being external and integration regulated. This depended on the context of the competition. The external regulation of competition occurred when a triathlete made the conscious choice to rival against teammates or other triathletes in a race. The women who had strategies for overcoming another triathlete enjoyed and often giggled at their thoughts of how they would view the other triathletes during a race. For Brooklyn Diva, it was a production where she was the hero going after the villain, entitled 'Superhero'. "I go into a different mindset like I'm in a movie. I'm following this person. I gotta keep up and I'm just thinking the entire time, 'You gotta catch them,' and I just play a movie in my head." Competition also contained an element of integration of setting a goal and essentially creating a personal and internal competition. Nita believed that, "The only person that I'm competitive against, is myself."

Introjection regulated. The researcher postulated the SDT scales recognition and self-esteem to be regulated through introjection. Most participants stated they were not concerned about what others thought of their participation in triathlons and did not participate for approval. All but one participant said recognition did not directly motivate them; yet, they all appreciated receiving recognition in the form of encouragement, compliments, respect, or motivation for other women to participate. Achieving different feats within the sport is cause for celebration but the level of celebration is not defined by the distance of the race. For example, the new sprinter who completed her first triathlon spoke of how much recognition she received just like the three-time Ironman finisher did. Their eyes lit up with such pride and a smile cut across their faces, as though they could recall every encouraging word they received during training.

Medals (i.e., bling) were a form of recognition that were regulated as introjection. The medals serve as 'proof' that the triathletes had completed a course and were most often displayed by the participants. They also serve as a reminder of the participants' past experiences and accomplishment. In this way, medals are also be described as external regulated because some triathletes would not participate in certain races if they knew they would not receive, at least, a finisher's medal. Hanna, explicitly said, "I do it for the bling—but that's about it."

The MOMS-T scale, self-esteem, was marked by two themes, confidence and fear. Confidence can change over time and is built based on experience. The women who had not been racing as long expressed that participating increased their confidence. The older women expressed that they overcame self-esteem issues years earlier so now self-esteem is, "like the cherry ... it's like that added little benefit," said Melle.

Fear, a theme which described a mental to physical paralysis, could occur while training or during a race if it was not overcome. While there was some type of fear in all three disciplines, fear of swimming was discussed the most. There were levels of fear of the swimming including: (1) fearing the pool; (2) fearing the deep end of the pool; (3) fearing the fresh open water; (4) fearing the animals (i.e., fish) that might be in the fresh open water; (5) fearing the saltwater; (6) fearing the bigger animals that might be in the saltwater (e.g., alligators). The two fears in the cycling portion of triathlon were falling off the bike or getting hit by a vehicle while riding. The fear of getting hit by a vehicle was synonymous with running too, as well as not being fast enough to get away from a dog chase. The location of the dog did not matter either because dogs live everywhere—in the city and the country. Recognition and self-esteem were not one-dimensional regulated scales due to the differences in the how the themes were regulated.

Integration regulated. The researcher speculated integration to regulate the SDT scales of personal goal achievement, health orientation, and psychological coping. Every one of the participants found personal goals important as there was a sense of pride with setting goals and achieving them. The themes related to personal goal achievement had equal weight. It was motivating to finish the course, no matter the obstacles. Additionally, it was equally important to improve in either one's personal time in one or all the disciplines, or in one's finish time. Draya expressed, "What's ... important is to ... see if I can beat the time I had before on that same course." There is a difference between the personal goal achievement themes of finishing the course and accomplishment. Accomplishment occurred after completing the race and the feeling was reported to carry into other parts of life. Finishing the course simply meant they crossed the finish line; however, crossing the line did not have the overflow into other parts of life.

The theme of physical awareness represented the scale, health orientation. The process of awareness was personal and for an athlete's health to be integrated, a synthesis of meaningful aspects related to triathlon occurred. Experiences made the older triathletes realize how necessary having good health is. Awareness was described as being integrated into their motive for training; once training started, they could experience the effects physically, spiritually, socially and psychologically.

Psychological coping was also regulated through integration as triathlons were described as a coping mechanism to get through life by the majority of the participants. They reported using the physical aspect (i.e., health orientation) to cope with anger and the stressors of life. One of the three disciplines was a favorite or the 'go-to' form of exercise for the women. Eve stated, "Whenever I'm upset or angry, I take it out on the pavement." In addition, Marissa jokingly expressed that, "This world is a safer place because I'm doing triathlons. I just need to tell you that right now, there are people who are walking around alive today because I'm doing triathlons." Similar to what was experienced with fear, the theme depression was either a barrier or served as a motivator to complete goals. However, depression was more integrated because it directly regulated behavior (rather than being an external regulator like fear). Several of the women used triathlon to free themselves from negative behavior caused by their diagnosis of depression. Elle was the first to explain, "I do have depression but [when] taking medication ... I just didn't like the side effects ... so, I just did my research. Exercising was the thing that made me feel good."

Identified regulated. Identified is the final form of extrinsic regulators which the researcher had not previously thought to be a regulator among the SDT scales. Two themes, inspiration (under recognition) and transitions were analyzed to be identified regulators attached to a new proposed scale Triathlon lifestyle. The women spoke of how they were inspired to be triathletes and then recognized their own ability to be an inspiration. However, in order to maintain the ability to inspire others, the participants adopted a sense of accountability. Nora stated, "I just want to be an example to others, in terms of being in good physical shape and looking the part." While they experienced their autonomy of continuing to practice the sport, it became a practice that engaged more women to participate, thus benefitting others as well.

The theme, transition, was the self-identification of owning the title 'triathlete.' This was not as easily adopted by some of the women because of the more socially accepted and described views of what a triathlete should look like. However, as the women furthered their pursuit of adopting the lifestyle of a triathlete, they also came to identify themselves as a triathlete—regardless of their personal looks.

Triathlon lifestyle. The new theme of triathlon lifestyle emerged from the interviews. It is described as a 'motivation that is or is perceived to be sustainable over time, as opposed to motivation that is temporal'. The lifestyle, itself, is a journey one takes when they begin the sport, continues through participation in the sport and looks forward toward aspirations for the sport in later life.

When beginning the sport, there are those who do are 'one and done'. This is a person who has likely checked off 'triathlon' from their bucket list. However, a person who 'catches the bug' has the potential to become a junkie who is addicted to the lifestyle. The lifestyle triathlete, however, recognizes that after they have spent weeks or months to prepare for a race, they must continue to live this lifestyle because completing one race is not enough. To continue to be successful, the triathlete's preparation becomes a lifestyle. Some of the women of this study thought triathlon would be a onetime event in their lives, too, but they felt differently after their first experience. For Letti, the transition to recognizing her lifestyle change occurred when she came to respect what triathlon did for her beyond the physical. "When I first started ... I did not really appreciate – did not recognize the healing of stress, of problem solving. It does so much for you. But, at the beginning? I didn't recognize that." The usage of the words being 'hooked' or 'junkie' and 'crazy' became descriptor words the women heard from others and proudly adopted for themselves. Lexi recognized that making triathlon a lifestyle and being part of the triathlon family is fine because it was, " ... encouraging that I'm not [the only] crazy person. Here's a group of people that have a similar goal and so it's been encouraging me to continue and work on that. When everybody is crazy, nobody is."

4. Discussion

Motivation to participate in triathlons is gaining exploration, lending to a variety of motivation constructs that vary across populations. This study adds to the knowledge of diversity of triathletes by including a group of minority women. Using dual methods, the motivations and regulators of triathlon participation were examined among 121 Black women, aged 36 and older. The theoretical focus on extrinsic motivation was characterized by Self Determination Theory (SDT), a theory of human motivation that addresses issues such as psychological needs, goals, and other issues related to well-being [3]. The sub-theory of SDT, the Organismic Integration Theory (OIT), defines those barriers or facilitators in behavior regulation [5]. To measure motivation, the researcher used the Motivations of Marathoners Scale for Triathletes (MOMS-T) as a survey to collect the motivational thought and then developed questions from the MOMS-T for semi-structured interviews which explored participants' motivational thought for descriptive and narrative data.

Using the SDT keywords and OIT regulators to identify how the scales in the MOMS-T are regulated is novel. Other surveys, like the Sport Motivation Scale II, have also used the SDT to understand the regulators of sport motivation [2]. Unlike the SMS II, the MOMS-T did not have statements hypothesized to be identified. In the SMS II, 'develop myself' is a phrase consistently used with statements related to the identified regulator. The idea of personal development, in the MOMS-T, is directly related to measurable racing goals (e.g., To try to run faster) within personal goal achievement. Identified was not believed to be a regulator with this population. However, themes extracted from the MOTIG helped with the development of the new scale, Triathlete Lifestyle. This scale was also directly related to the regulator, identified. The women self-identified as triathletes because their lifestyle differed from other athletes who may only perform one of the three disciplines (e.g., marathoners) or do another form of exercise (e.g., yoga). Like the study by Armentrout, which described that Ironman triathletes go through a process of change—where they adopt a healthy lifestyle—the same holds true for all the women of this study, regardless of the distance. All transitioned into recognizing their life as a triathlete [27].

Integration was identified as the strongest SDT motivational regulator for the quantitative and qualitative methods. Quantitatively, more than 50% of the women believed it was the integration of the sport which motivated their participation. This suggests that the women's motivations were more personal in nature and were not motivated by others' views of their accomplishments. While the MOMS-T, alone, provided more of 'what' motivates a person to participate, the interviews provided 'how' they were regulated. The interviews revealed integration regulating four of the MOMS-T scales (Psychological Coping, Health Orientation, Personal Goal Achievement, and Triathlete Lifestyle).

Another key finding was the interpretation of the scale, Competition. The MOMS-T defines competition as competing with others and being faster than someone else. The statements were insignificant for the survey participants with an overall mean of 2.67. However, when the women were interviewed, they provided a richer explanation as to why this mean scale was low. The items did not ask about competition with themselves. Similar items that could be described as self-competition, were found under the scale Personal Goal Achievement. Statements including, 'to push myself beyond my current limits,' and 'to compete with myself,' could be considered as a form of self-competition. Yet, when the women discussed their personal goals, the themes of finishing the race, having feelings of accomplishment, is what was gleaned from the interviews—not a form of self-competition.

Using a survey of motivational factors for triathletes (i.e., MOMS-T) was a strength. Findings were comparable to previous studies on triathletes [10,28,29]. However, using the novel method of survey transformation for the dual-method approach provided additional qualitative explanations of the survey answers not previously noted. Using a secondary method of gathering data through interviews, as a follow-up to gathering survey data, was feasible for providing further understanding about certain constructs. For example, the lack of assessment of triathlon medals, as a form of external regulation, was not measured in the MOMS-T but was important to these triathletes.

Limitations to the study include methodological issues, participant representativeness, and potential misrepresentation. The sampling resulted in participant self-selection, which suggests that those who participated in this study may differ from those who did not. The surveys were only made available through computer access; it is possible that the computer sampling techniques did not reach as many subjects as possible. The researcher used convenience and snowball sampling techniques, making it difficult for the triathlon affiliated networks (e.g., USAT) to verify the legitimacy of samples' participation rates. Due to self-reporting, the demographic survey asked questions could have been answered incorrectly (e.g., weight/height).

The results of the study lay the foundation for considering expanding the scope of analysis related to the SDT. Multiple studies, in varying disciplines, have used the SDT to understand motivation. However, self-determination has been most applied to sport, education, and health care [3,28]. Therefore, to understand how people are further motivated, the SDT regulators and how they intersect with motivation requires additional mixed-methods analysis.

One way to expand the scope of analysis of the SDT and possibly affect policy related to exercise would be to use of the Short Form (SF-12) Health Survey in additional studies. The SF-12 has most recently been used to evaluate the validity and reliability of a questionnaire developed to measure the influence of competitive sport participation on lifespan health and well-being [29]. The use of such an instrument in combination with surveys of exercise levels and motivation, like the MOMS-T, may help in understanding the effect of exercise on health status.

5. Conclusions

This study is a first to explore the motivations of Black women who participate in a sport dominated by white men in the United States. Understanding the motivations for Black women who participate in triathlons is important to the pursuit of health equity, as Black adults are the racial/ethnic group least likely to meet physical activity guidelines, and Black women are less active than Black men [30,31]. Although researchers have identified barriers of exercise for women, this information, not previously highlighted in research, may assist in identifying the factors to motivate Black women to exercise regularly [32].

The novel method of using survey transformation allowed researchers to glean previously uninterpreted information from a quantitative survey through the interview process. Previous research on motivation has not used a qualitative version of the MOMS; therefore, the interpretation of competition in previous studies, or other surveys like the SMS II, were not able to identify competition as a personal motivation but rather, as a motivation based on rivalry in sport. This is useful knowledge when considering previous research revealed that young girls, who abandon the sport, may not if they receive support through change of the rules of competition [33].

The interviews also confirmed that the MOMS-T survey should be revised and revalidated after including of questions relevant to the newly emerged 'Triathlon Lifestyle' scale. Not previously seen in studies related to motivation using the MOMS, this scale can provide a separate dimension of understanding motivation from the perspective of it being a sport maintained throughout life. Additionally, the interviews of this study also supported earlier research that stated expanding analysis to the MOMS-T by measuring the fun or enjoyment as motivation for participating triathlons [20].

The survey transformation method confirmed an adaptable approach to using surveys, in future settings, to other populations when there are insufficient resources to redo formative qualitative work that informed the initial survey. Triathlon programs, like those which have been implemented into school physical education programs [34], can be designed to motivate minorities to participate in triathlon races and may find it useful to include some motivation statements identified in this study. Future research also might seek to identify extrinsic motivations in other demographic groups, by utilizing the mixed-methods research approaches as in the present study.

Funding: This research received no external funding.

Acknowledgments: Special thanks to J. James Cotter; Diane Dodd-McCue; Tracey L. Gendron; Amy G. Huebschmann; and Kevin S. Masters for their guidance to complete this project. Special thanks to Greg Samanez-Larkin for his support to complete the manuscript.

Conflicts of Interest: The authors declare no conflict of interest.

Appendix A

Table A1. Descriptive Statistics of the seven Scales.

Scales	N	Mean	SD	Min	Max
Health Orientation	115	32.03	7.975	6	42
Weight Control	118	18.17	6.597	4	28
Personal Goal Achievement	118	32.20	6.789	6	42
Competition	117	10.75	5.914	4	28
Recognition	113	14.57	7.306	6	42
Psychological Coping	112	30.15	14.33	9	63
Self-Esteem	116	22.05	10.63	7	49

Appendix B

Table A2. Descriptive Statistics of Regulators by Age, BMI, and Distance.

Category	Regulator	N	Mean	SD	Min	Max
Age						
35–50	External	90	39.54	13.31	11	77
	Introjection	87	49.29	16.47	14	98
	Integration	85	92.02	24.08	21	141
50+	External	23	43.83	15.25	20	77
	Introjection	21	51.29	14.58	22	74
	Integration	20	105.70	18.32	74	147
BMI						
Normal	External	36	37.33	14.50	11	77
	Introjection	34	47.12	19.11	14	84
	Integration	31	93.10	27.26	21	147
Overweight	External	34	41.56	13.92	16	71
	Introjection	34	48.35	13.37	20	74
	Integration	33	96.00	24.35	39	141
Obese	External	31	43.19	14.50	13	77
	Introjection	28	55.39	16.34	32	98
	Integration	29	96.14	20.91	57	141

Table A2. *Cont.*

Category	Regulator	N	Mean	SD	Min	Max
Distance completed						
Not completed	External	10	39.20	18.65	13	71
	Introjection	9	43.11	15.96	20	64
	Integration	10	90.90	25.93	57	130
Sprint	External	57	40.23	13.93	11	77
	Introjection	55	49.62	17.20	14	98
	Integration	53	93.47	24.51	21	141
Olympic	External	14	40.36	13.39	20	59
	Introjection	13	50.54	17.62	22	77
	Integration	13	92.62	17.37	66	132
Half-Ironman	External	15	35.93	10.52	16	51
	Introjection	15	47.33	13.70	26	72
	Integration	14	94.29	25.29	39	131
Ironman	External	17	45.65	12.84	30	77
	Introjection	16	56.38	11.44	30	74
	Integration	15	102.00	24.63	72	147

Appendix C

Table A3. Interview Participant Characteristics.

Participant	Age	Preferred Triathlon Distance	BMI
Brooklyn Diva	45	Olympic	normal
Lexi	51	Sprint	normal
Eve	45	Half-Ironman	normal
Elle	44	Sprint	obese
Letti	56	Sprint	normal
Nita	50	Sprint	overweight
Marissa	43	Ironman	overweight
Draya	58	Olympic	overweight
Melle	54	Half-Ironman	overweight
Rado	49	Ironman	obese
Nora	60	Half-Ironman	overweight
Hanna	39	Sprint	obese

References

1. Weinberg, R.; Gould, D. *Foundations of Sport and Exercise Psychology*; Human Kinetics: Champaign, IL, USA, 2011; p. 51.
2. López-Fernández, I.; Merino-Marbán, R.; Fernández-Rodríguez, E. Examining the Relationship between Sex and Motivation in Triathletes. *Percept. Mot. Ski.* **2014**, *119*, 42–49. [CrossRef] [PubMed]
3. Deci, E.L.; Ryan, R.M. Self-Determination Theory: A Macrotheory of Human Motivation, Development, and Health. *Can. Psychol.* **2008**, *49*, 182–185. Available online: http://www.anitacrawley.net/Resources/Articles/Deci%20and%20Ryan.pdf (accessed on 12 December 2018). [CrossRef]
4. Teixeira, P.J.; Carraça, E.V.; Markland, D.; Silva, M.N.; Ryan, R.M. Exercise, physical activity, and self-determination theory: A systematic review. *Int. J. Behav. Nutr. Phys. Act.* **2012**, *9*, 78. [CrossRef]
5. Wilson, P.M.; Sabiston, C.M.; Mack, D.E.; Blanchard, C.M. On the nature and function of scoring protocols used in exercise motivation research: An empirical study of the behavioral regulation in exercise questionnaire. *Psychol. Sport Exerc.* **2012**, *13*, 614–622. [CrossRef]
6. Clancy, R.B.; Herring, M.P.; MacIntyre, T.E.; Campbell, M.J. A review of competitive sport motivation research. *Psychol. Sport Exerc.* **2016**, *27*, 232–242. Available online: https://www.researchgate.net/publication/308078234_A_review_of_competitive_sport_motivation_research (accessed on 17 December 2018). [CrossRef]

7. La Gerche, A.; Prior, D. Exercise—Is it possible to have too much of a good thing? *Heart Lung Circ.* **2007**, *16*, S102–S104. Available online: https://www.researchgate.net/publication/6232047_Exercise-Is_it_Possible_to_Have_Too_Much_of_a_Good_Thing (accessed on 20 July 2019). [CrossRef] [PubMed]
8. Bell, G.J.; Howe, B.L. Mood State Profiles and Motivations of Triathletes. *J. Sport Behav.* **1988**, *11*, 66.
9. Cronan, M.; Scott, D. Triathlon and women's narratives of bodies and sport. *Leis. Sci.* **2008**, *30*, 17–34. Available online: https://www.tandfonline.com/doi/abs/10.1080/01490400701544675?journalCode=ulsc20 (accessed on 30 July 2016). [CrossRef]
10. Lamont, M.; Kennelly, M. A qualitative exploration of participant motives among committed amateur triathletes. *Leis. Sci.* **2012**, *34*, 236–255. [CrossRef]
11. USA Triathlon Membership Survey Report. Available online: https://www.teamusa.org/USA-Triathlon/News/Articles-and-Releases/2017/December/18/USA-Triathlon-Membership-Survey-Report (accessed on 28 December 2018).
12. Clarke, T.C.; Norris, T.; Schiller, J.S. Early Release of Selected Estimates Based on Data from the 2016 National Health Interview Survey. U.S. Department of Health and Human Services. Available online: https://www.cdc.gov/nchs/data/nhis/earlyrelease/earlyrelease201705.pdf (accessed on 2 April 2018).
13. Brown, C.S.; Masters, K.S.; Huebschmann, A.G. Identifying Motives of Midlife Black Triathlete Women Using Survey Transformation to Guide Qualitative Inquiry. *J. Cross Cult. Gerontol.* **2018**, *33*, 1–20. [CrossRef]
14. Pathak, E.B. 'Is Heart Disease or Cancer the Leading Cause of Death in United States Women? *Women Health Issues* **2016**, *26*, 89–594. Available online: https://www.ncbi.nlm.nih.gov/pubmed/27717539 (accessed on 22 January 2019). [CrossRef] [PubMed]
15. Brown, C.S.; Collins, S. African American triathletes: An exercise regimen for the aging woman. In Proceedings of the Poster Session, Gerontological Society of America Annual Meeting, Atlanta, GA, USA, 18–22 November 2009.
16. Masters, K.S.; Ogles, B.M.; Jolton, J.A. The development of an instrument to measure motivation for marathon running: The Motivations of Marathoners Scales (MOMS). *Res. Q. Exerc. Sport* **1993**, *64*, 134–143. [CrossRef] [PubMed]
17. LaChausse, R.G. Motives of competitive and non-competitive cyclists. *J. Sport Behav.* **2006**, *29*, 304–314.
18. Rundio, A.; Heere, B.; Newland, B. Cause-related versus non-cause-related sport events: Differentiating endurance events through a comparison of athletes' motives. *SMQ* **2014**, *23*, 17.
19. Croft, S.J.; Gray, C.C.; Duncan, J.F. Motives for participating in triathlon: An investigation between elite and non-elite competitors in an Australian setting. *Health* **2007**, *34*, 3–6. Available online: http://www.geocities.ws/CollegePark/5686/su99p12.htm (accessed on 7 September 2019).
20. Lovett, M.; Barnes, J.; Marley, S. An Examination of the motives to participate in sprint-distance triathlon. *J. Sport Behav.* **2018**, *41*, 424–450. Available online: http://www.southalabama.edu/psychology/journal.htm (accessed on 30 December 2018).
21. Ryan, R.M.; Deci, E.L. Self-Determination Theory and the Facilitation of Intrinsic Motivation, Social Development, and Well-Being. *Am. Psychol.* **2000**, *55*, 68–78. Available online: https://selfdeterminationtheory.org/SDT/documents/2000_RyanDeci_SDT.pdf (accessed on 22 June 2018). [CrossRef] [PubMed]
22. Solberg, P.A.; Halvari, H. Perceived autonomy support, personal goal content, and emotional well-being among elite athletes: Mediating effects of reasons for goals. *Percept. Mot. Skills* **2009**, *108*, 721–743. Available online: https://selfdeterminationtheory.org/SDT/documents/Solberg,%20P.%20A.%20&%20Halvari,%20H.%20(2009).pdf (accessed on 9 April 2019). [CrossRef] [PubMed]
23. World Health Organization Physical Activity. Available online: http://www.who.int/dietphysicalactivity/pa/en/index.html (accessed on 12 February 2019).
24. Knechtle, B.; Knechtle, P.; Lepers, R. Participation and performance trends in ultra- triathlons from 1985 to 2009. *Scand. J. Med. Sci. Sports* **2010**, *21*, 82–90. [CrossRef]
25. Gillet, N.; Vallerand, R.J.; Amoura, S.; Baldes, B. Influence of coaches' autonomy support on athletes' motivation and sport performance: A test of the hierarchical model of intrinsic and extrinsic motivation. *Psychol. Sport Exerc.* **2010**, *11*, 155–161. [CrossRef]
26. Bowen, G.A. Naturalistic inquiry and the saturation concept: A research note. *Qual. Res.* **2008**, *8*, 137–152. Available online: https://journals.sagepub.com/doi/10.1177/1468794107085301 (accessed on 22 September 2017). [CrossRef]

27. Armentrout, S.M. Exploring motives of Ironman triathletes using the transtheoretical model. *Athl. Insight* **2014**, *6*, 35–62. Available online: https://login.proxy.lib.duke.edu/login?url=https://search-proquest-com.proxy.lib.duke.edu/docview/1623319303?accountid=10598 (accessed on 14 January 2019).
28. Brummett, B.; Babyak, M.; Grønbæk, M.; Barefoot, J.C. Positive emotions associated with 6-year change in functional status in individuals aged 60 and older. *J. Posit. Psychol.* **2011**, *6*, 216–223. [CrossRef]
29. Sorenson, S.C.; Romano, R.; Azen, S.P.; Schroeder, E.T.; Salem, G.J. Life span exercise among elite intercollegiate student athletes. *Sports Health* **2015**, *7*, 80–86. Available online: https://doi-org.proxy.lib.duke.edu/10.1177%2F1941738114534813 (accessed on 12 January 2019). [CrossRef] [PubMed]
30. Paschal, A.M.; Lewis-Moss, R.K.; Sly, J.; White, B.J. Addressing health disparities among African Americans: Using the stages of change model to document attitudes and decisions about nutrition and physical activity. *J. Community Health* **2009**, *35*, 10–17. [CrossRef] [PubMed]
31. Hillier, A.; Tappe, K.; Cannuscio, C.; Karpyn, A.; Glanz, K. In an urban neighborhood, who is physically active and where? *Women Health* **2014**, *54*, 194–211. [CrossRef]
32. Pekmezi, D.; Marcus, B.; Meneses, K.; Baskin, M.L.; Ard, J.D.; Martin, M.Y.; Demark-Wahnefried, W. Developing an intervention to address physical activity barriers for African-American women in the Deep South (USA). *Women Health* **2013**, *9*, 301–312. Available online: https://www.ncbi.nlm.nih.gov/pmc/articles/PMC3816507/ (accessed on 20 February 2019). [CrossRef] [PubMed]
33. Vilchez, M.P. Analisis de la participation en el triathlon en edad escolar de la Region de Murcia (tempradas 2011, 2012 y 2013). *SPORT TK Rev. Eur. Am. Cincias Deporte* **2015**, *4*, 11–22. Available online: https://revistas.um.es/sportk/article/view/239781/182691 (accessed on 21 August 2019). [CrossRef]
34. Machota Blas, V.E. Triathlon: An innovative approach in Secondary School Physical Education. *SPORT TK Rev. Eur. Am. Cincias Deporte* **2016**, *5*, 55–64. Available online: https://revistas.um.es/sportk/article/view/249121 (accessed on 21 August 2019). [CrossRef]

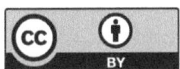

© 2019 by the author. Licensee MDPI, Basel, Switzerland. This article is an open access article distributed under the terms and conditions of the Creative Commons Attribution (CC BY) license (http://creativecommons.org/licenses/by/4.0/).

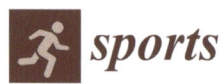

Article

Core Temperature in Triathletes during Swimming with Wetsuit in 10 °C Cold Water

Jørgen Melau [1,2,3,*], Maria Mathiassen [4], Trine Stensrud [5], Mike Tipton [6] and Jonny Hisdal [1,2]

1. Institute of Clinical Medicine, University of Oslo, 0316 Oslo, Norway; jonny.hisdal@medisin.uio.no
2. Department of Vascular surgery, Oslo University Hospital, 0424 Oslo, Norway
3. Prehospital Division, Vestfold Hospital Trust, 3103 Toensberg, Norway
4. Department of Cardiology, Telemark Hospital Trust, 3710 Skien, Norway; maria.mathiassen@gmail.com
5. Department of Sports Medicine, Norwegian School of Sport Sciences, 0806 Oslo, Norway; trine.stensrud@nih.no
6. Extreme Environments Laboratory, Department of Sport and Exercise Science, University of Portsmouth, Portsmouth PO1 2ER, UK; michael.tipton@port.ac.uk
* Correspondence: jorgen@melau.no; Tel.: +47-911-73-629

Received: 18 April 2019; Accepted: 24 May 2019; Published: 28 May 2019

Abstract: Low water temperature (<15 °C) has been faced by many organizers of triathlons and swim-runs in the northern part of Europe during recent years. More knowledge about how cold water affects athletes swimming in wetsuits in cold water is warranted. The aim of the present study was therefore to investigate the physiological response when swimming a full Ironman distance (3800 m) in a wetsuit in 10 °C water. Twenty triathletes, 37.6 ± 9 years (12 males and 8 females) were recruited to perform open water swimming in 10 °C seawater; while rectal temperature (Tre) and skin temperature (Tskin) were recorded. The results showed that for all participants, Tre was maintained for the first 10–15 min of the swim; and no participants dropped more than 2 °C in Tre during the first 30 min of swimming in 10 °C water. However; according to extrapolations of the results, during a swim time above 135 min; 47% (8/17) of the participants in the present study would fall more than 2 °C in Tre during the swim. The results show that the temperature response to swimming in a wetsuit in 10 °C water is highly individual. However, no participant in the present study dropped more than 2 °C in Tre during the first 30 min of the swim in 10 °C water.

Keywords: swimming; core temperature; skin temperature; wetsuit; triathlon; endurance

1. Introduction

Long distance triathlon is rising in popularity [1]. In 2003, the first "Norseman Xtreme Triathlon" was arranged in Norway, and the race soon became known as one of the toughest triathlons in the world [2]. Athletes swim 3800 m in the Hardangerfjord, bike 180 km with approximately 3000 m of vertical ascent and then run 42 km, to finish at the peak of Mt. Gaustadoppen at 1883 m above sea level [3]. The low water temperature (<15 °C) has generally been a challenge for the organizers. In 2015, the participants faced a water temperature of 10 °C, and the swim was then shortened to half the distance [4].

Low water temperature has been faced by many organizers of triathlons [5] and swim-runs [6] in the northern part of Europe during recent years, and more knowledge about how cold water affects athletes swimming in wetsuits is warranted.

The International Triathlon Union (ITU) has taken this into account in their regulations of racing water temperature and wetsuit usage in ITU sanctioned races [7]. Recently, scientific inquiries into the rationale behind these regulations have been made, and the rules have been modified accordingly [8]. The International Swimming Federation (FINA) has specified 16 °C as their lowest water temperature in their

Open Water Swimming Rules [9]. In a recent study [8], Saycell J, Lomax M, Massey H, et al. identified lean swimmers and cold water as significant risk factors for hypothermia. This has also been elucidated further, with new minimum water temperature limits for open water marathon swim racing [10].

Despite this, the knowledge of how deep body temperature is affected in triathletes swimming in wetsuits in cold water down to 10 °C is limited. For the vast majority of triathletes, the swim portion is completed in <2 h.

The aim of this study was therefore to investigate the physiological response to swimming in a wetsuit in 10 °C water. Based on previous experience, our hypothesis was that the deep body temperature (Tre) would decrease less than 1 °C·h^{-1} during swimming in 10 °C water with a properly fitting wetsuit, suggesting that the Tre would not drop more than 2 °C (or below 35 °C) during a full swim in an Ironman competition.

2. Materials and Methods

2.1. Participants

The study protocol was evaluated by the Regional Ethics Committee (REC) (ref 2015/1533/REK Sør-Øst), according to the principles of the declaration of Helsinki. Before inclusion, all participants provided written informed consent. Twenty participants (12 males, 8 females) were recruited for the present study. All were active triathletes, at elite- or recreational level. Recruitment took place via social media, and the individuals had to be able to swim 3800 m non-stop in less than 1h and 45 min, not have any history of cardiovascular disease or arrhythmias and have their own wetsuit.

2.2. Measurements

Prior to the tests, medical screening was performed by the study doctor and a nurse. The screening included a medical survey and an ECG test (Cardiovit AT102 Plus, Schiller Handelsgesellschaft m.b.H., Sveits) in accordance with the recommendation of the European Society of Cardiology [11,12].

Baseline measurements, including weight, height, DXA-scan (Lunar Prodigy densitometer, GE Medical Systems, WI, USA) were performed 2 h before the start of the swim at the Norwegian School of Sport Sciences (NIH) in Oslo. Maximal oxygen uptake (VO$_{2max}$) was measured at NIH, within one week after the test by a Oxycon Pro analyzer (Jaeger Instrument, Carefusion/BD, San Diego, CA, USA) using a graded (5.3%) running test on a treadmill (Bari-Mill, Woodway, WI, USA) with gradually increasing running speed each minute until exhaustion, according to Astrand, Rodahl et al. 2003 [13].

All participants had a warm-up of easy running (10 min) on the treadmill before the test started. During the test, all participants wore a nose clip (9015 Reusable Series, Hans Rudolph Inc., Kansas City, MI, USA) and used a silicone rubber mouthpiece (9060 Reusable Series, Hans Rudolph Inc., Shawnee Mission, KS, USA).

VO$_{2max}$ was identified when a plateau (a rise of less than 2 mL·kg^{-1}·min^{-1} in VO$_2$, despite increasing running speed) was observed. In addition, two more criteria of VO$_{2max}$ were applied, a respiratory exchange ratio (*RER*) > 1.05 and heart rate of >95% of maximum heart rate.

After testing, the participants were transferred to the test site in the Oslofjord at Høvik, 20 min outside of Oslo city, where the temperature sensors were mounted on the participants. A skin sensor (YSI 400) was mounted on the upper left side of the chest (approximately 8 cm below *clavicula*) and a rectal probe (YSI 400, YSI Incorporated, Yellow Springs, OH, USA) was self-inserted by the athletes after instruction from the scientists. The rectal probe was inserted 10 cm past the anal sphincter. The sensors were connected to a logging device (Veriteq Spectrum Precision Thermistor Logger 1400, Surrey, BC, Canada) and temperatures were logged every minute from 15 min prior to the swim until a minimum of 45 min after the swim. No rewarming intervention was incorporated in this study. The logger was mounted in a custom-made waterproof box (length 12 cm, width 7 cm and height 4 cm) that was taped to the back of the outside of the participant's wet suit. The logging system did not affect swimming technique.

2.3. Swim Test

The testing was very time consuming, and due to safety reasons, we were not able to have more than one test subject in the water at a time. The swim test was therefore performed over a period of three consecutive days. Mean (SD) water temperature was 10.0 (0.7 °C) and air temperature 7.4 (2.1 °C) during the three test days. On day one, six participants swam 3800 m (82 (14) min), and on day 2 and 3, the swim time was shortened to a maximum of 55 min. In total, 13 participants performed 46 (5) min of swimming. To ensure the optimal fit of the wetsuit, the participants used their personal wetsuits, approved in accordance with the ITU Competition Rules for triathlon [7]. The thickness of the wetsuit should not exceed 5 mm of thickness anywhere, and have long arms and legs. In addition, a standard silicone swim cap was used, with no other aid for warming the body during the swim. During the first day, six participants were tested, and all of them swam a full Ironman distance (3800 m). After the first day of testing, we observed a rectal temperatrue (Tre) below 35 °C in one of the participants, and we therefore decided to reduce the swim time to a maximum of 55 min the next two days to prevent a fall in Tre below 35 °C. In none of the athletes who participated in the last 2 days of testing did the Tre fall below 35 °C. The participants were swimming one at a time, a maximum of five meters from the pier and were constantly monitored by five paramedics and a rescue swimmer. A medical doctor was present at the test site at all times during the three days of testing. All rescue personnel where updated and trained in the latest protocols regarding hypothermia [14] and advanced cardiopulmonary resuscitation [15]. Mandatory rescue- and medical equipment was located on the pier for the paramedics and medical doctor to use if needed [16].

2.4. Data Analysis and Statistics

The study was powered to be able to detect a drop in core temperature >0.5 °C during the swim. Given a significance level of 0.05 and a power of 80%, 16 participants were needed, given a start temperature at 37.5 ± 0.5 °C. Further, to compensate for a 20% dropout rate, a total of 20 participants were recruited to the study. Statistical analyses and all graphics were performed in SigmaPlot 10.0 (Systat Software, Inc., GmbH, Erkrath, Germany). Pearson Product Moment Correlation was performed to evaluate correlation between variables. Data are reported as mean (standard deviation) unless otherwise stated. A *p*-value <0.05 was considered statistically significant.

3. Results

One participant was excluded before swimming due to failing the medical screening, and in two participants, Tre was not recorded during the swim due to equipment failure. Seventeen participants (6 women) were therefore included in the final analysis (Table 1).

Table 1. Demographic, anthropometric and physiological characteristics of the study sample; as a total and for both women and men separately. Values are given as mean ± SD.

	Total	Women	Men
Number (n)	17	6	11
Age (yrs.)	37.6 ± 9.0	37.5 ± 10.3	37.6 ± 8.8
Body composition			
Weight (kg)	77.9 ± 7.4	66.4 ± 8.0	84.3 ± 12.9
Height (cm)	177.6 ± 7.4	173.4 ± 5.6	179.9 ± 7.3
LBM (kg)	58.3 ± 11.5	46.2 ± 5.4	65.0 ± 7.8
%BF (%)	23.3 ± 9.0	27.7 ± 6.6	20.9 ± 9.6
FM (kg)	17.2 ± 7.4	17.8 ± 5.3	16.7 ± 8.6
VO_{2max}			
Relative (mL·kg^{-1}·min^{-1})	57.5 ± 11.0	49.3 ± 6.6	62.4 ± 10.3
Absolute (L·min^{-1})	4.5 ± 1.1	3.3 ± 0.5	5.2 ± 0.7

Table 1. *Cont.*

	Total	Women	Men
Training per week (hh:min)	9:30 ± 4:06	8:18 ± 4:54	10:18 ± 3:42
Total Swimming pool	1:36 ± 1:18	1:36 ± 1:24	1:36 ± 1:12

LBM is lean body mass; %BF is percentage body fat; FM is fat mass and VO_{2max} is maximal oxygen uptake.

3.1. Rectal Temperature (Tre)

Before the swim, average Tre was 36.6 (0.1) °C. The Tre of all participants was maintained for the first 10 min of the swim. In 13 of the 17 participants, Tre dropped below starting value during the swim, with a statistically significant drop in Tre of 0.9 (1.1) °C in the group ($p < 0.001$). For all 13 participants that displayed a fall in Tre, a further fall ("afterdrop") in Tre was observed after the swim (0.6 (0.3) °C). The average (SD) time from exiting the water until lowest temperature was 25 (12) min. Tre for the participants that swam 3800 m (n = 4) are displayed in Figure 1, panel A, and panel B shows results for 13 athletes that swam for a maximum of 55 min.

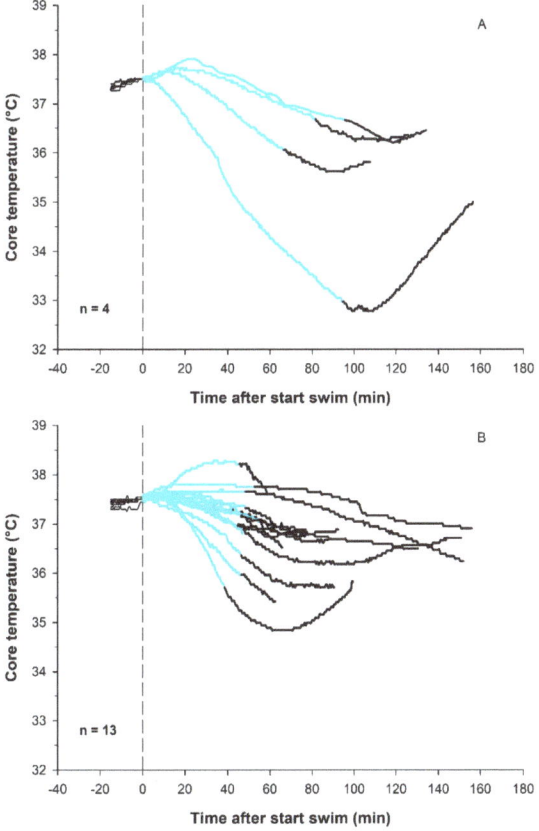

Figure 1. Tre before (black line), during (blue line) and after (black line) swimming in 10 °C water. Panel A shows results for the athletes that swam 3800 m in 82 (14) min (n = 4), and panel B shows results after the shortened swim to 46 (5) min (n = 13). For comparison, all temperature curves are adjusted to start at 37.5 °C at swim start.

The slope for the drop in Tre was on average 1.38 (1.24) °C·h^{-1}. The results show that with an exposure time of 135 min, 47% (8/17) of the athletes would experience a drop in Tre larger than 2 °C (Figure 2). However, at 30 min of swim time, none of the participants in the present study experienced a drop in Tre >2 °C.

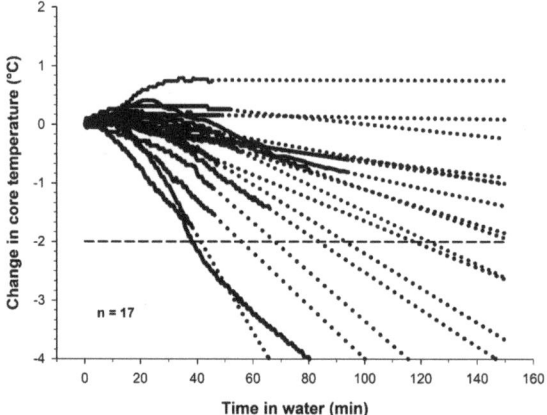

Figure 2. Solid line shows the development of Tre during swimming in 10 °C cold water. Dotted lines show extrapolated time course, based on the slope for Tre during the last 20 min of the swim (n = 17).

3.2. Skin Temperature (Tsk)

Due to technical problems with the skin sensors on three of the athletes, Tsk was successfully recorded during the swim in 14 of 17 athletes where Tre were recorded. Average Tsk beneath the wet suit was 33.3 (0.3) °C before the swim and was significantly reduced to 19.2 (1.7) °C during the first 30 min of the swim ($p < 0.001$). Tsk before, during and after the swim for all athletes are shown in Figure 3.

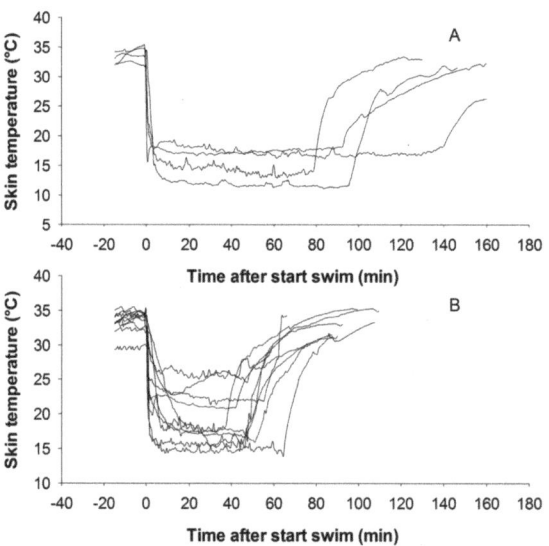

Figure 3. Tsk before, during and after swimming in 10 °C water with a wet suit. Panel A shows results for the 4 athletes that swam 3800 m in 82 (14) min (n = 4), and panel B shows results for 10 athletes that swam a shortened swim to 46 (5) min (n = 10).

3.3. Relation between Tre, Skin Temp, fat% and Gender

We observed a significant correlation between the slope for Tre during the swim and total fat mass (kg), ($r^2 = 0.25$, $p = 0.04$). There was a non-significant tendency for correlation between the slope for Tre during the swim and % bodyfat (%), ($r^2 = 0.21$, $p = 0.06$) and BMI ($r^2 = 0.13$, $p = 0.08$). No other significant correlations were observed between the slope for Tre during the swim and any of the other following relevant variables as; weight ($p = 0.33$), height ($p = 0.33$), age ($p = 0.51$), LBM ($p = 0.94$), average skin temp last 20 min of swim ($p = 0.86$), hours swimming training per week ($p = 0.47$) or gender ($p = 0.43$). In Figure 4, change in Tre, Tsk and, fat% and gender are shown for all participants.

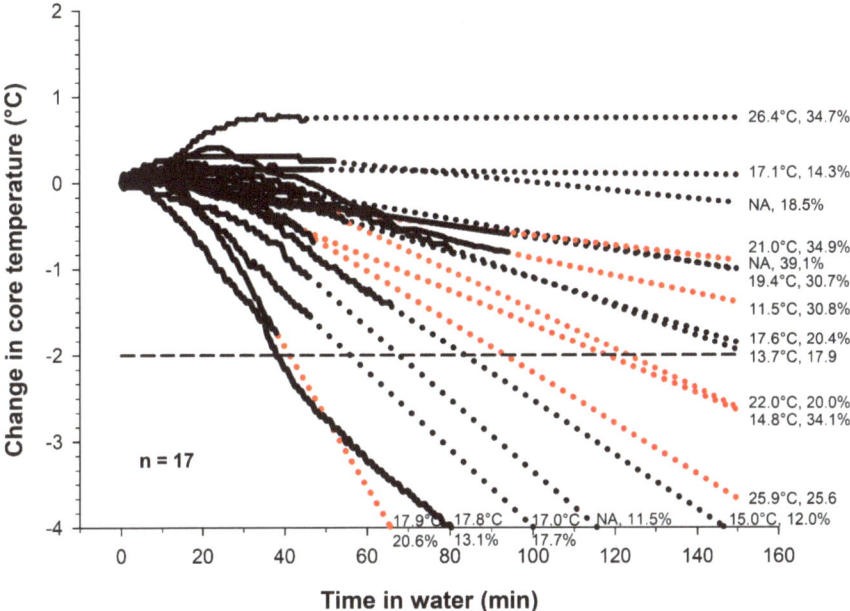

Figure 4. Solid line shows the Tre during swimming in 10 °C water. Dotted lines show the linearly extrapolated time course, based on the slope for Tre during the last 20 min of the swim (red dots = female). Average Tsk during swim and body fat % are presented for all participants (n = 17).

4. Discussion

The main finding in the present study was the heterogeneity in the temperature response to swimming in a wetsuit in cold water. However, for all participants, the Tre was maintained for the first 10–15 min of the swim, and no participants dropped more than 2 °C in Tre during the first 30 min of swimming in 10 °C water. However, given a swim time above 135 min, 47% (8/17) of the participants in the present study would be predicted to have greater than a 2 °C in Tre.

4.1. Rectal Temperature

The results from the present study showed that the participants were able to maintain the Tre for the first 10–15 min of the swim. An explanation for this is the cold-induced vasoconstriction at the skin's surface, and the time required to set up a conductive cooling gradient from the water to the deep body tissues. The conductive cooling gradient is dependent on the length of the conductive pathway (size/fatness of the individual) [17]. Further, after this initial period, Tre started to drop in 76% (13/17) of our test participants. The linear pattern of the temperature curve, made it possible to calculate a slope, and therefore the possibility to interpolate the curves and predict Tre if swimming had been prolonged. Several studies have shown the potential harmful effects of hypothermia [18–20]. One of the study participants in the present study had a Tre as low as 33.1 °C, classified as mild hypothermia. When this was discovered, we immediately took action to prevent similar cases, and the exposure time to cold water was therefore reduced during days 2 and 3 of the project.

The results from the present study displayed a large heterogeneity in the Tre response. One participant started to drop in Tre after 10.5 min, and another increased in Tre during the swim. The participant with the early drop had a body fat % of 13.1, and the one that increased had a fat % of 34.7. Further analysis also confirmed a significant correlation between low body fat % and drop in Tre. This is in line with previous findings in other studies [8,17]. This should be of interest for race organizers, as more elite athletes often have a lower body fat % and therefore are more prone to become hypothermic during swimming.

It is complicated to prescribe safe limits for swimming in cold water due to the interaction between many variables that may affect the cooling rate [8]. In addition to the absolute water temperature: exposure time, metabolic heat production, body composition, body mass and wetsuit construction (length and thickness) and fit may affect the cooling rate. One important research question in the present study was to estimate how long it would take before the athletes reached a Tre of 35 °C or below. Figure 2 shows an estimation of this, where we have extrapolated the Tre cooling curves to predict when Tre exceeds a 2 °C fall. The cut-off for the swim in Norseman Xtreme Triathlon is 135 min. The average swim time during the last 10 years was approximately 82 min. The fastest athletes completed the swim in 50 min. The results from the present study show that given a water temperature at 10 °C, 47% of the athletes that swam for 135 min would drop more than 2 °C in Tre.

Given a well-fitted wetsuit, our results indicate that to avoid hypothermia, the exposure time should be limited to a maximum of 30 min, in 10 °C water. For the slowest swimmers, this would probably correspond to a maximum swim distance of 1000 m under such conditions.

4.2. Tsk

The results from the present study showed that the Tsk dropped immediately on entering the cold water and stabilized at a constant level within a few minutes. A relatively large variation in Tsk was observed between the participants during the swim (12–26 °C), however no significant relationship between the drop in Tsk and Tre was observed.

In the present study, the athletes used their own personal wetsuit of different brands, thickness and fit and this could possibly be the explanation for the lack of correlation between Tsk and drop in Tre. Evidence suggests a relationship between wetsuit fit and cardiovascular response [21]. The relationship between drop in Tre, Tsk and type and fit of wetsuit needs to be elucidated in further studies.

4.3. Post-Immersion Cooling

The post-immersion cooling observed in our study was on average 0.6 °C, and the lowest temperature was observed on average 25 min after the swim. The fact that Tre may continue to fall post- open water swim should be of interest to organizers. It is also important for triathlon organizers and triathletes to expect that Tre can fall in T1 (Transition Zone 1—the shift from swimming to cycling during a triathlon) and during the first part of the cycling [8]. Race organizers and medical crew should have increased levels of alertness during these periods. Our findings on post-immersion cooling is also in accordance with previous published results from Nuckton et al. 2000 [22] who studied open water swimmers in 11.7 °C water. In that study, post-immersion cooling was observed in 10 of 11 test participants. The effect is possibly worsened by the fact that triathletes are affected by the wind chill factor [23,24] during cycling (continued cooling). The International Triathlon Union (ITU) has taken this into consideration, as they have incorporated both air temperature and water temperature into their competition rules [7]. According to ITU competition rules, the swim can be shortened or cancelled according to a combined water temperature and air temperature.

4.4. Practical Implications

From a safety perspective, athletes competing in a race should never be exposed to environmental conditions that induce mild hypothermia or worse. The Tre therefore should not drop more than 2.0 °C, or below 35 °C. Taking into account the post-immersion cooling, the maximum drop during the swim should be less than 1.5 °C to ensure athletes' body temperatures do not fall within hypothermic ranges during subsequent portions of the event. For those undertaking an open water swim only, it should be realised that the participants may have their lowest deep body temperature after the event when attempting, for example, to drive home.

4.5. Limitations

For practical reasons, the Tre continued to be measured 20–90 min after the swim. Ideally, the measurements should have been continued until the Tre was back to baseline values. Further, more details about the wetsuit (thickness, fit, conditions) is warranted. The surface temperature of the wet suit should also be measured to better explain the relationship between Tsk and the drop in Tre.

5. Conclusions

It is concluded that the temperature response to swimming in a wetsuit in 10 °C water is highly individual. However, the Tre of no participant in the present study cooled more than 2 °C during the first 30 min of the swim. To be on the safe side, this would probably correspond to a maximum swim distance of 1000 m in 10 °C water. One would expect even the least able swimmers to cover 1000 m in 30 min: with the caveat that they do not suffer swim failure due to neuromuscular cooling.

Author Contributions: Conceptualization, J.M. and J.H.; investigation, J.M., M.M., T.S., and J.H.; writing—original draft preparation, J.M.; writing—review and editing, J.M., M.M., T.S., M.T. and J.H.; visualization, J.H.; supervision, M.T. and J.H.

Funding: This research received external funding from Hardangervidda Triathlon Club and the Norwegian Triathlon Federation.

Acknowledgments: The authors would like to acknowledge paramedics Emilie Nordstrøm, Charlotte Engan, Oda Johanne Reiholm, Frida Klaudine Martiniussen Mæland, Tonje Lunde and Stine Bakken for medical safety during the cold water swim investigations. We would also like to acknowledge students from the Norwegian School of Sport Sciences, Julie Stang and Camilla Rønn Illidi, for helping with data collection.

Conflicts of Interest: The authors declare no conflict of interest.

References

1. Knechtle, B.; Knechtle, P.; Lepers, R. Participation and performance trends in ultra-triathlons from 1985 to 2009. *Scand. J. Med. Sci. Sport* **2011**, *21*, e82–e90. [CrossRef] [PubMed]
2. It's Grim up Norse: The World's Toughest Triathlon. The Telegraph. Available online: https://www.telegraph.co.uk/men/active/11231917/Its-grim-up-Norse-the-worlds-toughest-triathlon.html (accessed on 15 April 2019).
3. Athletes Guide—Norseman Xtreme Triathlon. Available online: https://nxtri.com/race-info/athlete-guide/ (accessed on 1 April 2019).
4. Norseman Swim Shortened. Slowtwitch.com. Available online: https://www.slowtwitch.com/News/2015_Norseman_swim_shortened_5243.html (accessed on 19 February 2019).
5. Be Prepared for a Cold Swim. Available online: https://nxtri.com/be-prepared-for-a-cold-swim/ (accessed on 1 April 2019).
6. Pressure is on for the ÖtillÖ World Championship. 2018. Available online: https://otilloswimrun.com/pressure-is-on-for-the-otillo-swimrun-world-championship/ (accessed on 5 November 2018).
7. International Triathlon Union. ITU Competition Rules. 2018. Available online: https://www.triathlon.org/uploads/docs/itusport_competition-rules_2019.pdf (accessed on 20 may 2019).

8. Saycell, J.; Lomax, M.; Massey, H.; Tipton, M. Scientific rationale for changing lower water temperature limits for triathlon racing to 12 °C with wetsuits and 16°C without wetsuits. *Br. J. Sports Med.* **2018**, *52*, 702–708. [CrossRef] [PubMed]
9. FINA. Fina Open Water Swimming Rules for 2017–2021. Available online: https://www.fina.org/sites/default/files/2017_2021_ows_12092017_ok.pdf (accessed on 1 September 2018).
10. Saycell, J.; Lomax, M.; Massey, H.; Tipton, M. How cold is too cold? Establishing the minimum water temperature limits for marathon swim racing. *Br. J. Sports Med.* **2019**. [CrossRef] [PubMed]
11. Corrado, D.; Pelliccia, A.; Heidbuchel, H.; Sharma, S.; Link, M.; Basso, C.; Biffi, A.; Buja, G.; Delise, P.; Gussac, I.; et al. Recommendations for interpretation of 12-lead electrocardiogram in the athlete. *Eur. Heart J.* **2009**, *31*, 243–259. [CrossRef] [PubMed]
12. Corrado, D.; Pelliccia, A.; Bjørnstad, H.H.; Vanhees, L.; Biffi, A.; Borjesson, M.; Panhuyzen-Goedkoop, N.; Deligiannis, A.; Solberg, E.; Dugmore, D.; et al. Cardiovascular pre-participation screening of young competitive athletes for prevention of sudden death: Proposal for a common European protocol—Consensus Statement of the Study Group of Sport Cardiology of the Working Group of Cardiac Rehabilitation an. *Eur. Heart J.* **2005**, *26*, 516–524. [CrossRef] [PubMed]
13. Åstrand, P.O.; Rodahl, K.; Dahl, H.A.; Strømme, S.B. *Textbook of Work Physiology: Physiological Bases of Exercise*; Human Kinetics: Windsor, ON, Canada, 2003.
14. Filseth, O.M.; Fredriksen, K.; Gamst, T.M.; Gilbert, M.; Hesselberg, N.; Næsheim, T. Veileder for håndtering av aksidentell Hypothermi i Helse Nord. Guidelines for handling of accidental hypothermia, Northern Norway Regional Health Authority. Available online: http://h24-files.s3.amazonaws.com/90181/663578-X0gAY.pdf (accessed on 1 September 2018).
15. Soar, J.; Perkins, G.D.; Abbas, G.; Alfonzo, A.; Barelli, A.; Bierens, J.J.; Brugger, H.; Deakin, C.D.; Dunning, J.; Georgiou, M.; et al. European Resuscitation Council Guidelines for Resuscitation 2010 Section 8. Cardiac arrest in special circumstances: Electrolyte abnormalities, poisoning, drowning, accidental hypothermia, hyperthermia, asthma, anaphylaxis, cardiac surgery, trauma, pregna. *Resuscitation* **2010**, *81*, 1400. [CrossRef] [PubMed]
16. International Triathlon Union. Guidelines for Management of Triathlon Related Medical Emergencies. Available online: https://www.triathlon.org/uploads/docs/itusport_2013_medical_guidelines-for-management-of-medical-triathlon-emergencies.pdf (accessed on 1 may 2019).
17. Tipton, M.; Bradford, C. Moving in extreme environments: Open water swimming in cold and warm water. *Extreme Physiol. Med.* **2014**, *3*, 12. [CrossRef] [PubMed]
18. Brannigan, D.; Rogers, I.R.; Jacobs, I.; Montgomery, A.; Williams, A.; Khangure, N. Hypothermia is a significant medical risk of mass participation long-distance open water swimming. *Wilderness Environ. Med.* **2009**, *20*, 14–18. [CrossRef] [PubMed]
19. De Castro, R.R.T.; Da Nbrega, A.C.L. Hypothermia in open-water swimming events: A medical risk that deserves more attention. *Wilderness Environ. Med.* **2009**, *20*, 394–395. [CrossRef] [PubMed]
20. Diversi, T.; Franks-Kardum, V.; Climstein, M. The effect of cold water endurance swimming on core temperature in aspiring English Channel swimmers. *Extreme Physiol. Med.* **2016**, *5*. [CrossRef]
21. Prado, A.; Dufek, J.; Navalta, J.; Lough, N.; Mercer, J. A first look into the influence of triathlon wetsuit on resting blood pressure and heart rate variability. *Biol. Sport* **2017**, *34*, 77–82. [CrossRef] [PubMed]
22. Nuckton, T.J.; Claman, D.M.; Goldreich, D.; Wendt, F.C.; Nuckton, J.G. Hypothermia and afterdrop, following open water swimming: The Alcatraz/San Francisco Swim study. *Am. J. Emerg. Med.* **2000**, *18*, 703–707. [CrossRef] [PubMed]
23. Bluestein, M. An evaluation of the wind chill factor: Its development and applicability. *J. Biomech. Eng.* **1998**, *120*, 255–258. [CrossRef] [PubMed]
24. Moore, G.W.K.; Semple, J.L. Freezing and Frostbite on Mount Everest: New Insights into Wind Chill and Freezing Times at Extreme Altitude. *High Alt. Med. Biol.* **2011**, *12*, 271–275. [CrossRef] [PubMed]

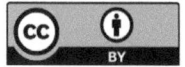

© 2019 by the authors. Licensee MDPI, Basel, Switzerland. This article is an open access article distributed under the terms and conditions of the Creative Commons Attribution (CC BY) license (http://creativecommons.org/licenses/by/4.0/).

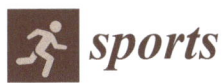

Article

Effectiveness of Manual Therapy, Customised Foot Orthoses and Combined Therapy in the Management of Plantar Fasciitis—A RCT

Casper Grim [1,*], Ruth Kramer [2], Martin Engelhardt [1], Swen Malte John [3], Thilo Hotfiel [1,4] and Matthias Wilhelm Hoppe [1,5]

1. Department of Orthopaedic, Trauma, Hand and Neuro Surgery, Klinikum Osnabrueck GmbH, 49076 Osnabrueck, Germany; martin.engelhardt@klinikum-os.de (M.E.); thilo.hotfiel@klinikum-os.de (T.H.); matthias.hoppe@klinikum-os.de (M.W.H.)
2. Physiopraxis Kramer, 49492 Westerkappeln, Germany; ruth@physiopraxis-kramer.de
3. Department of Dermatology, Environmental Medicine and Health Theory, University of Osnabrueck, 49076 Osnabrueck, Germany; sjohn@uos.de
4. Department of Orthopedic Surgery, Friedrich-Alexander-University Erlangen-Nuremberg, 91054 Erlangen, Germany
5. Department of Movement and Training Science, University of Wuppertal, 42119 Wuppertal, Germany
* Correspondence: casper.grim@klinikum-os.de

Received: 30 March 2019; Accepted: 26 May 2019; Published: 28 May 2019

Abstract: Background: Plantar fasciitis (PF) is one of the most common causes of plantar heel pain. Objective: To evaluate the effectiveness of three different treatment approaches in the management of PF. Methods: Sixty-three patients (44 female, 19 men; 48.4 ± 9.8 years) were randomly assigned into a manual therapy (MT), customised foot orthosis (FO) and a combined therapy (combined) group. The primary outcomes of pain and function were evaluated using the American Orthopaedic Foot and Ankle Society-Ankle Hindfoot Scale (AOFAS-AHS) and the patient reported outcome measure (PROM) Foot Pain and Function Scale (FPFS). Data were evaluated at baseline (T0) and at follow-up sessions after 1 month, 2 months and 3 months (T1–T3). Results: All three treatments showed statistically significant ($p < 0.01$) improvements in both scales from T0 to T1. However, the MT group showed greater improvements than both other groups ($p < 0.01$). Conclusion: Manual therapy, customised foot orthoses and combined treatments of PF all reduced pain and function, with the greatest benefits shown by isolated manual therapy.

Keywords: plantar fasciitis; heel pain; manual therapy; joint mobilization; customised orthoses; insoles; back pain

1. Introduction

Plantar fasciitis (PF) is reported as the most common cause of plantar heel pain and is referred to as plantar fasciosis or fasciopathy, because these terms more accurately describe the inflammatory degenerative nature of the disease [1–5]. The prevalence rate ranges from 4% in general to 7% in older populations, and from 8% in athletes to 25% in runners [6]. In non-athletes, women are more frequently affected [1,7,8] and have a higher risk of persisting symptoms [9] than men.

The aetiology is largely unknown [2] and risk factors remain unclear. Obesity, prolonged standing, running, limited ankle dorsiflexion, shortened triceps surae, hindfoot malalignment and increased age are all considered as potential risk factors [2,4,6,10,11]; however, their scientific evidence is weak. The high occurrence rate and level of impairment require a better understanding not only of the diagnosis, but also of evidence-based recommendations for the therapy. Concerning the latter, the quality of the studies is heterogeneous and often several forms of therapy are carried out simultaneously [1,2,6]. This makes it difficult to determine the effectiveness of any individual therapy or to rank therapies in order of their effectiveness [4]. Many patients report having persisting or recurrent pain following treatment [12]. In addition to night splints, resistance training, corticoid injections and extracorporeal shockwave therapy, manual therapy and foot orthoses are commonly recommended interventions [13,14].

Due to limited research, there are however no clear arguments for the use of foot orthoses. The theoretical underpinning for their use includes improvement of the hindfoot alignment, the relief in plantar pressure to the origin of the PF and modification in heel pitch, which may alter the mechanical loading of the plantar fascia [15]. A lack of high quality evidence was found for the use of foot orthoses [6,16]. Statistically significant differences were not found between customised or prefabricated foot orthoses or soft and firm foot orthotic materials [2,6,13,17]. A longer duration of foot orthoses use was associated with impairment in the plantar fascia and toe flexor muscle function [12]. There are no two studies that used the same type of orthoses, which limits the comparisons between studies and suggestions as to which orthoses features may be most effective. What is considered most important is whether foot orthoses are beneficial to patients by effectively alleviating their symptoms [6].

There is only weak [1] or moderate evidence for short-term treatment [18,19] using manual therapy interventions. However, compared to physical therapy, patients needed fewer sessions, thereby reducing treatment costs [20]. Stretching of the calf muscles and improvement of the ankle dorsiflexion is often recommended [13]; however, this additional mobilisation was no more effective than stretching and ultrasound treatment alone [21]. In a study comparing customised foot orthoses versus mobilisation of the foot and stretching, the mobilisation group had better results after two weeks, but not after one or two months [17]. In only two of the reviewed studies [7,22], a single treatment was applied in isolation in the experimental group. The other two well-rated studies reporting significant improvements [1,23] used multiple interventions simultaneously. Thus, the studies did not allow conclusions to be drawn with regards to the effectiveness of manual therapy alone [4]. In an osteopathic study, the overall results were not significantly improved with three treatments [24].

After receiving conservative treatments, nearly 50% of patients still had symptoms when interviewed after nine years [9,25]. Patients with plantar heel pain had a high prevalence of lumbar back pain. Compared to the control group, more than twice as many patients with plantar heel pain had lumbar back pain with the corresponding risk being five times higher. Treatment of local and proximal restrictions, including those associated with back pain, may be justified for improving the management of PF [25]. Hence, in the current study, the spine was also evaluated and treated. To date, there has been no prospective, randomised, controlled trial in which manual therapy and customised foot orthoses were investigated in relation to back pain in patients with PF.

Thus, the aim of this study was to compare the effectiveness of manual therapy, customised foot orthoses and combined therapy in the management of PF.

2. Materials and Methods

The Ethics Committee of the University of Osnabrueck approved and accepted all procedures involved in this study (4/7/1043.5). The patients were consecutively recruited over a 36-month period. Patients were screened for eligibility by a foot and ankle surgeon. Inclusion criteria were: a clinical diagnosis of PF with symptoms for <6 months and an age ≥18 years. Exclusion criteria were: red flags for manual therapy interventions, previous surgeries, fractures, rheumatoid diseases, tumours and other forms of therapy during the study. All patients were informed about the procedures involved in the study and signed an informed consent form. Based on order of appearance, the patients were randomly assigned into one of the three groups: (i) manual therapy (MT) group, (ii) customised foot orthosis (FO) group and (iii) combined therapy (combined) group. The patients were then referred to a manual therapist, an orthopaedic technician or to both, respectively.

2.1. Examination Procedures

All patients provided demographic information, medical history and previous treatments of PF. They received a physical examination at baseline (T0) and at follow-up sessions after 1 month, 2 months and 3 months (T1–T3). The primary outcomes of pain and function were evaluated using the American Orthopaedic Foot and Ankle Society-Ankle Hindfoot Scale (AOFAS-AHS) and the patient reported outcome measure (PROM) Foot Pain and Function Scale (FPFS). An intention to treat analysis was carried out using missing data from the last available value for the final evaluation [26,27]. Figure 1 shows the patient recruitment and sample sizes, drop-outs and intention to treat of the three groups.

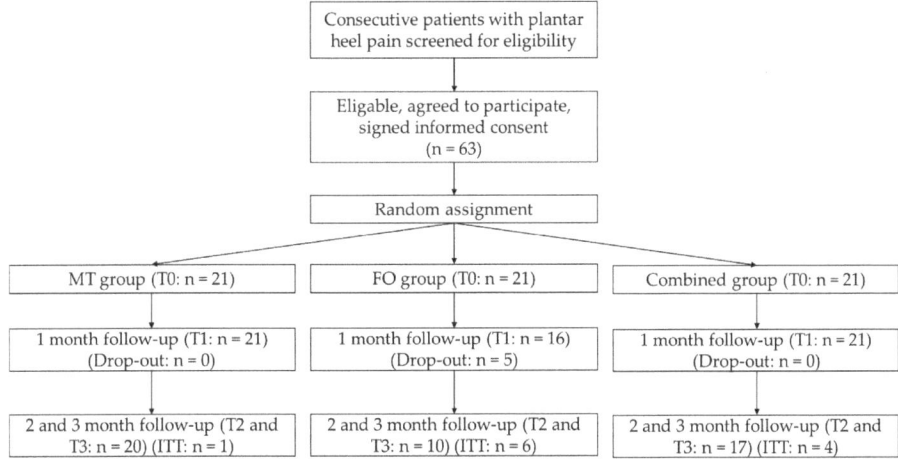

Figure 1. Flow-diagram of patient recruitment. Abbreviations: MT, manual therapy; FO, foot orthoses; ITT, Intention to treat; T0, baseline; T1–T3, follow-up sessions after 1–3 months.

2.2. Outcome Measures

The AOFAS-AHS includes both subjective, patient reported items in pain and function (60%) and objective, physician assessed items in function (40%). The AHS is scored from 0 to 100, where higher values indicate a better outcome [28,29]. The AHS was preferred over the commonly used Short Form 36 (SF-36), because the SF-36 has not been specifically studied in relation to foot and ankle disorders [4]. Additionally, the time required for the evaluation of the nine items of the AHS is lower than for the SF-36, which increases patient compliance in reporting data. Despite methodological criticisms, the AHS is an established and frequently used rating system, making it possible to compare the results with other studies [30,31]. The degrees of correlation and reliability provided an acceptable validity for the subjective scores; however, the reliability of the objective component of the AHS has yet to be reported [29,32]. There have been no reliable data published regarding the minimal clinically important difference (MCID) related to the AOFAS score [29]. The MCID of the AHS in hallux valgus surgery were indicated between 7.9 and 30.2, effect size derived 8.4 [33] or 8.9 out of 100 [34]. In the current study, the MCID was set at 10 out of 100. In the AHS, the subscale pain is one single item. Pain is however subjective, with PROM providing the most valid measure of the experience [35].

In order to obtain more differentiated values for the typical pain of PF, the Foot Pain and Function Scale (FPFS) was created with an 11-point numeric rating scale (NRS) from 0 to 10, where higher values indicate better outcomes. The low gradation of the NRS for pain compensates for the large variance in point values in the Ankle Hindfoot Scale [29]. The FPFS contains five questions on pain (first steps, during rest, on pressure, while standing, weight bearing) and five questions about function (limping, weakness, stiffness, restrictions in sports, at work). The highest possible total score is 100. The FPFS uses 20 questions from the Visual Analogue Scale Foot and Ankle (VAS FA) [31], all of which were validated against the SF-36 and the Hannover Questionnaire. VAS and NRS have a well-documented reliability and validity in a variety of populations [1,4]. Due to the heterogeneity between study results, no meaningful overall value for the MCID change can be determined. In the subgroup pain, the NRS median for the MCID was 15% [36], those considered as clinically important or "improved" ≥20%, clinically very important or "much improved" ≥30% and "very much improved" ≥40%, respectively [37–39].

Blinding is barely achievable with the application of manual therapy in interventional studies, making an even higher quality of the evaluation difficult [4]. Therefore, in the current study, assignment of the patients to treatment groups was blinded for the therapist. The form of intervention itself was recognisable to patients and therapists, though patients did not know if they were participating in an intervention or control group.

2.3. Interventions

The patients were treated with manual therapy twice during the first week and subsequently once per week for the remaining three-month period.

Patients in the manual therapy and combined group were evaluated with a standardised clinical examination. The therapist used pre- and post-tests for each joint of the foot and intervertebral segment of the spine. The order and type of treatment in therapy was standardised. The tests and joint mobilisations were performed talocrural for dorsiflexion, subtalar for eversion and inversion, and then tarsi transversal for pro- and supination. The sacroiliac joints and the symphysis pubica were assessed and mobilised as well as the intervertebral joints in the supine position, partially in lateral decubitus with rotation.

In the foot orthoses group, the orthopaedic technician used blueprints and foot scanners as measuring instruments for the production of the orthoses. The orthoses were checked with pedobarography and medilogic soles (T&T MediLogic Medizintechnik GmbH, Schoenefeld, Germany). With the data obtained from the pressure distribution measurement, the orthoses (Footpower, FSGmbH, Gummersbach, Germany) were milled with three layers (shore hardness A 50, A 25 and A 35) and an additive support layer from ethylene vinyl acetate using computer-aided design and computer-aided manufacturing techniques. To relieve pressure of the origin of the plantar fascia, a canal (referring to the medial tuber calcanei) was milled and filled with soft material and a cushion layer was applied to the heel. Subsequently, the footprints were produced, and the orthoses were individually manufactured (Figure 2). The underlying idea of this type of foot orthoses is to relieve the plantar fascia, reduce heel pressure and pain and obtain a positive, non-restrictive effect on joint mobility without compromising the muscle activity of the foot itself. At the highest point of the foot orthoses, a medial support for the sustentaculum tali was moulded. Through raising the toe berries and using a retrocapital edged pelotte, pre-tensioning of the plantar fascia was expected.

2.4. Statistical Analysis

The AOFAS-AHS and FPF Scale data were transferred into Microsoft Excel and were then analysed with a statistical software package (IBM, SPSS version 23, Chicago, IL, USA). Descriptive data were presented as relative frequency, mean and standard deviation. Differences in the distributions were investigated by chi-square tests. Levene tests were applied to examine the variance homogeneity between the three groups. Differences in the changes in scale values from T0 to T3 between the three groups were investigated using an analysis of variance (ANOVA) and Bonferroni post hoc tests. Differences between T0 and T3 within each group were calculated using dependent Student's t-tests. Differences in the numbers of physiotherapy and evaluation of the foot orthoses between the groups were investigated by independent Student's t-tests. A p-value of ≤0.05 was assumed to be statistically significant.

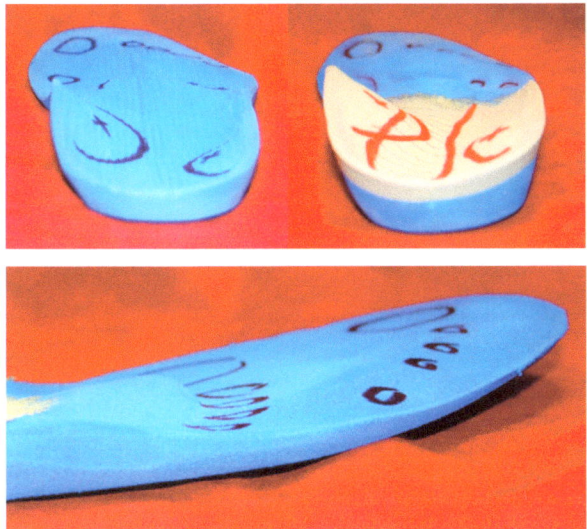

Figure 2. Customised foot orthoses.

3. Results

Sixty-three patients met the eligibility criteria. The mean age and duration of PF symptoms were 48.4 ± 9.8 years and 4.4 ± 1.3 months, respectively. There were no statistically significant differences for age, gender and body mass index between the three groups at T0 ($p > 0.05$). However, the patients of the FO group had statistically significant shorter duration of symptoms, fewer had back pain with shorter duration, lower FPFS values for work, and received fewer treatments and medications before starting the study than both other groups (Table 1).

Table 1. Demographic data, symptoms, and therapies of the three groups at T0.

Variable	MT Group (n = 21)	FO Group (n = 21)	Combined Group (n = 21)	p-Value
Female sex, n (%)	16 (76.2)	14 (66.7)	14 (66.7)	0.74[1]
BMI (kg/m^2)	28.3 ± 6.2	30.4 ± 4.8	29.4 ± 4.2	0.43[2]
Duration of PF symptoms (month)	5.3 ± 0.8	2.9 ± 1.8	5.0 ± 1.2	<0.01[2]
Back pain, n (%)	19 (90.5)	6 (28.6)	17 (81.0)	<0.01[2]
Duration of back pain (years)	11.0 ± 8.1	2.5 ± 6.0	9.0 ± 8.6	<0.01[2]
Work: Standing, weight bearing, n (%)	11 (52.4)	7 (43.7)	13 (61.9)	0.02[2]
Sporting activities, n (%)	17 (81.0)	12 (57.1)	18 (85.7)	0.08[2]
Therapy pre-study, n (%)	17 (81.0)	8 (38.1)	17 (81.0)	<0.01[1]
Duration of therapy pre-study (month)	3.4 ± 2.4	1.2 ± 2.1	3.5 ± 2.4	<0.01[2]
Medications at the start of the study, n (%)	12 (57.1)	6 (28.6)	14 (66.7)	0.02[1]

Abbreviations: MT, manual therapy; FO, foot orthoses; BMI, body mass index; n, number; PF, plantar fasciitis; [1] Chi square tests; [2] ANOVA.

A total of 58 (92%) patients appeared for the follow-up assessment after one month (T1). Five patients from the FO group were counted as drop-outs (Figure 1). A total of 47 (75%) patients completed the three-month follow-up (T0). Intention to treat was applied in the MT, FO and combined group for one (5%), six (29%) and four (19%) patients, respectively. There were statistically significant changes for the AOFAS-AHS ($p < 0.01$) and the FPFS ($p < 0.01$).

Between-group differences in the AOFAS-AHS and its subscales showed a greater improvement from T0–T3 in the MT group ($p < 0.01$) than the FO and combined group (Figure 3, Table 2).

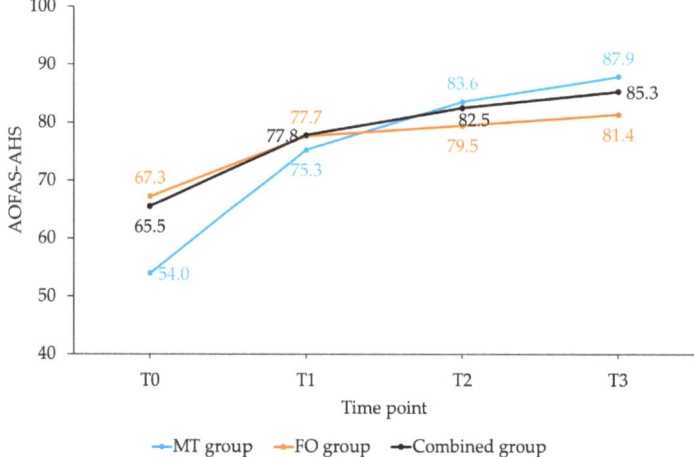

Figure 3. Changes in American Orthopaedic Foot and Ankle Score-Ankle Hindfoot Scale (AOFAS-AHS) for the three groups from T0–T3. Abbreviations: MT, manual therapy; FO, foot orthoses; T0, baseline; T1–T3, follow-up sessions after 1–3 months.

Table 2. Comparison of the mean improvements in American Orthopaedic Foot and Ankle Score-Ankle Hindfoot Scale (AOFAS-AHS), Foot Pain and Function Scale (FPFS) and their subscales for the three groups from T0–T3.

Variable	MT Group (n = 21)	FO Group (n = 16)	Combined Group (n = 21)
AOFAS-AHS	33.9*	14.1	19.1
Pain subscale	48.8*	26.3	26.3
Function subscale	24.5*	6.1	6.1
FPFS	37.2*	14.6	22.9
Pain subscale	48.4*	28.4	28.4
Function subscale	32.8*	19.0	19.0

Abbreviations: MT, manual therapy; FO, foot orthoses; * Statistically significant higher ($p < 0.01$) than in the other groups.

Likewise, between-group differences in the FPFS and in its subscales showed that the MT group improved more from T0–T3 ($p < 0.01$) than the FO and combined group (Figure 4, Table 2).

Besides the statistically significant differences, all three groups showed clinically meaningful improvements over time. Differences in AHS from T0–T3 for the MT, FO and combined group were 35% ("much improved"), 15% ("minimally improved") and 21% ("improved"), respectively. The corresponding FPFS changes were 37% ("much improved"), 18% ("minimally improved") and 24% ("improved"), respectively. The FO and combined group did not reach the MCID in AHS subscale function. In all groups, the improvement in subscale pain was higher than in subscale function.

One FPFS question was "first step" pain after a period of rest. The improvement of the values in the MT, FO and combined group were 50%, 32% and 43%, respectively. Effectiveness on pressure pain and weight bearing were similar; in the MT group for 56% and 59%, in the FO group for 41% and 41% and in the combined group for 45% and 42%. The values for pain during rest and while standing were lower, just as in the subscale function for weakness and stiffness. Restrictions in sports and work had an improvement of 51% and 30% in the MT group, 26% and 31% in the FO group and 28% and 20% in the combined group. The improvements in limping varied greatly between the groups; 41% in the MT group, 36% in the FO group and 16% in the combined group.

The number of treatments did not differ between the MT and combined group ($p > 0.05$).

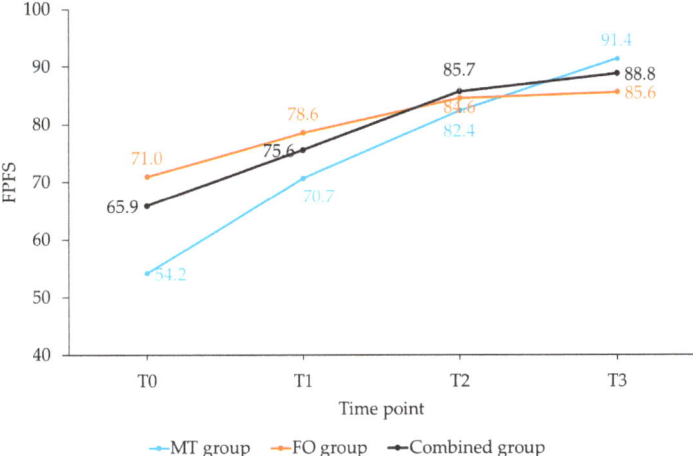

Figure 4. Changes in Foot Pain and Function Scale (FPFS) for the three groups from T0–T3. Abbreviations: MT, manual therapy; FO, foot orthoses; T0, baseline; T1–T3, follow-up sessions after 1–3 months.

4. Discussion

The results of our study showed that all three interventions for PF achieved both a statistically and clinically significant improvement over time. Furthermore, it suggests that manual therapy offers greater clinical benefits, reducing pain and improving function compared to customised foot orthoses and combined therapy. The application of manual techniques was standardised, and no additional forms of therapy were used, making the therapy reproducible and comparable to other studies with multiple concurrent therapies.

4.1. Comparison with Previous Studies

Cleland and colleagues [1] conducted a study in which 30 patients of a manual therapy group underwent a five minute aggressive soft tissue mobilisation directed at the triceps surae and insertion of the plantar fascia as well as a rear foot eversion mobilisation. It included an impairment-based manual therapy at the hip, knee, ankle and foot on the clinical decision making of the treating therapist. The other group with 30 patients was treated with electrophysical agents and exercises. Three outcome measures were reported: Lower Extremity Functional Scale (LEFS), Foot and Ankle Ability Measures (FAAM) and a numerical pain rating scale (NPRS). The overall group-by-time interaction showed significantly better results for the manual therapy group. In comparison to the Cleland study, the improvement reported in the pain subscale was greater at the three month follow-up than the six month follow-up, and the AHS and FPFS total scores were higher than in LEFS of Cleland et al. [1]. The underlying mechanism for improvements related to manual physical therapy in the study of Cleland et al. [1] could not be determined as a first level of standardised intervention was used in addition to a second level of intervention that utilised an impairments-based approach. Hence, it could not be determined with any certainty which specific manual therapy and exercise technique was most advantageous.

In our study, the focus was placed on treating local impairments of the joint structures of the foot and the proximal impairments of the spine. No stretching of the soleus and gastrocnemius muscle or plantar fascia took place, and no additional treatments of the knee and hip joints were performed. McClinton and colleagues [25] also reported an association between PF and lumbar back pain. The result of our study suggests that a therapy integrating the spine may help to alleviate the often long-lasting symptoms of PF and ultimately achieve a better result.

The Burmeister study [24] used a similar intervention methodology. In addition to the spine, a treatment of internal organs was conducted with 15 patients. Three osteopathic treatments were conducted within a three-week period. Despite improvement on some items, no significant difference could be detected between the verum and control group. It is possible that a higher number of treatments could have led to a further improvement; however, this was not tested.

In our study, many patients actually required three months of therapy with a mean of 10.6 treatments to be symptom free. Cleland et al. [1] also questioned whether more than six therapies would have resulted in a further improvement in function. The dosage also remained unclear in the included studies of the clinical practise guidelines of Martin and colleagues [13]. The majority of the studies selected by Mischke and colleagues in their review [4] evaluated the short-term effects of a treatment. This might be less meaningful in the often long-lasting course of PF.

Custom made foot orthoses versus a combined treatment of manipulation and mobilisation of the foot and stretching exercises with 10 patients per group were compared in a study by Dimou and colleagues [40]. A review by Hawke and colleagues [17] reported that both groups in the Dimou study had statistically significant reductions in pain on the NPRS. After only two weeks, there was a statistically significant difference in foot pain favouring mobilisation of the foot versus stretching, with no significant difference after one month and two months. The review indicated that the customised foot orthoses did not reduce foot pain more than non-customised or sham foot orthoses, including when combining them with stretching exercises or night splints. However, it is suggested that using customised foot orthoses and night splints together may reduce foot pain. The foot orthoses in our study complied with Hawke and colleague's definition [17] of customised orthoses: fabricated according to practitioner-prescribed specifications, the orthoses should be contoured, removable in-shoe devices that are moulded or milled from an impression of the foot. In our study, customised foot orthoses were found to be less effective compared to manual therapy or combined treatment. The result also showed that wearing the foot orthoses over three months did not reduce the number of manual therapies required in comparison to the MT group.

Overall, PF still remains a "black box". Besides insoles and manual therapy, different treatment options (e.g. resistance training, corticoid injections and extracorporeal shockwave therapy) seem to be reasonable in the treatment of PF. It is, however, unclear what the underlying mechanisms are. Additionally, it is important to highlight that individuals may respond differently to the various treatment options, meaning that there is no general or overall recommendation for the treatment of PF. In particular, the results of manual therapy for treating PF suggest that the pathophysiology seems to be more complex and not fully understood. Our study shows that joint mobility and low back pain play a role in treating PF. Joint dysfunction treated with manual therapy seems to lead to a functional improvement and a relief of symptoms. If these dysfunctions lead directly to altered mechanical loading of the plantar fascia or indirectly via the myofascial slings remains unclear. We found in our study that only a one- to two-week manual therapy intervention altered the symptoms of PF. It is unclear [41] if this easy-to-implement treatment can be used for preventive purposes, e.g. in athletes, as it requires more research.

4.2. Strength and Limitations

In this study, manual therapy and customised foot orthoses treatments were carried out in isolation, meaning that the methodology is reproducible, and any differences clearly assigned to the treatment condition. Based on experience from other studies in which 3–6 weeks of therapy were reported to be insufficient, the duration of treatment in our study was set at three months. Since the disease is often long-lasting with severe discomfort, patients should receive treatment in the control group, rather than to being exposed to placebo treatment over such a long period. The entire sample population of our study was recruited from one clinical practice, which could be seen as a possible limitation. As a limitation of our study, we did not perform a power analysis prior to the upcoming recruitment. However, it must be considered that we were the first to investigate the effectiveness of these three different treatment approaches in the management of PF within a randomised controlled trial and that we nevertheless found statistically significant differences in our data.

The baseline outcome scores of the foot orthoses group were significantly higher at the beginning of the study than those of the manual therapy and combined group. So, selection bias may have occurred. High scores at baseline generally complicate an improvement over the course of the study or even make it impossible. To enable an improvement, a limitation of the input values set on the scales in the inclusion criteria would have been useful. An attrition bias occurred, because participation in the follow-up assessment in the FO group with 10 patients, versus 20 in MT, respectively 17 in MT and FO (combined group) was significantly lower. To counteract possible bias, we performed an intention to treat analysis. The weekly treatment in the manual therapy group represented a more intense support for the patients over three months. In contrast, the patients of the foot orthoses group had one appointment with the orthopaedic technician for the footprints and a second to receive the fabricated foot orthoses. After receiving their orthoses, patients may have seen little reason for clinical follow-up appointments, resulting in a performance bias. This may have reduced the success rate, because a higher number of FO patients no longer participated in the evaluation compared to the manual therapy group.

The combination of manual therapy and customised foot orthoses should demonstrate whether two simultaneously applied interventions would improve the outcome more than one treatment in isolation. According to our study design, we intended to mobilise the local restrictions of the foot before producing the foot orthoses. This was however not possible in all cases. The actual procedure in the combination therapy could have contributed to the fact that the combined group hardly achieved any improvements in the items function and alignment of the foot axis, whereas in the manual therapy group, the results increased in both items. Some patients of the combined treatment group reported foot pain, possibly caused by the fact that the orthoses no longer fitted optimally after mobilisation of the restrictions of the feet. Therefore, differences were smaller in the manual therapy group than in the foot orthoses group. Caution should be applied when interpreting these results, as patients in the manual therapy group had significantly more complaints of accompanying back pain, which could be another explanation as to why manual therapy was more successful in this group.

4.3. Clinical Implications

A meaningful overall minimal clinically important change (MCID) could not be reported for NRS or AOFAS-AHS PHP (plantar heel pain) [36]. Additionally, it is a problem to calculate the mean difference in pain score for the treatment group and to compare it to the MCID, because MCID is a metric based on longitudinal differences in individuals and should be used in the same context [39]. Analyses of the relationships between changes in NPRS scores demonstrated a reduction of two points, or 30%, to be clinically important and were measured using a standard seven-point patient Global Impression of Change [37]. These results are similar to results that were found in lower back pain patients compared after physical therapy using a 15-point Global Rating of Change scale [42]. The Global Rating of Change scale has been criticised because it is a transitional scale that requires recall of prior health status [43]. The Global Rating of Change scale is not temporally stable, with a finding in one week not associating to functional results the following week. The Global Rating of Change scale is only correlated to functional measures up to three weeks [44], so it was not included as an additional measure in the current study.

5. Conclusions

Manual therapy, customised foot orthoses and the combined treatments achieved statistically and clinically significant improvements over time, with the greatest effect for the treatment of PF being found in the manual therapy group. In addition, the results indicate that integrating spinal treatment for patients experiencing back complaints together with PF could improve treatment outcome.

Author Contributions: C.G., R.K., and M.E. designed the manuscript. C.G., R.K. and M.W.H. have made major contributions in section "Results". T.H., M.E. and S.M.J. have made major contributions in drafting and writing the section "Discussion". All authors read and approved the final manuscript.

Funding: This research received no external funding.

Acknowledgments: The authors would like to thank Joana Brochhagen for her linguistic revisions.

Conflicts of Interest: The authors declare no conflict of interest.

References

1. Cleland, J.A.; Abbott, J.H.; Kidd, M.O.; Stockwell, S.; Cheney, S.; Gerrard, D.F.; Flynn, T.W. Manual physical therapy and exercise versus electrophysical agents and exercise in the management of plantar heel pain: A multicenter randomized clinical trial. *J. Orthop. Sports Phys. Ther.* **2009**, *39*, 573–585. [CrossRef] [PubMed]
2. Landorf, K.B. Plantar heel pain and plantar fasciitis. *BMJ Clin. Evid.* **2015**, *2015*, 1–46.
3. McMillan, A.M.; Landorf, K.B.; Barrett, J.T.; Menz, H.B.; Bird, A.R. Diagnostic imaging for chronic plantar heel pain: A systematic review and meta-analysis. *J. Foot. Ankle Res.* **2009**, *2*, 32. [CrossRef] [PubMed]
4. Mischke, J.J.; Jayaseelan, D.J.; Sault, J.D.; Emerson Kavchak, A.J. The symptomatic and functional effects of manual physical therapy on plantar heel pain: A systematic review. *J. Man. Manip. Ther.* **2017**, *25*, 3–10. [CrossRef] [PubMed]
5. Pollack, Y.; Shashua, A.; Kalichman, L. Manual therapy for plantar heel pain. *Foot* **2018**, *34*, 11–16. [CrossRef] [PubMed]
6. Whittaker, G.A.; Munteanu, S.E.; Menz, H.B.; Tan, J.M.; Rabusin, C.L.; Landorf, K.B. Foot orthoses for plantar heel pain: A systematic review and meta-analysis. *Br. J. Sports Med.* **2018**, *52*, 322–328. [CrossRef]
7. Ajimsha, M.S.; Binsu, D.; Chithra, S. Effectiveness of myofascial release in the management of plantar heel pain: A randomized controlled trial. *Foot* **2014**, *24*, 66–71. [CrossRef]
8. Renan-Ordine, R.; Alburquerque-Sendin, F.; de Souza, D.P.; Cleland, J.A.; Fernandez-de-Las-Penas, C. Effectiveness of myofascial trigger point manual therapy combined with a self-stretching protocol for the management of plantar heel pain: A randomized controlled trial. *J. Orthop. Sports Phys. Ther.* **2011**, *41*, 43–50. [CrossRef]
9. Hansen, L.; Krogh, T.P.; Ellingsen, T.; Bolvig, L.; Fredberg, U. Long-term prognosis of plantar fasciitis: A 5- to 15-year follow-up study of 174 patients with ultrasound examination. *Orthop. J. Sports Med.* **2018**, *6*, 2325967118757983. [CrossRef]
10. Goff, J.D.; Crawford, R. Diagnosis and treatment of plantar fasciitis. *Am. Fam. Physician* **2011**, *84*, 676–682.
11. Van Leeuwen, K.D.; Rogers, J.; Winzenberg, T.; van Middelkoop, M. Higher body mass index is associated with plantar fasciopathy/'plantar fasciitis': Systematic review and meta-analysis of various clinical and imaging risk factors. *Br. J. Sports Med.* **2016**, *50*, 972–981. [CrossRef] [PubMed]
12. McClinton, S.; Collazo, C.; Vincent, E.; Vardaxis, V. Impaired foot plantar flexor muscle performance in individuals with plantar heel pain and association with foot orthosis use. *J. Orthop. Sports Phys. Ther.* **2016**, *46*, 681–688. [CrossRef] [PubMed]
13. Martin, R.L.; Davenport, T.E.; Reischl, S.F.; McPoil, T.G.; Matheson, J.W.; Wukich, D.K.; McDonough, C.M.; American Physical Therapy Association. Heel pain-plantar fasciitis: Revision 2014. *J. Orthop. Sports Phys. Ther.* **2014**, *44*, 1–33. [CrossRef] [PubMed]
14. Huffer, D.; Hing, W.; Newton, R.; Clair, M. Strength training for plantar fasciitis and the intrinsic foot musculature: A systematic review. *Phys. Ther. Sport* **2017**, *24*, 44–52. [CrossRef] [PubMed]
15. Hotfiel, T.; Hotfiel, K.H.; Gelse, K.; Engelhardt, M.; Freiwald, J. Einlagenversorgung im leistungssport – indikationen, wirkungsweise, sportspezifische versorgungsstrategien [The use of insoles in competitive sports – Indications, effectiveness, sport specific treatment strategies]. *Sports Orthop. Traumatol.* **2016**, *32*, 250–257. [CrossRef]
16. Whittaker, G.A.; Munteanu, S.E.; Menz, H.B.; Landorf, K.B. Should foot orthoses be used for plantar heel pain? *Br. J. Sports Med.* **2018**, *52*, 1224–1225. [CrossRef] [PubMed]
17. Hawke, F.; Burns, J.; Radford, J.A.; du Toit, V. Custom-made foot orthoses for the treatment of foot pain. *Cochrane Database Syst. Rev.* **2008**, *16*, 1–131. [CrossRef]

18. Brantingham, J.W.; Bonnefin, D.; Perle, S.M.; Cassa, T.K.; Globe, G.; Pribicevic, M.; Hicks, M.; Korporaal, C. Manipulative therapy for lower extremity conditions: Update of a literature review. *J. Manipul. Physiol. Ther.* **2012**, *35*, 127–166. [CrossRef] [PubMed]
19. Brantingham, J.W.; Globe, G.; Pollard, H.; Hicks, M.; Korporaal, C.; Hoskins, W. Manipulative therapy for lower extremity conditions: Expansion of literature review. *J. Manipul. Physiol. Ther.* **2009**, *32*, 53–71. [CrossRef]
20. Fraser, J.J.; Glaviano, N.R.; Hertel, J. Utilization of physical therapy intervention among patients with plantar fasciitis in the united states. *J. Orthop. Sports Phys. Ther.* **2017**, *47*, 49–55. [CrossRef]
21. Shashua, A.; Flechter, S.; Avidan, L.; Ofir, D.; Melayev, A.; Kalichman, L. The effect of additional ankle and midfoot mobilizations on plantar fasciitis: A randomized controlled trial. *J. Orthop. Sports Phys. Ther.* **2015**, *45*, 265–272. [CrossRef] [PubMed]
22. Wynne, M.M.; Burns, J.M.; Eland, D.C.; Conatser, R.R.; Howell, J.N. Effect of counterstrain on stretch reflexes, hoffmann reflexes, and clinical outcomes in subjects with plantar fasciitis. *J. Am. Osteopath. Assoc.* **2006**, *106*, 547–556. [PubMed]
23. Saban, B.; Deutscher, D.; Ziv, T. Deep massage to posterior calf muscles in combination with neural mobilization exercises as a treatment for heel pain: A pilot randomized clinical trial. *Man. Ther.* **2014**, *19*, 102–108. [CrossRef] [PubMed]
24. Burmeister, S. Osteopathie und ihr Effektivität bei Fasciitis Plantaris. Master's Thesis, Donau Universität Krems, Krems, Germany, 2012.
25. McClinton, S.; Weber, C.F.; Heiderscheit, B. Low back pain and disability in individuals with plantar heel pain. *Foot* **2018**, *34*, 18–22. [CrossRef] [PubMed]
26. Armijo-Olivo, S.; Warren, S.; Magee, D. Intention to treat analysis, compliance, drop-outs and how to deal with missing data in clinical research: A review. *Phys. Ther. Rev.* **2009**, *14*, 36–45. [CrossRef]
27. Gupta, S.K. Intention-to-treat concept: A review. *Perspect. Clin. Res.* **2011**, *2*, 109–112. [CrossRef]
28. Kitaoka, H.B.; Alexander, I.J.; Adelaar, R.S.; Nunley, J.A.; Myerson, M.S.; Sanders, M. Clinical rating systems for the ankle-hindfoot, midfoot, hallux, and lesser toes. *Foot Ankle Int.* **1994**, *15*, 349–353. [CrossRef]
29. Madeley, N.J.; Wing, K.J.; Topliss, C.; Penner, M.J.; Glazebrook, M.A.; Younger, A.S. Responsiveness and validity of the sf-36, ankle osteoarthritis scale, aofas ankle hindfoot score, and foot function index in end stage ankle arthritis. *Foot Ankle Int.* **2012**, *33*, 57–63. [CrossRef]
30. Kostuj, T.; Schaper, K.; Baums, M.H.; Lieske, S. Eine Validierung des aofas-ankle-hindfoot-scale für den deutschen Sprachraum [German Validation of the AOFAS ankle hindfoot scale]. *Foot Ankle* **2014**, *12*, 100–106.
31. Richter, M.; Zech, S.; Geerling, J.; Frink, M.; Knobloch, K.; Krettek, C. A new foot and ankle outcome score: Questionaire based, subjective, visual-analogue-scale, validated and computerized. *Foot Ankle Surg.* **2006**, *12*, 191–199. [CrossRef]
32. Ibrahim, T.; Beiri, A.; Azzabi, M.; Best, A.J.; Taylor, G.J.; Menon, D.K. Reliability and validity of the subjective component of the american orthopaedic foot and ankle society clinical rating scales. *J. Foot Ankle Surg.* **2007**, *46*, 65–74. [CrossRef] [PubMed]
33. Chan, H.Y.; Chen, J.Y.; Zainul-Abidin, S.; Ying, H.; Koo, K.; Rikhraj, I.S. Minimal clinically important differences for american orthopaedic foot & ankle society score in hallux valgus surgery. *Foot Ankle Int.* **2017**, *38*, 551–557. [PubMed]
34. Dawson, J.; Doll, H.; Coffey, J.; Jenkinson, C. Responsiveness and minimally important change for the manchester-oxford foot questionnaire (moxfq) compared with aofas and sf-36 assessments following surgery for hallux valgus. *Osteoarthr. Cartil.* **2007**, *15*, 918–931. [CrossRef] [PubMed]
35. Katz, J.; Melzack, R. Measurement of pain. *Surg. Clin. North Am.* **1999**, *79*, 231–252. [CrossRef]
36. Olsen, M.F.; Bjerre, E.; Hansen, M.D.; Hilden, J.; Landler, N.E.; Tendal, B.; Hrobjartsson, A. Pain relief that matters to patients: Systematic review of empirical studies assessing the minimum clinically important difference in acute pain. *BMC Med.* **2017**, *15*, 35. [CrossRef]
37. Farrar, J.T.; Young, J.P., Jr.; LaMoreaux, L.; Werth, J.L.; Poole, R.M. Clinical importance of changes in chronic pain intensity measured on an 11-point numerical pain rating scale. *Pain* **2001**, *94*, 149–158. [CrossRef]

38. Hawker, G.A.; Mian, S.; Kendzerska, T.; French, M. Measures of adult pain: Visual analog scale for pain (vas pain), numeric rating scale for pain (nrs pain), mcgill pain questionnaire (mpq), short-form mcgill pain questionnaire (sf-mpq), chronic pain grade scale (cpgs), short form-36 bodily pain scale (sf-36 bps), and measure of intermittent and constant osteoarthritis pain (icoap). *Arthrit. Care Res.* **2011**, *63* (Suppl. 11), S240–S252.
39. Katz, N.P.; Paillard, F.C.; Ekman, E. Determining the clinical importance of treatment benefits for interventions for painful orthopedic conditions. *J. Orthop. Surg. Res.* **2015**, *10*, 24. [CrossRef]
40. Dimou, E.; Brantingham, J.; Wood, T. A randomized, controlled trial (with blinded observer) of chiropractic manipulation and achilles stretching vs orthotics for the treatment of plantar fasciitis. *J. Am. Chiropr. Assoc.* **2004**, *41*, 32–42.
41. Stecco, C.; Corradin, M.; Macchi, V.; Morra, A.; Porzionato, A.; Biz, C.; De Caro, R. Plantar fascia anatomy and its relationship with achilles tendon and paratenon. *J. Anat.* **2013**, *223*, 665–676. [CrossRef]
42. Childs, J.D.; Piva, S.R.; Fritz, J.M. Responsiveness of the numeric pain rating scale in patients with low back pain. *Spine* **2005**, *30*, 1331–1334. [CrossRef] [PubMed]
43. Michener, L.A.; Snyder, A.R.; Leggin, B.G. Responsiveness of the numeric pain rating scale in patients with shoulder pain and the effect of surgical status. *J. Sport Rehabil.* **2011**, *20*, 115–128. [CrossRef] [PubMed]
44. Garrison, C.; Cook, C. Clinimetrics corner: The global rating of change score (groc) poorly correlates with functional measures and is not temporally stable. *J. Man. Manip. Ther.* **2012**, *20*, 178–181. [CrossRef] [PubMed]

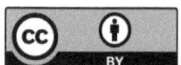

© 2019 by the authors. Licensee MDPI, Basel, Switzerland. This article is an open access article distributed under the terms and conditions of the Creative Commons Attribution (CC BY) license (http://creativecommons.org/licenses/by/4.0/).

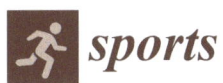

Article

Effects of Cycling on Subsequent Running Performance, Stride Length, and Muscle Oxygen Saturation in Triathletes

Guillermo Olcina [1,*], Miguel Ángel Perez-Sousa [1,2], Juan Antonio Escobar-Alvarez [3] and Rafael Timón [1]

1. Sports Sciences Faculty, University of Extremadura, Cáceres 10003, Spain; perezsousa@gmail.com (M.Á.P.-S.); rtimon@unex.es (R.T.)
2. Education, Psychology and Sports Sciences Faculty, University of Huelva, Huelva 21007, Spain
3. HE Department, South Essex College, Southend-on-Sea SS1 1ND, UK; juan.escobaralvarez@southessex.ac.uk
* Correspondence: golcina@unex.es; Tel.: +34-927-257540

Received: 27 February 2019; Accepted: 14 May 2019; Published: 16 May 2019

Abstract: Running performance is a determinant factor for victory in Sprint and Olympic distance triathlon. Previous cycling may impair running performance in triathlons, so brick training becomes an important part of training. Wearable technology that is used by triathletes can offer several metrics for optimising training in real-time. The aim of this study was to analyse the effect of previous cycling on subsequent running performance in a field test, while using kinematics metrics and SmO_2 provided by wearable devices that are potentially used by triathletes. Ten trained triathletes participated in a randomised crossover study, performing two trial sessions that were separated by seven days: the isolated run trial (IRT) and the bike-run trial (BRT). Running kinematics, physiological outcomes, and perceptual parameters were assessed before and after each running test. The running distance was significantly lower in the BRT when compared to the IRT, with a decrease in stride length of 0.1 m ($p = 0.00$) and higher $\%SmO_2$ ($p = 0.00$) in spite of the maximal intensity of exercise. No effects were reported in vertical oscillation, ground contact time, running cadence, and average heart rate. These findings may only be relevant to 'moderate level' triathletes, but not to 'elite' ones. Triathletes might monitor their $\%SmO_2$ and stride length during brick training and then compare it with isolated running to evaluate performance changes. Using wearable technology (near-infrared spectroscopy, accelerometry) for specific brick training may be a good option for triathletes.

Keywords: SmO_2; wearable; stride length; monitoring; NIRS

1. Introduction

Triathlon is characterised by integrating three sports disciplines: swimming, cycling, and running. Triathletes include workouts in their training plans that stack two disciplines, one after the other, with minimal to no breaks in between, which is called a brick. This is because one of the most important aspects of this sport is the transition from cycling to running, which is a key factor in achieving a good result [1]. In the last decade, the bibliography on this topic has grown quickly.

There is a range of studies that identify the alterations of different physiological and biomechanical variables that occur during running after cycling or during running in triathlon competitions. In this sense, several alterations in biomechanical and neuromotor patterns that may modify running economy, and consequently the performance and final results of a race, have been described. In several studies comparing the effects of isolated runs versus running after cycling, it has been shown that biomechanical variables, such as stride length and step cadence, may affect the metabolic cost [2,3]. Some researchers have found a decrease in stride length and step cadence [4–6]. However, others have not found any change in these parameters [7].

An increase in muscle recruitment activity has also been observed, as measured by EMG correlated with an increase in oxygen consumption (VO_2) [8,9]. In this way, the alterations in biomechanical parameters that are mentioned above modify muscular recruitment, changing motor patterns, as well as produce decreases in running economy. These detrimental effects are directly related to the changes in physiological aspects, as described in numerous studies in which an increase in heart rate (HR) occurred during running after cycling, due to the accumulated fatigue in the cycling component, and also because of the stresses that are involved in the cycle-run transition [10–12]. Running after cycling also produced an increase in cycle minute ventilation and breathing frequency, which therefore result in an intensification of oxygen uptake [2,13,14]. All of these increases in physiological variables during the second transition and subsequent running induce an increase in energy cost [13], thereby affecting the running economy and performance in a variety of triathletes [3,7,15].

All of the above suggests that some biomechanical alterations may modify the physiological aspects and thus change the running economy, which ultimately cause a decrease in the performance of triathletes. Consequently, it seems imperative to evaluate the ability of running in triathlon concerning running kinematics and physiological aspects that link cycling and running. However, the majority of these investigations have been performed under laboratory conditions [16,17] using costly equipment that is difficult to transport. As a result, this methodology is difficult to implement for coaches and scientists who want to obtain accurate data in the field.

During the last few years, several wearable devices to assess run kinematics through accelerometry and muscle oxygen saturation (SmO_2) by near-infrared spectroscopy (NIRS) have been developed. NIRS has been suggested as a sensitive measure to assess local muscle oxygen delivery and utilisation during dynamic muscle work in response to exercise and training [18]. It may also help to discern small changes (<1%) in muscle oxygenation during different running conditions or fatigue, as well as being useful in metabolic exercise studies and movement monitoring by accelerometers [19]. In this regard, NIRS is an effective method for assessing the SmO_2 during cycling [20,21] and running [22], which makes it an applicable tool for monitoring interval efforts in athletes [23]. This device is characterised by its feasibility, portability, ease of use, and low cost [24,25]. However, to the best of our knowledge, there have not been any studies to date that have evaluated running segments in triathlons or running after cycling using NIRS as a tool to provide information regarding muscle tissue O_2 saturation.

Therefore, the aim of this study was to analyse the effect of previous cycling on subsequent running performance using wearable technology in a field test, through well-studied kinematics parameters and an emergent variable, such as SmO_2 in triathletes.

2. Materials and Methods

2.1. Participants

Ten trained Sprint/Olympic distance triathletes, including eight males and two females, participated in this study (training volume 16.4 ± 6.8 h per week). The participants were all regular competitors in regional and national triathlon events. The mean and standard deviation (SD) age, height, and body mass were 25.7 ± 8.9 years, 174.6 ± 10.1 cm, and 71.3 ± 9.8 kg, respectively. Ten days before the experimental test, the participants carried out a tapering period. Twenty-four hours before conducting each test, the athletes were only permitted to perform low volume and low intensity training. The subjects agreed to participate by signing the informed consent form. The experimental procedures received ethical approval from the University Committee on Human Research, University of Extremadura, Spain, and followed the Declaration of Helsinki (register code 135/2015).

2.2. Design and Procedures

This study was a randomised crossover. The triathletes performed session A or B and with an interval of seven days, and then performed the other session as stipulated (Figure 1). Forty-eight hours before each trial, the triathletes followed a diet rich in CHO (8 gr/kg/day) to ensure sufficient muscle glycogen for tests. Furthermore, they were instructed on hydration habits to ensure proper hydration status.

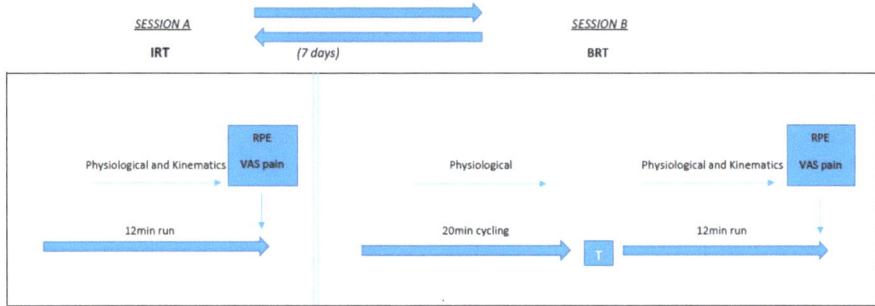

Figure 1. Testing protocol.

Isolated Run Trial (IRT). Height and weight were registered and a sociodemographic questionnaire was completed to know the athlete's profile. The IRT was carried out after 10 minutes of a standard warm up. The IRT consisted of a maximal running 12-min. Cooper test on a 400 m track. Cooper's 12-min run is one of the most commonly used VO_{2max} field tests in adults [26] and has demonstrated high validity coefficients in aerobically fit populations (r >0.90) [27,28]. During the test, the cardiovascular response in terms of HR, %SmO_2, and running kinematics (stride length, step cadence, vertical oscillation of the centre of gravity, and ground contact time) were collected. At the end of the test, the perceptual measures Rating of Perceived Exertion (RPE) and Visual Analogue Scale for pain (VAS pain 0–10) were taken [29].

Bike-Run Trial (BRT). This consisted of a 12-min Cooper test that was identical to that implemented within IRT, but it was preceded by a 20-min time trial on a trainer (Hammer CycleOps, Madison, WI, USA) with the triathletes' own bikes. Relative power (W/kg), mean, and maximal heart rate were measured to ensure proper intensity developed for a time trial. During the time trial, the triathletes drank 500 mL of a mixed drink with water, electrolytes, and 30 gr of carbohydrates, following the same protocol to that used in their triathlon races in order to avoid dehydration and minimise glycogen sparing. The transition period between bike and run was 60 seconds, to enable the triathletes to dismount the ergometer and change footwear. The following information was obtained during the running test: cardiovascular response in terms of HR, %SmO_2, and running kinematics (stride length, step cadence, vertical oscillation of the centre of gravity, and ground contact time). Following the running test, perceptual measures (RPE and VAS pain 0–10) were taken.

2.3. Measurements

Body weight. This was measured to the nearest 0.1 kg using a Tanita SC-330, (Tanita Corp., Japan). Height was estimated with an aluminium stadiometer Seca 713 model, (Seca GmbH, Hamburg, Germany) to the nearest 1 mm.

Heart rate. A HR-Run strap assessed this (Garmin Ltd., Olathe, KS, USA), with a frequency of 2.4 GHz and ANT+ wireless communication. This was paired to a Garmin Forerunner 735XT SmartWatch (Garmin Ltd., Olathe, KS, USA). Heart rate is expressed in beats per minute (bpm).

Running kinematics data. These were assessed with the same HR-Run strap, which includes a triaxial accelerometer, to measure step cadence expressed in steps by minute, vertical oscillation of the centre of gravity (VO) expressed in cm, ground contact time (GCT) expressed in ms, and stride length (SL) expressed in metres. Data for each variable were registered during both 12 min running tests and they were expressed as the average of the whole test. Several studies have examined the validity and reliability of these devices, showing satisfactory results [30].

Perceptual measures. The Borg 6–20 Scale was used to assess the triathletes' RPE, where 6 was no exertion and 20 denoted the maximum [31]. It was also recorded through VAS pain 0–10, which was employed to determine the muscular pain as perceived by the subjects in a 90° knee-bending position after trials. Zero (0) on the scale represents that there is no pain experienced, while ten (10) means that it is extremely painful. This method of evaluation has been used in other studies as a non-invasive method of monitoring the changes in muscular pain perception after exercising, and the consequent muscle damage [32].

SmO_2. Muscle oxygenation was measured second-by-second in the vastus lateralis muscle during both test (IRT and BRT) trials using NIRS (Moxy, Fortiori Design LLC, Minneapolis, MN, USA) [23]. An average was taken every minute for the analysis. The spectroscopy measurement quantified variation in optical transmission by sequentially sending light waves (630–850 nm) from four light emitting diodes into the tissue beneath the device and recording the amount of returned, scattered light at two detectors that were positioned 12.5 and 25 mm from the light source. An algorithm that combines a tissue light propagation model processes the scattered light and, via the Beer-Lambert Law, determined the amount of light absorbed at wavelengths relative to oxygenated and deoxygenated Hb. This allows for the percentage of haemoglobin + myoglobin containing O_2 (%SmO_2) to be calculated. The sensor was applied to the vastus lateralis muscle about 15 cm above the knee and was held tightly in position by a flexible polyurethane skirt that blocks sunlight. The %SmO_2 average of the entire test was calculated, as well as for every minute during both of the running test conditions.

2.4. Statistical Analysis

Statistical analyses were carried out with the statistical analysis software SPSS v.20 for Mac (IBM, New York, NY, USA). Standard statistical methods were used for the calculation of the mean and standard deviations. Additionally, absolute change and the percentage change from pre- to post-test were calculated for all of the variables for each group. A Kolmogorov–Smirnov test was conducted to show the distribution of the studied variables, as was a Levene test for homogeneity of variance. The statistical significance of the different paired samples that are shown in Table 2 was estimated with a Students' T. Moreover, an ANOVA repeated measures test was performed to compare the kinetics of %SmO_2 between the two trials. The value $p < 0.05$ was used to establish statistical significance. Effect size (ES), which represents the magnitude of the difference between two conditions in terms of SD, was calculated by dividing the change in the mean by the average SD of the two conditions. An ES of <0.2 was classified as trivial; d < 0.5 was classified as small, d = 0.51 to d = 0.8 was considered moderate, and d > 0.8 was large [33].

3. Results

Table 1 shows the data from the time trial that preceded running in BRT trials. They show the high intensity performed by triathletes. The RPE values were close to the values that were reported after running. The heart rate was lower than that achieved during the running tests.

Table 1. Kinematics, physiological, and perceptual measures from time trial.

Variables	BRT
Relative power (w/kg)	3.4 ± 0.4
Cadence (revolutions per min)	95.8 ± 7.4
HR average (bpm)	162 ± 12.8
HR peak (bpm)	175 ± 12.7
RPE (units)	16.5 ± 2.5
VAS pain 0–10 (units)	5.9 ± 2.1

BRT as mean ± SD.

The distance covered during the 12-min running test, and kinematic and physiological parameters, as well as perceived measurements after performing an IRT, as compared to the BRT, are shown in Table 2.

Table 2. Kinematics, physiological and perceptual measures changes from IRT to BRT.

Variables	IRT	BRT	% (CL 90%)	ES (CL 90%)	p-Value
12-min run (m)	3345 ± 306	3150 ± 296	−5.8 (−8.2 to −3.4)	0.6 (0.3 to 0.8)	0.00
Cadence (step per min)	178 ± 8.5	177 ± 8.8	−0.3 (−2.6 to 2.0)	0.0 (−0.3 to 0.4)	0.81
Vertical Oscillation (cm)	9.5 ± 1.3	9.7 ± 1.3	2.1 (−1.9 to 6.3)	0.1 (−0.4 to 0.1)	0.34
Ground contact time (ms)	206± 16.6	209 ± 19.2	1.6 (−0.1 to 3.2)	0.1 (0.0 0.3)	0.12
Stride Length (m)	1.64 ± 0.11	1.52 ± 0.11	−4.2 (−6.2 to −2.1)	0.4 (0.1 to 0.5)	0.00
SmO_2 average (%)	41.5 ± 6.4	55.1 ± 3.3	35.7 (22.7 to 46.4)	1.63 (1.16 to 2.26)	0.00
HR average (bpm)	175 ± 11.0	173 ± 10.5	−0.9 (−1.7 to 0.0)	0.1 (0.0 to 0.2)	0.09
HR peak (bpm)	184 ± 12.2	181 ± 11.3	−1.7 (−2.6 to −0.9)	0.2 (0.1 to 0.3)	0.00
RPE (units)	17.4 ± 1.8	17.2 ± 1.7	−1.1 (−9.3 to 7.9)	0.0 (−0.6 to 0.8)	0.80
VAS pain 0–10 (units)	5.4 ± 2.7	6.2 ± 2.1	22.6 (−1.8 to 53.1)	0.3 (0.0 to 0.7)	0.25

IRT–BRT as mean ± SD % (CL 90%) = percentage of change with 90% confidence limits. ES (CL 90%) = Effect size and 90% confidence limits.

3.1. Running Performance

The distance that was covered in the Cooper's test by triathletes was greater in the IRT than the BRT, reaching statistical significance with a moderate ES from Cohen's standardised differences.

3.2. Kinematic Parameters

Running cadence was similar in both of the trials, as were the vertical oscillation and ground contact time. Stride length was statistically significantly higher in the IRT than the BRT, but with a trivial size effect.

3.3. Physiological Parameters

Peak heart rate was higher during the IRT test when compared with BRT trials, with a small size effect. There were no differences in average heart rate between the two tests.

The average SmO_2 registered during each run test was lower in those that were performed without previously cycling (IRT). The size effect was large, reaching statistical significance.

For a better understanding of SmO_2 kinetics during running, Figure 2 shows the bias of SmO_2 in the two experimental conditions. The decrease in the slope of %SmO_2 from the IRT to BRT after minute 2 of running until the end of the test is statistically significant.

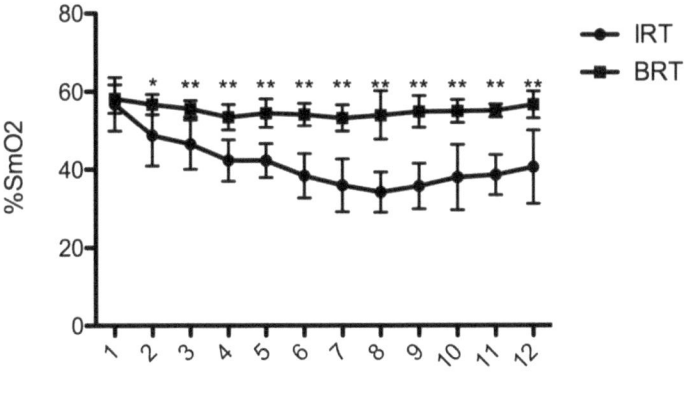

Figure 2. %SmO_2 slope between Isolated Run Trial (IRT) and Bike-Run Trial (BRT). * $p < 0.05$ ** $p < 0.01$.

3.4. Perceptual Variables

Table 2 shows RPE and VAS pain 0–10 reported by triathletes at the end of the IRT and BRT. It seems that previous cycling does not affect RPE after running, because the data were similar under both of the conditions, with no statistical significance and a trivial effect size for RPE and small size for VAS pain 0–10.

4. Discussion

The purpose of this study was to examine the effects of cycling on running after transitioning when compared with an isolated run in field tests using wearable technology that is potentially used by the triathletes for assessment.

The main findings confirmed the adverse effects that prior cycling has on running performance in a brick session in the field when compared with an isolated run, with a large impact on $\%SmO_2$, small effect on kinematic parameters, such as stride length and a trivial or no effect on other kinematics, physiological, or perceptual parameters.

The characteristics of the triathletes and their physiological responses in both of the tests support the fact that the participants were well trained but not elite triathletes. The distance covered was 3.345 m in the IRT; therefore, the running pace was 3:30 min:sec/km, which is higher than in professional triathletes over sprint and Olympic distances [34].

The performance in the 12-min maximal run after transitioning from biking to running significantly decreased when compared to isolated runs, where they were able to run an average of 195 m further. Therefore, the detrimental effects of cycling before running are verified. Our results are supported by previous findings in studies that were performed in laboratory conditions [7,35,36] or in outdoor conditions with cycling and running distances that are similar to those in our investigation [37]. The damaging effects of cycling prior to running might be due to accumulated muscular fatigue in the bike segment and could be attributed to an increase in neural fatigue, causing alterations in the neuromotor pattern [10,38], as has been argued in previous studies. Consequently, the importance of brick training in triathletes is highlighted.

Some running kinematic variables, such as ground contact time, step cadence, or vertical oscillation, do not appear to be affected by previous biking under the conditions of this study, which supports the findings of previous researches, and suggesting that bike-run transitioning will affect physiological parameters more than biomechanical parameters [7,37]. However, the running kinematics after cycling might be impaired when compared to isolated run kinematics, with a significant decrease in terms of stride length, which significantly reduces after cycling transition.

Triathletes shortened their strides by an average of 0.1 m after cycling as compared to in isolated runs. This finding is consistent with previous studies, where there was a trend towards a decrease in stride length after biking due to muscle fatigue [6,7,39], but not in well trained triathletes [40]. In fact, this worsening stride length after cycling has been shown to mainly occur in low-level triathletes [41].

Speed is the product of running cadence and stride length, which suggests a possible inverse relationship between them. Running cadence was optimal in both of the trials [42] and it did not change after biking. Therefore, our findings emphasise the importance of maintaining stride length during brick sessions or working on factors that cause stride length reductions, in order to avoid a worsening of performance in running after biking.

The biggest magnitude of change in the variables studied during running affected by previous cycling was for $\%SmO_2$, which was much lower, on average, during the isolated run; this was confirmed by the longitudinal analysis of the average SmO_2 every minute. This indicates that triathletes start running with a similar $\%SmO_2$, but after minute 2 during BRT trials, they are not able to decrease it, as well as during the IRT. If more oxygen is being demanded than is being delivered, as indicated by the lower dissolved oxygen levels in the tissue, oxygen saturation will decrease. This means that the muscles involved in exercise are able to use more oxygen to obtain energy to produce movement or go faster. This situation occurs better during the IRT trials.

The cause of higher %SmO$_2$ during the run after cycling might be neuromuscular fatigue accumulated during cycling, which generates an inability to use circulating intramuscular oxygen and making it impossible to increase exercise intensity. This hypothesis is consistent with previous studies that found the highest SmO$_2$ during a run, preceded by moderate-to-high intensity exercise, as compared to an isolated run [43].

Other physiological outcomes, such as average heart rate, did not achieve significant changes. This was similar in of the both trials, while peak heart rate was trivially higher. However, the magnitude of change in the running performance between both conditions of the study was much higher. This means that heart rate might not explain the differences in the running performance between trials, or, in accordance with previous studies, suggests that NIRS could be an alternative for monitoring exercise intensity instead of HR in some situations, since the HR devices are not able to detect sudden changes in intensity and/or fatigue states [44], and because HR is systemic while NIRS is local.

Finally, regarding perceptual parameters, running RPE is similar, independent of whether the triathletes had previously been cycling or not. This means that they perceived themselves to be very fatigued after running in both trials, even though they ran faster in the IRT. The VAS pain 0–10 results support this finding, as there were no differences between the trials. Therefore, these subjective variables might not help to set differences between running sessions and brick sessions in triathletes.

One of the strengths of the study was the use of wearable devices, which are not expensive in comparison with laboratory equipment and they meet the validity and reliability standards. Therefore, our study applied a proposal method to measure running after biking performance in middle level and age group triathletes, whose characteristics are similar to the majority of participants in these competitions.

On the other hand, this research presents certain limitations. One is that the samples for this study were not homogeneous in terms of gender and age, with a mixture of eight males and two females. It would be necessary to observe whether the results obtained are similar when independently comparing men and women, and using groups of similar ages. Another limitation is that athletes were given recommendations on what to eat and drink, but formal diet logs were not used and the hydration status was never directly measured; therefore, it is possible that the athletes did not follow the recommendations.

Future research should focus on evaluating high performance triathletes and/or performing different brick protocols, simulating sprint and Olympic distance triathlon races or middle/long distance triathlons in terms of pace and distance.

5. Conclusions

It can be concluded that intense cycling prior to running in triathletes may impair running performance due to a reduction in stride length and the inability to peripherally utilise oxygen in muscles presenting higher %SmO$_2$.

These findings could be useful for coaches and triathletes to develop brick training programmes in triathlon. Using wearable technology that allows for stride length data and %SmO$_2$ to be monitored in real-time and the analysis after training could help to control changes in running performance after cycling by comparing the data with those from isolated running.

Author Contributions: G.O. conceived and designed the experiments; M.Á.P.-S. and J.A.E.-A. performed the experiments; G.O. and M.Á.P.-S. analysed the data; R.T. contributed reagents/materials/analysis tools; G.O., R.T. and M.Á.P.-S. wrote the paper.

Funding: This research was funded by COUNCIL OF EXTREMADURA, grant number GR 18003.

Conflicts of Interest: The authors declare no conflict of interest. The funding sponsors had no role in the design of the study, in the collection, analyses, in the interpretation of data, in the writing of the manuscript, or in the decision to publish the results.

References

1. Cejuela, R.; Cortell-Tormo, J.M.; Chinchilla-Mira, J.J.; Pérez-Turpin, J.A.; Villa, J.G. Gender differences in elite Olympic distance triathlon performances. *JHSE* **2012**, *7*, 434–445. [CrossRef]
2. Hausswirth, C.; Bigard, A.X.; Berthelot, M.; Thomaïdis, M.; Guezennec, C.Y. Variability in energy cost of running at the end of a triathlon and a marathon. *Int. J. Sports Med.* **1996**, *17*, 572–579. [CrossRef]
3. Hausswirth, C.; Bigard, A.X.; Guezennec, C.Y. Relationships between running mechanics and energy cost of running at the end of a triathlon and a marathon. *Int. J. Sports Med.* **1997**, *18*, 330–339. [CrossRef]
4. Gottschall, J.; Palmer, B. Acute Effects of Cycling on Running Step Length and Step Frequency. *J. Strength Cond. Res.* **2000**, *14*, 97–101.
5. Hausswirth, C.; Lehénaff, D. Physiological demands of running during long distance runs and triathlons. *Sports Med.* **2001**, *31*, 679–689. [CrossRef]
6. Landers, G.J.; Blanksby, B.A.; Rackland, T. Cadence, Stride Rate and Stride Length during Triathlon Competition. *Int. J. Exerc. Sci.* **2011**, *4*, 40–48.
7. Hue, O.; Le Gallais, D.; Chollet, D.; Boussana, A.; Préfaut, C. The influence of prior cycling on biomechanical and cardiorespiratory response profiles during running in triathletes. *Eur. J. Appl. Physiol. Occup. Physiol.* **1998**, *77*, 98–105. [CrossRef] [PubMed]
8. Burnley, M.; Doust, J.H.; Ball, D.; Jones, A.M. Effects of prior heavy exercise on VO_2 kinetics during heavy exercise are related to changes in muscle activity. *J. Appl. Physiol.* **2002**, *93*, 167–174. [CrossRef] [PubMed]
9. Saunders, M.J.; Evans, E.M.; Arngrimsson, S.A.; Allison, J.D.; Warren, G.L.; Cureton, K.J. Muscle activation and the slow component rise in oxygen uptake during cycling. *Med. Sci. Sports Exerc.* **2000**, *32*, 2040–2045. [CrossRef] [PubMed]
10. Bentley, D.J.; Millet, G.P.; Vleck, V.E.; McNaughton, L.R. Specific aspects of contemporary triathlon: Implications for physiological analysis and performance. *Sports Med.* **2002**, *32*, 345–359. [CrossRef]
11. Guezennec, C.Y.; Vallier, J.M.; Bigard, A.X.; Durey, A. Increase in energy cost of running at the end of a triathlon. *Eur. J. Appl. Physiol. Occup. Physiol.* **1996**, *73*, 440–445. [CrossRef] [PubMed]
12. Walsh, J.A.; Stamenkovic, A.; Lepers, R.; Peoples, G.; Stapley, P.J. Neuromuscular and physiological variables evolve independently when running immediately after cycling. *J. Electromyogr. Kinesiol.* **2015**, *25*, 887–893. [CrossRef]
13. Millet, G.P.; Millet, G.Y.; Hofmann, M.D.; Candau, R.B. Alterations in running economy and mechanics after maximal cycling in triathletes: Influence of performance level. *Int. J. Sports Med.* **2000**, *21*, 127–132. [CrossRef]
14. Yoshida, T.; Kamiya, J.; Hishimoto, K. Are oxygen uptake kinetics at the onset of exercise speeded up by local metabolic status in active muscles? *Eur. J. Appl. Physiol. Occup. Physiol.* **1995**, *70*, 482–486. [CrossRef] [PubMed]
15. Millet, G.P.; Bentley, D.J. The physiological responses to running after cycling in elite junior and senior triathletes. *Int. J. Sports Med.* **2004**, *25*, 191–197. [PubMed]
16. Schabort, E.J.; Killian, S.C.; St Clair Gibson, A.; Hawley, J.A.; Noakes, T.D. Prediction of triathlon race time from laboratory testing in national triathletes. *Med. Sci. Sports Exerc.* **2000**, *32*, 844–849. [CrossRef]
17. Zhou, S.; Robson, S.J.; King, M.J.; Davie, A.J. Correlations between short-course triathlon performance and physiological variables determined in laboratory cycle and treadmill tests. *J. Sports Med. Phys. Fit.* **1997**, *37*, 122–130.
18. Perrey, S.; Ferrari, M. Muscle oximetry in sports science: A systematic review. *Sports Med.* **2018**, *48*, 597–616. [CrossRef]
19. Steimers, A.; Vafiadou, M.; Koukourakis, G.; Geraskin, D.; Neary, P.; Kohl-Bareis, M. Muscle Oxygenation During Running Assessed by Broad Band NIRS. *Adv. Exp. Med. Biol.* **2016**, *876*, 41–47.
20. Skovereng, K.; Ettema, G.; van Beekvelt, M.C.P. Oxygenation, local muscle oxygen consumption and joint specific power in cycling: The effect of cadence at a constant external work rate. *Eur. J. Appl. Physiol.* **2016**, *116*, 1207–1217. [CrossRef] [PubMed]

21. Skovereng, K.; Ettema, G.; van Beekvelt, M. The Effect of Cadence on Shank Muscle Oxygen Consumption and Deoxygenation in Relation to Joint Specific Power and Cycling Kinematics. *PLoS ONE* **2017**, *12*, 1–13. [CrossRef]
22. Oueslati, F.; Boone, J.; Ahmaidi, S. Respiratory muscle endurance, oxygen saturation index in vastus lateralis and performance during heavy exercise. *Respir. Physiol. Neurobiol.* **2016**, *227*, 41–47. [CrossRef]
23. Bortolotti, H.; Pasquarelli, B.N.; Soares-Caldeira, L.F.; Altimari, L.R.; Nakamura, F.Y. Repeated sprint ability evaluation in soccer. *Mot. Rev. De Educ. Fis.* **2010**, *16*, 1006–1012.
24. Crum, E.M.; O'Connor, W.J.; Van Loo, L.; Valckx, M.; Stannard, S.R. Validity and reliability of the Moxy oxygen monitor during incremental cycling exercise. *Eur. J. Sport Sci.* **2017**, *17*, 1037–1043. [CrossRef]
25. McManus, C.J.; Collison, J.; Cooper, C.E. Performance comparison of the MOXY and PortaMon near-infrared spectroscopy muscle oximeters at rest and during exercise. *J. Biomed. Opt.* **2018**, *23*, 1–14. [CrossRef] [PubMed]
26. Reilly, T. Assessment of performance team games. In *Kinanthropometry and Exercise Physiology Lab Manual: Tests, Procedures, and Data*; Eston, R., Reilly, T., Eds.; Routledge: New York, NY, USA, 2001; pp. 171–182.
27. Cooper, K.H. A means of assessing maximal oxygen intake. Correlation between field and treadmill testing. *JAMA* **1968**, *203*, 201–204. [CrossRef] [PubMed]
28. Safrit, M.J.; Glaucia-Costa, M.; Hooper, L.M.; Patterson, P.; Ehlert, S.A. The validity generalization of distance run tests. *Can. J. Sport Sci.* **1988**, *13*, 188–196.
29. Hawker, G.A.; Mian, S.; Kendzerska, T.; Rrench, M. Measures of adult pain: Visual Analog Scale for Pain (VAS Pain), Numeric Rating Scale for Pain (NRS Pain), McGill Pain Questionnaire (MPQ), Short-Form McGill Pain Questionnaire (SF-MPQ), Chronic Pain Grade Scale (CPGS), Short Form-36 Bodily Pain Scale (SF-36 BPS), and Measure of Intermittent and Constant Osteoarthritis Pain (ICOAP). *Arthritis Care Res.* **2011**, *63*, 240–252.
30. Adams, D.; Pozzi, F.; Carroll, A.; Rombach, A.; Zeni, J. Validity and reliability of a commercial fitness watch for measuring running dynamics. *J. Orthop. Sports Phys. Ther.* **2016**, *46*, 471–476. [CrossRef] [PubMed]
31. Borg, G.A. Psychophysical bases of perceived exertion. *Med. Sci. Sports Exerc.* **1982**, *14*, 377–381. [CrossRef]
32. Vaile, J.M.; Gill, N.D.; Blazevich, A.J. The effect of contrast water therapy on symptoms of delayed onset muscle soreness. *J. Strength Cond. Res.* **2007**, *21*, 697–702.
33. Cohen, J. *Statistical Power Analysis for the Behavioral Sciences*, 2nd ed.; Psychology Press: New York, NY, USA, 2009.
34. Rüst, C.A.; Lepers, R.; Stiefel, M.; Rosemann, T.; Knechtle, B. Performance in Olympic triathlon: Changes in performance of elite female and male triathletes in the ITU World Triathlon Series from 2009 to 2012. *SpringerPlus* **2013**, *2*, 685. [CrossRef]
35. Beneke, R.; Hütler, M.; Leithäuser, R.M. Maximal lactate-steady-state independent of performance. *Med. Sci. Sports Exerc.* **2000**, *32*, 1135–1139. [CrossRef]
36. Paavolainen, L.; Nummela, A.; Rusko, H.; Häkkinen, K. Neuromuscular characteristics and fatigue during 10 km running. *Int. J. Sports Med.* **1999**, *20*, 516–521. [CrossRef]
37. Bernard, T.; Vercruyssen, F.; Grego, F.; Hausswirth, C.; Lepers, R.; Vailler, J.-M.; Brisswalter, J. Effect of cycling cadence on subsequent 3 km running performance in well trained triahtletes. *Br. J. Sports Med.* **2003**, *37*, 154–159. [CrossRef]
38. Hopker, J.G.; O'Grady, C.; Pageaux, B. Prolonged constant load cycling exercise is associated with reduced gross efficiency and increased muscle oxygen uptake. *Scand. J. Med. Sci. Sports* **2017**, *27*, 408–417. [CrossRef]
39. Millet, G.P.; Vleck, V.E. Physiological and biomechanical adaptations to the cycle to run transition in Olympic triathlon: Review and practical recommendations for training. *Br. J. Sports Med.* **2000**, *34*, 384–390. [CrossRef]
40. Tew, G. The effect of cycling cadence on subsequent 10 km running performance in well-trained triahtletes. *J. Sports Sci. Med.* **2005**, *4*, 342–353.
41. Díaz, V.; Peinado, A.B.; Vleck, V.E.; Alvarez-Sánchez, M.; Benito, P.J.; Alves, F.B.; Calderon, F.J.; Zapico, A.G. Longitudinal Changes in Response to a Cycle-Run Field Test of Young Male National "Talent identification" and Senior Elite Triathlon Squads. *J. Strength Cond. Res.* **2012**, *26*, 2209–2219. [CrossRef]
42. Leberman, D.E.; Warrener, A.G.; Wrang, J.; Castillo, E.R. Effects of stride frequency and foot position at landing on braking force, hip torque, impact peak force and the metabolic cost of running in humans. *J. Exp. Biol.* **2015**, *218*, 3406–3414. [CrossRef]

43. Buchheit, M.; Laursen, P.B.; Ahmaidi, S. Effect of prior exercise on pulmonary O2 uptake and estimated muscle capillary blood flow kinetics during moderate-intensity field running in men. *J. Appl. Physiol.* **2009**, *107*, 460–470. [CrossRef] [PubMed]
44. Born, D.-P.; Stöggl, T.; Swarén, M.; Björklund, G. Near-Infrared Spectroscopy: More Accurate Than Heart Rate for Monitoring Intensity in Running in Hilly Terrain. *Int. J. Sports Physiol. Perform.* **2017**, *12*, 440–447. [CrossRef] [PubMed]

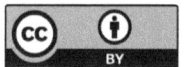

© 2019 by the authors. Licensee MDPI, Basel, Switzerland. This article is an open access article distributed under the terms and conditions of the Creative Commons Attribution (CC BY) license (http://creativecommons.org/licenses/by/4.0/).

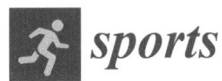

Communication

The Rise of Elite Short-Course Triathlon Re-Emphasises the Necessity to Transition Efficiently from Cycling to Running

Joel A. Walsh

Illawarra Health and Medical Research Institute, University of Wollongong, Wollongong, NSW 2522, Australia; joelw@uow.edu.au; Tel.: +61-2-4298-1962

Received: 24 March 2019; Accepted: 26 April 2019; Published: 29 April 2019

Abstract: Transitioning efficiently between cycling and running is considered an indication of overall performance, and as a result the cycle–run (C–R) transition is one of the most researched areas of triathlon. Previous studies have thoroughly investigated the impact of prior cycling on running performance. However, with the increasing number of short-course events and the inclusion of the mixed relay at the 2020 Tokyo Olympics, efficiently transitioning from cycle–run has been re-emphasised and with it, any potential limitations to running performance among elite triathletes. This short communication provides coaches and sports scientists a review of the literature detailing the negative effects of prior variable-cycling on running performance experienced among elite, short-course and Olympic distance triathletes; as well as discussing practical methods to minimise any negative impact of cycling on running performance. The current literature suggests that variable-cycling negatively effects running ability in at least some elite triathletes and that improving swimming performance, drafting during cycling and C–R training at race intensity could improve an athlete's triathlon running performance. It is recommended that future research clearly define the performance level, competitive format of the experimental population and use protocols that are specific to the experimental population in order to improve the training and practical application of the research findings.

Keywords: cycle–run; transition; triathlon; performance; elite; training

1. Introduction

Triathlon comprises several different racing formats (Table 1.) that can be generally categorised as short-course (super sprint/sprint); Olympic distance (short-distance/standard); or long-course (70.3/Ironman). Each category of triathlon places substantially different physical demands on the athletes [1], such as short-course triathlon (super-sprint/sprint distance) involving producing repetitive, high-intensity efforts due to the technical courses [2] changing the physiological demands of this type of triathlon [3], compared to the consistent, steady-state paced efforts required during long-course triathlon. However, all formats of triathlon require an athlete to transition from cycling-to-running. Subjective descriptions of perceived incoordination are commonly reported among triathletes of all levels during the cycle–run (C–R) transition [4], leading to a potential competitive advantage to athletes that can minimise the presence of impaired movement coordination during the C–R transition. Indeed, successful performance in triathlon is considered to be largely dependent on the ability of an athlete to overcome the specific physiological [5], neuromuscular [6] and biomechanical [7] complications associated with transitioning from cycling to running. Furthermore, recent evidence also suggests that specific effects of the C–R exist between elite male and female triathletes [8]. As a result of the recent increase in the number of short-course events held throughout the 2018/19 International Triathlon Union (ITU) World Triathlon Series (WTS), as well as the advent of the Super League Triathlon series (variable short-course distances), and the inclusion of the mixed relay event at the 2020 Tokyo Olympics, the relative importance of efficiently transitioning from C–R during triathlon, particularly during short-course formats, is re-emphasised and with it, any potential limitations to running performance.

Table 1. Commonly raced formats of triathlon.

Event	Swim	Bike	Run	Course Structure	Event Characteristics
Super sprint [†]	400 m (0.25 mi)	10 km (6.2 mi)	2.5 km (1.6 mi)	Short circuit racing, highly technical	Repetitive, high-intensity accelerations, high power/speed, technical courses, highly tactical, drafting/non-drafting, emphasis on C–R transition.
Sprint [†]	750 m (0.47 mi)	20 km (12 mi)	5 km (3.1 mi)	Circuit racing, criterium-style bike leg, relatively technical	Repetitive, high-intensity accelerations, high power/speed, technical courses, highly tactical, drafting/non-drafting, emphasis on C–R transition.
Olympic [*]	1.5 km (0.93 mi)	40 km (25 mi)	10 km (6.2 mi)	Often circuit racing, draft/non drafting bike leg, some technical aspects	Repetitive, high-intensity accelerations, high power/speed, technical courses, highly tactical, drafting/non-drafting, emphasis on C–R transition energy conservation/minimising physical effort.
70.3 [§]	1.9 km (1.2 mi)	90 km (56 mi)	21.1 km (12 mi)	Long course, non-drafting bike leg, out-and-back courses, non-technical	Prolonged, submaximal steady-state efforts, management of energy consumption and effort, non-drafting cycle leg, non-technical course.
Ironman [§]	3.9 km (2.4 mi)	180 km (112 mi)	42.2 km (26.2 mi)	Long course, non-drafting bike leg, out-and-back courses, non-technical	Prolonged, submaximal steady-state efforts, management of energy consumption and effort, non-drafting cycle leg, non-technical course.
Mixed relay [*,†]	300 m (0.19 mi)	8 km (5.0 mi)	2 km (1.2 mi)	Short circuit racing, highly technical, similar to super sprint events	Repetitive, high-intensity accelerations, high power/speed, technical courses, highly tactical, drafting/non-drafting, emphasis on C–R transition.

[*] denotes Tokyo 2020 event; [†] denotes short-course event; [§] denotes long-course event.

2. The Influence of Cycling on Running Performance in Elite Triathletes

2.1. The Disparity Between Cycle–Run Testing Protocols and Race Demands

Previous research has indicated that among highly-trained triathletes competing in short-course and Olympic-distance triathlon, any negative impact of prior cycling on running performance is minimal, compared to effects experienced by lesser trained, recreational triathletes [1,9–11]. However, a majority of research investigating the C–R use constant/steady state or incremental cycling protocols, prior to running. As a result, these findings may lack practical and training specificity for triathletes competing in draft-legal short-course and Olympic distance triathlon where cycling is highly variable with respect to both power output and cadence ranges [3] that would therefore, have a substantially different impact on running performance [2]. Subsequent studies have aimed to replicate the metabolic demand of cycling experienced during short-course triathlon, by prescribing constant cycling intensities based on a percentage of maximal aerobic power (~72% MAP) [12] or above the ventilatory threshold (~80% VO_{2max}) [13]. Exercising at such intensities may reflect the average metabolic cost of the cycle leg of short-course and Olympic distance triathlon however, considering the variable nature of cycling during these formats of triathlon such testing protocols lack specificity, at least concerning elite draft-legal short-course and Olympic distance triathlon. As a result, it could be argued that non-specific testing protocols contribute to the lack of clarity regarding the understanding of the effects of prior cycling on running performance specific to elite short-course and Olympic distance triathlon. Alternatively, others [11] have used a run-cycle–run protocol to determine the differences between elite short-course versus elite long-course [12] and elite junior (male and female) versus elite senior triathletes [10,14]. While the findings of these experiments provide valuable information relating to identifying the physiological characteristics of select cohorts of elite triathletes, potentially aiding talent identification and monitoring training progression, they do not specifically outline potential changes among elite short-course and Olympic distance triathletes transitioning from C–R; that is a primary aim of this short communication. Therefore, discussions of past research in Section 2 and summarised in Table 2 of this short communication, will be limited to those articles that recruited elite triathletes and used a variable-cycling protocol [15] (i.e., variable power output and/or cadence) prior to running or a protocol that reflected the workload of a short-course triathlon [11] (Table 2).

2.2. The Effects of Variable-Cadence Cycling Protocols on Running Performance in Elite Triathletes

In order to specifically understand the impact of prior cycling on running performance previous researchers developed a protocol to determine the effects of cycling on the movement pattern of subsequent running (Table 2) [15]. These authors designed a moderate-intensity protocol aimed at minimising the impact of fatigue. In particular, they identified typical cadence ranges from data collected from elite triathletes competing at an international level to create their cycling protocol. Using this variable-cadence protocol (i.e., individually preferred cadence, 55–60, 75–80, and 95–100 rpm), on-going studies involving elite triathletes aimed to identify changes to the neuromuscular control [16], muscle recruitment patterns [17,18], kinematics [17,19], biomechanics [11] and economy [6,20] of subsequent running performance (Table 2).

Alternatively, others [21] have used moderate-intensity (variable-cadence) and high-intensity (power profile test) protocols to quantify changes to the neuromuscular control between an isolated/control run (IR) and C–R using electromyography (EMG) and joint angle waveforms (kinematics) sampled from the muscles of the lower limb (i.e., quadriceps, hamstrings and gastrocnemius and tibialis anterior) in elite triathletes (Table 2). Using the high-intensity, power profile test [21], these authors reported that overall, cycling minimally affects the stride-to-stride reproducibility of joint angles (<1.9°) or muscle recruitment patterns (<5.1%) during the early phase of subsequent running. Although, one participant did demonstrate altered muscle recruitment of biceps femoris following moderate-intensity, variable-cadence cycling, suggesting that adaptation to the C–R may be individual-specific. These results are in agreement with similar findings [6,17,19] indicating that most elite triathletes are able to effectively replicate pre-cycling running patterns when transitioning from moderate-intensity (variable-cadence) cycling. Moreover, using the same moderate-intensity, variable-cadence cycling protocol, no significant change in average muscle recruitment patterns or kinematics during the C–R, compared with an IR are evident [17,18]. However, among some elite triathletes (5/14 participants), muscle recruitment patterns recorded from the tibialis anterior muscle during the C–R closely reflect those recorded during cycling, and not the IR [17]. Alterations seen in some elite triathletes could be reflective of previous evidence that associates elite triathletes with a history of exercise-related leg pain (ERLP—5/10) with substantial (≥10%) alterations in EMG muscle patterns during C–R [19]. These authors suggested that those elite triathletes with a history of ERLP are ~2.4× more likely to have difficulty replicating neuromuscular control during running after variable-cadence cycling. Similarly, increased variability in muscle recruitment patterns recorded in the lower limb (coefficient of variation range = 18–37% has been observed during the early phase of C–R, i.e., 0–180 s), compared to IR [18]. These findings may suggest the presence of neuromuscular interference or the crossover of a generalised movement pattern that affects the control of running due to the prior, repetitive performance of the cycling movement pattern [15,16]. Furthermore, the changes in muscle recruitment patterns observed among some elite triathletes during the C–R, compared to an IR, have been associated with a reduction in running economy (3.7 ± 0.9%) [6]. Similarly, significant increases to the cost of running, respiratory exchange ratio, breathing frequency and heart rate have been reported among elite triathletes during the early phase of C–R, compared to an IR using the same moderate-intensity, variable-cadence cycling protocol (Table 2) [20]. These authors also reported an overall decrease in mean stride length (IR = 2.64 ± 0.18 v. C–R = 2.53 ± 0.17 m) and increase in mean stride frequency at the mean response time, ~63% of time to steady-state (IR = 85.7 ± 2.7 v. C–R = 87.0 ± 2.6 strides·min^{-1}) and at 180 s (IR = 85.4 ± 2.6 v. C–R = 87.3 ± 2.7 strides·min^{-1}) when running at the same self-selected velocity (13.5 ± 0.9 km·h^{-1}) during the IR and C–R condition. Furthermore, changes in running mechanics suggest that leg stiffness increases in elite triathletes during running after a bout of fatiguing cycling [11]. Increased leg stiffness during C–R may indicate superior elastic energy storage and improved efficiency of repetitive stretch-shortening cycle movements during C–R [11]. Such biomechanical changes observed in elite triathletes, coupled with decreased stride length and increased stride rate, may act to counter-balance the potential negative changes to other physiological and neuromuscular variables in order to meet the demands of C–R.

2.3. The Effects of Variable-Power Cycling Protocols on Running Performance

The aforementioned research provides evidence to suggest that even at moderate-intensity variable-cadence cycling can have a negative effect on subsequent running performance in at least some elite triathletes. To date, no research has investigated the effects of variable-power cycling, at any intensity, on subsequent running in elite triathletes. However, results of a previous study suggest that variable-power cycling (i.e., 10–90 s intermittent efforts between 40–140% maximal aerobic power) had a greater negative impact on C–R performance, compared to constant-power cycling (i.e., 65% maximal aerobic power) among well-trained triathletes [22]. These authors reported significantly higher levels of blood lactate at the start of the C–R after variable-power cycling (64 ± 61%) compared to that after constant power cycling. The elevated blood lactate levels reflected a reduced running velocity at lactate threshold (~4 mM) of 0.6 ± 0.9 km·h^{-1} during the C–R following variable-power cycling. Furthermore, increased central and peripheral fatigue of knee extensor muscles after variable-power, compared to constant power cycling, have also been reported in well-trained triathletes [23]. The participants in this study did not complete any subsequent running after cycling however, the increased neuromuscular fatigue that reflected a reduced strength output of the knee extensors of 12.8 ± 6.1% that would likely contribute to a decrement in running performance.

Overall, variable-cycling does not appear to heavily affect muscle recruitment patterns and joint kinematics in most elite triathletes competing in draft-legal short-course and Olympic distance triathlon, during the C–R period. Despite this, it is well acknowledged that the physiological cost of running during triathlon is substantially greater compared to IR [24], particularly during the early phase of C–R (0–180 s) [18]. Moreover, among those elite triathletes whose running performance is impacted by prior cycling, the effects are likely to have a substantially negative influence on overall performance; while increased variability of muscle recruitment patterns and altered stride mechanics during the early phase of C–R is evident among some elite triathletes and is more likely to be present in athletes with a history of ERLP.

Table 2. Physiological, neuromuscular and biomechanical effects of prior cycling on running performance specific to elite short-course and Olympic distance triathletes.

Participants	Protocol	Effects	Conclusions	Reference
8 elite triathletes (1 male) —international level (top 50 world ranking)	Run-cycle-run - 7-min run at sprint distance race-pace (18 and 15.1 ± 0.6 km·h^{-1}) - maximal incremental cycle (70 W increments/3-min from 70–280 W, 35 W increments/2-min to volitional exhaustion) - 7-min run at sprint distance race-pace (18 and 15.1 ± 0.6 km·h^{-1})	- ↑ [La-] between 1st and 2nd 7-min run - mean 3.7% ↓ C_R during 2nd 7-min run v. 1st 7-min run - mean 4.2% ↓ ΔH_{STRIKE} during 2nd 7-min run v. 1st 7-min run. - Small mean (4.3%) ΔC_M during 2nd 7-min run v. 1st 7-min run.	- Cost of running is not significantly affected by a fatiguing bout of cycling in elite triathletes, despite changes in [La-] between 7-min run bouts. - reduced mechanical changes during the 2nd 7-min run suggest that leg stiffness is better preserved in elite triathletes.	Millet, Millet, Hofmann and Candau (2000)
8 elite triathletes (1 male) —international level (top 50 world ranking)	see Millet et al. (2000)	- No significant Δ the mechanical or kinetic cost of running pre- and post-fatiguing cycling	- A prior bout of high- intensity, fatiguing cycling does not affect the subsequent running mechanics in elite triathletes.	Millet, Millet and Candau (2001)
16 elite triathletes —national/international level	see Chapman et al. (2009) - 10-min CR - 20-min variable-cadence cycling followed by a 30-min TR	- No Δ TA EMG patterns CR v TR - No Δ SL, SD or kinematic joint angles CR v TR - 5/14 did show ↓ EMG amplitude of TA during TR	- Short periods of variable-cadence, moderate-intensity cycling does not affect running kinematics or SL among elite triathletes. - However, cycling may influence muscle activation patterns during TR in some elite triathletes.	Chapman, Vicenzino, Blanch, Dowlan and Hodges (2008)
34 elite/highly-trained triathletes —national/international level —World championship qualified —Olympic distance specialisation	see Chapman et al. (2009) - 10-min CR - 20-min variable-cadence cycling followed by a 30-min TR	- No Δ joint kinematics or EMG muscle patterns in most triathletes (70%) - 30% of triathletes showed Δ EMG patterns during TR - Δ EMG muscle patterns associated with 3.7 ± 0.9% ↓ R_E (↑ VO$_2$)	Prior variable-cadence cycling impairs neuromuscular control on some elite triathletes that are associated with reduced TR economy	Chapman, Vicenzino, Hodges, Dowlan, Hahn, Alexander and Milner (2009)
34 elite/highly-trained triathletes —national/international level —World championship experience —Olympic distance specialisation	see Chapman et al. (2009) - 10-min CR - 20-min variable-cadence cycling followed by a 30-min TR	- No Δ joint kinematics - EMG patterns differed by ≥10% between CR and TR in 5/24 control triathletes and 5/10 triathletes with a history of ERLP	Potential association between ERLP and neuromuscular control during TR in elite triathletes with a history of ERLP	Chapman, Hodges, Briggs, Stapley and Vicenzino (2010)

Table 2. Cont.

Participants	Protocol	Effects	Conclusions	Reference
7 elite triathletes (3 female) —international level —national representatives at world level	Low-intensity - see Chapman et al. (2009) High-intensity cycling - see Quod et al. (2010)	- No Δ R_E or neuromuscular control of the left leg during TR following low and high intensity cycling. - No Δ lower limb kinematics - No Δ EMG patterns following high-intensity cycling - 1/7 triathletes showed altered EMG patterns during TR following low-intensity cycling	- Low and high intensity variable cycling does not adversely impact TR neuromuscular control of R_E in elite triathletes	Bonacci, Saunders, Alexander, Blanch and Vicenzino (2011)
6 triathletes —National/international level —ITU Olympic distance race experience	see Chapman et al. (2009)	- No mean Δ lower limb EMG muscle activity patterns between CR and TR - ↑ variability of EMG activity during TR	- lower limb EMG activity patterns are not substantially influenced by variable-cadence cycling in elite triathletes	Walsh, Stamenkovic, Lepers, Peoples and Stapley (2015)
8 triathletes —National/international level —ITU Olympic distance race experience	see Chapman et al. (2009)	- ↑ C_R, RER and HR at MRT and 10th minute of TR v CR - ↓ SL, ↑ SR during TR v CR	- moderate-intensity variable-cadence cycling significantly affects physiological and stride pattern variables during TR, compared to CR.	Walsh, Dawber, Lepers, Brown and Stapley (2017)

3. Minimising the Effects of Cycling on Running Performance in Draft-Legal Short-Course and Olympic Distance Triathlon

3.1. The Role of Fatigue during Draft-Legal Short-Course and Olympic Distance Triathlon

Fatigue has been defined as "the failure to maintain force output, leading to a reduced performance" [25,26], "failure to maintain the required of expected power output" [27] and "any decline in muscle performance associated with muscle activity" [28]. Fatigue can be classified based on duration (acute/chronic), mental (cognitive or perceptual) and physical, referring to human motor performance [29,30]. A form of physical fatigue effecting performance in muscle fatigue that is considered the reduction in maximal force output and production of power in response to activity involving muscle contractions [31]. Muscle fatigue is often a primary factor in limiting athletic performance during high-intensity and/or prolonged exercise and is predicated by both central and peripheral mechanisms [30]. Peripheral fatigue involves changes at or beyond the neuromuscular junction independent of the central nervous system (CNS), involving mechanisms that impede or impair neuromuscular transmission, impulse propagation, calcium release and uptake in the sarcoplasm, substrate depletion (i.e., muscle glycogen depletion that precipitates fluid loss and increasing cardiovascular and metabolic strain), and contraction coupling [32,33]. Meanwhile, central fatigue occurs within the CNS resulting in a reduced neural drive to skeletal muscles [30,31] and is thought to be due to changes in serotonin, dopamine and noradrenaline (norepinephrine) in specific brain regions due to prolonged exercise [33]. It is important to note that the exact understandings of the mechanisms involved in central fatigue are still being debated.

Every triathlete that has competed in elite-level draft-legal short-course and Olympic distance triathlon is likely to have experienced fatigue and as such, it is reasonable to suggest that increased fatigue, due to central and peripheral mechanisms, during elite draft-legal short-course and Olympic distance triathlon has a significant impact on running and overall performance. More specifically, the relatively duration and discipline distances of short-course and Olympic distance triathlon, relative to long-course formats, lends itself to higher intensity racing that exacerbates particular central and peripheral mechanisms responsible for fatigue. Indeed, the well reported increases in the energy cost, blood lactate concentrations, heart rate and oxygen uptake during the swim-cycle transition [34]; coupled with the documented increased oxygen cost [24,35–37], depletion of glycogen stores [24,35,36], muscle fatigue [24] and fluid loss [24,35,38], as well as loss of coordination [7,15], impairing neuromuscular control [6,17,18] and gait patterns [20,39] during the C–R transition is likely due to the complex build-up of central and peripheral fatigue mechanisms that significantly affects an elite triathlete's physical performance, as evidenced by the progressive reduction in pace during short-course triathlon [40]. Therefore, it is necessary for elite triathletes, to limit the fatigue-related changes to physiological, neuromuscular or biomechanical variables that impact their performance by adopting strategies that attempt to minimise the build-up of fatigue and the accompanying negative impact on their performance [1,40]. Strategies (i.e., drafting, positioning and pacing) that would likely limit the fatigue-related changes to physiological, neuromuscular or biomechanical variables are discussed in the following section. Adopting such strategies would likely minimise effects of cycling on running performance during draft-legal short-course and Olympic distance triathlon, resulting in the conservation of energy that could translate in to an improved C–R transition and therefore, overall performance.

3.2. Impact of Drafting during Cycling on Running Performance

Typically, the energy expended in order to overcome rolling and frontal air resistance contributes to the increased cost of running after prior cycling during triathlon [1]. As such, the most effective means of minimising the effect of cycling on running performance is by drafting that involves riding behind one or several riders during cycling. Riding in a tightly formed group of riders (i.e., peloton/bunch) increases the drafting effect as the larger number of riders provides shelter from frontal air resistance (i.e., wind) [41]. Indeed minimising the wind resistance can lower the aerodynamic drag down to 50–70%, compared to riding isolated [42,43]. Moreover, sheltering in the mid-rear of a peloton can see drag reduced down to 5–10% [41], resulting in a substantially reduced energy expenditure [41,44]. In order to best maximise drag reduction when drafting, a rider can adopt a more aerodynamic road cycling position (i.e., riding in the drops) on the bike by decreasing their torso angle (i.e., between 0–16°) to reduce their frontal area [45] and therefore, aerodynamic drag by up to 20% [45,46]. Adopting a more aerodynamic cycling position does result in altered muscle activation patterns [47] and could potentially increase the physiological cost of cycling [48]. However, it appears that the benefits of maximising aerodynamics in order to improve the drafting effect outweigh any physiological cost [48]. Moreover, previous reviews have highlighted the benefits of drafting during triathlon that minimises the performance decrement during the C–R, contributing to a better overall race performance [1,2,7,40,49]. In particular, VO_2 (~14%), ventilation (~30.8%), heart rate (~7.5%) and blood lactate concentrations are all reduced when drafting during 20 km of cycling at average speed of 39.5 km·h^{-1}, compared to isolated cycling, resulting in a 4% improvement (running speed; 17.8 versus 17.1 km·h^{-1}) in running performance during a sprint triathlon [50]. An even greater decrease in the energy cost of cycling has been shown when drafting behind a larger number of cyclists (eight versus, one, two and four cyclists) and has a significant influence on subsequent running performance [50].

3.3. The Importance of Positioning during Cycling on Running Performance

A triathlete can effectively improve their subsequent running performance by drafting to minimise energy expenditure, especially during the cycle leg of draft-legal, short-course and Olympic distance triathlon. However, the benefits of drafting are dependent on the number of athletes, their formation during cycling and the ability of the athlete to position and handle their bike within the bunch [40]. Indeed, it has been suggested that cycling speed increases substantially during the last kilometre of the cycle leg during elite triathlon due to athletes trying to attain a good position [7] toward the front of the bunch. Entering transition two (cycle–run: T2) at the front of the bunch would improve an athletes chance of minimising time in transition and may result in a better race performance [7]. Furthermore, the ability of a rider to maintain a good position at specific points during the race would likely result in conserving energy that could improve C–R performance. For example, riding at least 8 riders back from the front of the bunch during the early-latter parts of the cycle leg would maximise the drafting effect [50]. Additionally, moving in to the top 8 riders within the final kilometre(s) of cycling would reduce the intensity and number of accelerations performed [51] resulting in conservation of energy [2] and a better chance of moving through T2 more effectively than a rider positioned further back. Indeed, in road sprinting, positioning within the final kilometre(s) of a race (i.e., no less than 9 riders back) translates into a greater chance of winning, compared to a rider not positioned toward the front of the bunch [52]. As such, an athlete competing in draft-legal short-course and Olympic distance triathlon would benefit from having the skills necessary to navigate a bunch in order to effectively position themselves at certain points of the cycling leg to maximising the benefits of drafting in order to improve their running performance. Therefore, working on bunch riding and handling skills (i.e., cornering technique, rider-to-rider contact, effective braking, moving through gaps) to improve the athletes' ability to maximise the drafting effect, while maintaining an optimal pedaling frequency and conservative pacing strategy, would be beneficial.

3.4. Effects of Pedalling Frequency during Cycling on Running Performance

Despite the reported energy saving benefits of drafting during elite short-course and Olympic distance triathlon [50], it is suggested that variability of power output and cadence increases as a by-product of drafting [53]. In particular, pedalling frequency (PF) influences the physiological cost and running performance during the C–R [13,54–56]. It has been reported that higher PF (cadence range 80–120 rpm) increases the oxygen cost and negatively affects subsequent running performance [55,56]. In order to combat the negative effects of high PF cycling and maximise running performance, it has been suggested that triathletes cycle at cadences between 70 and 80 rpm [1,57] and focus on reducing physical effort (power output) during the final minutes of the cycle leg [1]. However, a freely chosen cadence of ~90 rpm during submaximal cycling is considered biomechanically optimal [58,59]. Ideally, it is recommended that elite triathletes competing in draft-legal short-course and Olympic distance triathlon can minimise the effects of PF on C–R performance by maintaining a freely chosen PF close to ~90 rpm. Despite the understanding of the effects of PF on C–R performance, the underlying mechanisms of the physiological, biomechanical and neuromuscular adaptations are not thoroughly understood [2].

3.5. Effects of Pacing Strategies on Short-Course and Olympic Distance Triathlon Performance

The minimisation of energy expenditure through drafting and effective positioning during draft-legal short-course and Olympic distance triathlon could be complimented by adopting an efficient pacing strategy, that is a conscious plan to regulate physical effort [40], during the cycle leg. Furthermore, carrying a pacing strategy in to the subsequent run leg of a triathlon can substantially improve an athlete's overall performance [5,60–62]. Triathletes of all levels, competing across most disciplines typically adopt a fast-start pacing strategy at the beginning of each new discipline (i.e., swim, cycle, run) during a race [40,61]. The fast-start strategy is thought to be due to high intensity of the swim leg in order to gain a good drafting positioning, "race dynamics" and environmental conditions [40]. However, the analysis of race pacing during elite ITU competition would indicate that a fast-start strategy is not the most efficient form of pacing [5,40,49,60–63]. However, differing pacing strategies may be required for certain disciplines of triathlon and between male and females triathletes [63]. Indeed, the current evidence suggests that top overall performers complete the first 400–500 m of the swim significantly faster than slower swimmers (i.e., positive pace strategy) [49]. This allows these athletes better positioning during the swim, among the top swimmers, maximising the drafting effect and resulting in a better swim exit that would lead to a more efficient cycle leg [40,61,62]. Alternatively, slower swimmers exit onto the bike further back and therefore, have to cycle faster, leading to an increased energy output that is inversely related to running performance [49,61]. However, it should be noted that previous research suggests that reducing swim speed (80–85% of mean swim speed) resulted in faster cycling performance [64]. Reducing swim speed during a race-situation may be detrimental to overall performance therefore, improving swimming ability that enables a triathlete to start-fast during the first 400–500 m and then maintain a steady swim pace below 90% of their maximal speed [40,64] could be seen as a preferred pacing strategy.

As previously mentioned, cycle pacing during draft-legal triathlon is heavily dependent on the number of riders in the pack, its configuration and the tactical location of other athletes [40]. Additionally, the importance of maintaining a position at the front of the bunch in an attempt to maximise the drafting effect and the pace of the leading athlete influence the pacing strategy of the cycle discipline [40]. As such, a fast-start pacing strategy is most commonly seen among all respective bunches, however, the pace of the "chasing" bunches likely remains higher than that of the front/lead bunch who often reduced their speed in the final few kilometres prior to the C–R [40]. Together, these "race dynamics" often results in variable-paced cycling.

Similar, to the swim and cycle disciplines, triathletes commonly adopt a reverse J-shaped pace during triathlon running [40,49,61], characterised by a fast-start that declines through the mid-race and then ramps during the final phase [40]. It is unknown whether this run pacing strategy is the most effective for overall performance; rather it is likely determined by "race dynamics". The reverse J-shaped pacing strategy contradicts the current evidence that advocates for an even-paced run strategy [5,60,61]. Specifically, adopting a running speed 5% slower than an athlete's average 10 km pace, during the first kilometre of the run, resulted in a superior run performance [5]. These authors suggested that the slower pace during the early C–R period reduced the development of fatigue, compared to a fast-start strategy, contributing the improved running performance. However, during short-course (i.e., sprint distance, super sprint, and mixed relay) a fast-start strategy may be more beneficial [40,65,66]. A fast-start pacing strategy has been shown to improve oxygen uptake kinetics during exercise lasting between 3–7 min, indicated by improve 3-min cycling performance [66].

Based on the current evidence the following pacing strategies for draft-legal short-course and Olympic distance triathlon are considered most efficient in order to achieve a high overall placing:

(a) Swim: fast 400–500 m, followed by adopting an even pace, below ~90% maximal swim speed, for the remainder of the swim.
(b) Cycle: despite the likelihood of a variable-paced cycle, athletes should aim to maximise the drafting effect through adopting an aerodynamic positioning and ensuring they are positioned efficiently at specific points during the cycle leg. Additionally, maintaining a PF of ~90 rpm and a constant pacing strategy, as well as decreasing their efforts during the latter phase (at least during the final 1 km) of the cycle discipline in order to conserve energy for the C–R. Alternatively, a fast-start strategy is recommended based on the previously reported superior performance during short duration cycling exercise.
(c) Run: athletes should aim to adopt a slightly slower pace (~5% below 10 km pace) during the first kilometre during the C–R and hold a constant pace throughout the run discipline. Alternatively, during short-course triathlon (i.e., sprint distance) a fast-start strategy is recommended.

It is acknowledged that the aforementioned pacing strategies are heavily dependent on other variables and as such athletes will need to react to specific race situations accordingly. However, the pacing strategies provided are based on data collected during elite draft-legal Olympic distance triathlon, namely the 2002 ITU Lausanne World Cup [61], 2007 ITU Beijing World Cup [63,67] and the 2009 European Triathlon Championships [60], and as such can be considered specific to draft-legal short-course and Olympic distance triathlon.

3.6. Effect of Swimming on Cycling Performance Prior to Running

Transitioning from swimming, a predominantly upper-body movement, to cycling that is a predominantly lower-body movement presents some difficulties, mainly blood pooling in the arms [2] that may delay redistribution of blood flow around the body when moving from a supine to upright posture. Moreover, it has been demonstrated that high-intensity swimming substantially increases the physiological cost during subsequent cycling [40,68]. In particular, reduced efficiency (~13%), increased [La-] (~56%) and elevated VO_2 (~5%) have been reported during the first 5-min of a 30-min bout of cycling [34]. However, in comparison to the C–R transition, it is reasonable to suggest that there is a relatively small amount of research investigating the effects of swimming on subsequent cycling and running performance. Apart from the difficulties of reliably conducting swim-based laboratory testing, the lack of focus on the swim-cycle transition, compared to the C–R, is likely due to the suggested weak correlation (r = 0.9730) between swim duration (~10% of total race time) and overall race time [69]. These authors suggested that run performance is considered a better overall predictor of triathlon performance (r = 0.97) and therefore, improving the C–R performance would likely contribute to a better race performance. However, the correlation between the time of the discipline (i.e., swim, cycle or run) may not be entirely reflective of performance, especially at an elite level [68]. Analysis of race data has shown that swimming performance has a substantial impact on an athlete's overall performance, particularly during draft-legal sprint and Olympic distance triathlon [1,49]. Analysing race data from an ITU World Cup event it was reported that the races' top performers swam significantly faster during the first 400–500 m putting them in to a better swim-exit position [49]. Consequently, the slower swimmers had to cycle significantly faster during the first 20 km of the cycle leg, likely compounding the negative effects of the C–R. These authors concluded that running performance largely determines overall performance and is inversely related to cycling speed in the early period of the cycle leg. These findings indicate that a superior swim performance can largely reduce the energy cost of cycling, contributing to an improved running performance. However, continued research by these authors demonstrates that pacing strategies during triathlon is different between sexes [61]. Interestingly, using similar ITU World Cup race data, these authors concluded that cycling performance is more important for elite female triathletes, compared to their male counterparts. It was reported that male triathletes who swam slower had to ride significantly faster in order to 'bridge' to the front group(s) prior to the C–R transition. Furthermore, those athletes in the first pack (superior swimmers) did, on average, run faster during the run leg compared to the athletes in packs two and three (slower swimmers). Alternatively, it has been proposed that elite female triathletes with superior swim and cycle performances significantly improve their chances of a higher overall finishing position compared to those athletes with a weaker swim/bike capacity [61]. Such findings have substantial training and race strategy implications in those elite female athletes with a superior swim/bike performance could isolate their competitors who possess a superior run performance but who are weaker swim/bikers. Overall, this race data indicates that superior swimming performance can substantially minimise the decrement in running performance during triathlon in both elite male and female athletes.

3.7. Specific Training Aimed at Minimising the Potential Effects of Cycling on Running Performance

Replicating race situations in training is a difficult task. However, for those elite triathletes whose running performance is affected by prior cycling, specific training aimed at adapting to the C–R transition should be considered. Common training modalities of elite triathletes has been previously reported however, the data suggests that C–R type sessions are not regularly used [70]. Furthermore, to the author's knowledge, only one previous study has looked at the effects of repetitive C–R training on performance [71]. These authors reported that six weeks of multicycle–run training sessions did not improve C–R performance however; improvements in the C–R transition were evident among the triathlete cohort. Despite the lack of evidence regarding C–R training in elite triathletes, such training may be beneficial for those elite triathletes identified as having difficulty replicating muscle recruitment patterns and neuromuscular control of running after cycling. This type of sequential "brick" training may serve to evoke a training effect that refines the central nervous system's use of a generalised movement strategy [72] that may govern cycling and running motor patterns among elite triathletes sensitive to the negative effects of the C–R [16]. Furthermore, the current literature suggests that variable-cycling does increase the physiological cost (i.e., [La-], R_E, C_R, RER and HR) of subsequent running in elite short-course and Olympic distance triathletes [11,20,73]. Incorporating multicycle–run training sessions in to the training programs of elite triathletes may assist with developing physiological adaptations to the C–R [71]. However, our current understanding of the training effects of back-to-back, "brick" or multicycle–run sessions on adaptation to the C–R are limited and requires further investigation.

However, should coaches and sports scientists use C–R training sessions as part of an elite short-course and Olympic distance triathlete's training program, the intensity should be reflective of the demands experienced during a race and completed as such. Currently, moderate-intensity variable-cycling appears sufficient enough to induce effects experienced during the C–R; however, to replicate race-specific demands during training, variable and repetitive high-intensity C–R efforts would likely be more beneficial [71]. The implementation of C–R training sessions that use variable-power/cadence cycling prior to running is likely to evoke a more specific training stimulus that may contribute to an improve ability to absorb repeated, high-intensity accelerations during draft-legal triathlon [74] and therefore, minimise any negative effect during the C–R period leading to a better overall performance. In addition, adopting a reverse J-shaped paced running strategy (i.e., fast-start, gradual decrease in speed, with a late acceleration of speed), commonly experienced during Olympic distance triathlon [40], would further exposure select elite triathletes to race-specific demands of the C–R transition and potentially improve adaptation. However, it should be noted that alternate pacing strategies are considered to be more efficient and may result in better overall performance. Another means of evoking the specific characteristics of the variable nature of cycling and running experienced during elite short-course and Olympic distance triathlon would include training with other elite triathletes where the pace of cycling and/or running is influenced by the individuals [40].

4. Future Recommendations

4.1. Considerations for Future Research

Currently, there is a limited amount of research investigating the effects of variable-cycling on running performance among elite triathletes and as a result, there is considerable scope to conduct further research within this area. However, based on the lack of clarity within the literature, it is recommended that future research should:

(I) More rigorously define the performance/ability level of the experimental population based on pre-defined criteria. For example, elite triathletes can be defined using a previously defined criteria [75] or based on an ITU world ranking inside the top 125 [2] or their current competitive level, i.e., national/international level (Table 2). Alternatively, using physiological characteristics, such as VO_{2max} or VO_{2peak}, to define the "trained" status of the triathlete population [76,77] may minimise the miscategorisation of the experimental cohort and therefore, improve the training implications of the research, specific to the target triathlete population.

(II) Define the format of triathlon that the testing populations competes. As previously outlined in this article (Table 1), there are various formats of triathlon that can be categorised as short-course, Olympic or long-course, each requiring differing skill sets and physiological output of triathletes. Defining the racing format of the testing population would largely improve the translation of the research findings.

(III) Implement testing protocols that are specific to the category of triathlon (i.e., short-course, Olympic or long-course) in which the testing population competes. For example, if the testing population predominantly competes in short-course triathlon, characterised by variable-, high-intensity cycling, the testing protocols should reflect this. Such testing protocols can be developed or refined using previously reported race data [49,61,78]. Although, within the current literature two field-based [79,80] and three laboratory-based [11,15,81] testing protocols have been reliably validated [15,82]. Therefore, should researchers not use any of the aforementioned protocols, they should at least adopt a testing protocol that resembles the changes a triathlete, male or female, elite or novice, is likely to experience.

(IV) Despite the previously mentioned changes in running performance after submaximal variable-cycling, experimental testing should be conducted using intensities that better reflect the demands that the triathlete cohort are likely to experience during racing.

(V) Investigate the use of alternative methodological techniques to help quantify the mechanisms influencing C–R performance. For example:

   a. Techniques including evoking compound motor action potential (M_{max}) in peripheral nerves (i.e., peripheral nerve stimulation), along with the use of transcranial magnetic stimulation and electrical stimulation can provide an understanding of the level of neuromuscular fatigue experienced during exercise [83,84]. In particular, these techniques have been used to detect changes in motoneuron excitability of the quadriceps muscles during exercise [84,85] and could be used to analyse the effect of the C–R on motoneuron excitability of the leg musculature as a way of identifying any potential neuromuscular fatigue.

   b. Previously, intra-individual variability of gait cycles and cycling patterns have been analysed using variance ratio formulae [86,87]. Such a formula could be used to analyse the reliability and consistency of replicating running gait patterns in order to quantify the reproducibility of efficient muscle activation patterns during C–R performance. For example, plotting muscle activation pattern across a time series during the C–R period would provide a visual representation of any athlete that has difficulty reproducing pre-cycling running patterns.

4.2. Incorporating New Technologies and Techniques into Triathlon Research

The increasing use of technology (i.e., power meters, GPS, blood lactate analysers, digital training platforms) in triathlon provides researchers with the ability to collect and analyse in-field data specific to the demands of each discipline. Access to such data could assist in the development of more specific laboratory-based experimental protocols and the refinement of analysis procedures that would carry a greater degree of practicality for the target triathlete populations. In particular, the use of power meters during cycling provides coaches and sports scientists with detailed power profiles of race course that can be used to develop specific training sessions that can be implemented during race-specific preparation. Meanwhile, the use of wearable GPS tracking units could be used to collate training load, paired with online training platforms, to minimise occurrence of soft tissue injuries [88–90]. Furthermore, the paired use of power meters and GPS can be used by the athlete and coaching staff to develop pacing strategies for specific races, as well as allowing the athlete to monitor their pacing throughout an event in order to maximise their overall performance. Additionally, other wearable motion analysis devices based for example on inertial measurement units (e.g., Leomo® TYPE-R, Leomo, Boulder, CO, USA) could be used to provide real-time data on power output, kinematics and biomechanical alterations outside of a controlled laboratory setting. Using such "live" and in situ motion analysis would likely improve the ability of coaches and researchers to more readily identify those triathletes susceptible to negative C–R performance and provide on-the-spot feedback to athletes that would provide considerable advancement in the specificity of training for triathlon. Additionally, this technology could be used "live" at races or as part of testing procedures in order to provide athletes with direct feedback of the physiological, kinematic and biomechanical changes they are experiencing during the C–R, and therefore, potentially assisting with them adopting different pacing strategies and/or adjusting their race tactics accordingly.

Investigating more sensitive measures of physiological, neuromuscular and biomechanical alterations surrounding the C–R transition should also be encouraged. For example, sagittal plane kinematic analysis suggests elite triathletes are able to replicate pre-cycling running patterns during the C–R transition [16]. However, analysing motor patterns using two-dimensional sagittal plane kinematics is typically limited to quantifying the excursion of individual joint angles and is limited in its ability to account for temporal changes or changes to the coordination of the segments of the leg during a gait cycle. Alternatively, analysing the coordination of the segments of the leg (i.e., thigh, shank and foot) together, using intersegmental coordination, has suggested that neural control of the leg is highly regulated in order to maintain equilibrium during walking and running [91–93]. Furthermore, the regulation of segmental coordination of the leg, during locomotion, has been linked to movement economy [91,92]. Applying such a measure may assist in the identification of those elite triathletes susceptible to kinematic and physiological changes induce during C–R performance.

5. Conclusions

In conclusion, the current evidence available shows that variable-cycling has minimal effect of running performance in elite triathletes. However, cycling does negatively affect running performance in some elite triathletes. Specifically, reductions in running economy, increased variation in muscle activation patterns and changes to stride patterns at intensities below that experienced during racing have been reported among affected elite triathletes. Furthermore, it is reasonable to estimate that these negative effects would be amplified under high-intensity conditions [16]. Meanwhile, pacing strategies employed during the swim and cycle disciplines appear to influence subsequent running and overall performance among all elite triathletes. Despite this, there are ways that an athlete and their coach can minimise the physiological, neuromuscular and biomechanical decrements associated with prior swimming and cycling on C–R performance, such as through drafting, effective bunch positioning, adopting efficient pacing strategies, pedaling frequency and C–R training. It is likely that short-course triathlon racing will continue to gain momentum as a specialty discipline within triathlon, similar to that of 70.3 and Ironman. In response, future research should apply specific criterion for defining the caliber of the experimental cohort in order to not miscategorise the ability of the athletes and use testing protocols that reflects the demands of racing experienced by the experimental population. Continued research should aim at refining and developing new laboratory analysis procedures and in-field testing methods that improve the ability of coaches and scientists to identify those elite triathletes susceptible to the negative effects of cycling on running performance, in order to improve specific training strategies. Additionally, a continued focus on the analysis of current race data will provide a more in-depth understanding of the ever-changing demands of draft-legal short-course and Olympic distance triathlon that will in-turn shape the direction of future research.

Author Contributions: All aspects of this article, including conceptualisation, methodology, investigation, writing—original draft preparation, writing—review and editing, where completed by J.A.W.

Funding: This research received no external funding.

Conflicts of Interest: The authors declare no conflict of interest.

References

1. Bentley, D.J.; Cox, G.R.; Green, D.; Laursen, P.B. Maximising performance in triathlon: Applied physiological and nutritional aspects of elite and non-elite competitions. *J. Sci. Med. Sport* **2008**, *11*, 407–416. [CrossRef] [PubMed]
2. Bentley, D.J.; Millet, G.G.P.; Vleck, V.N.E.; McNaughton, L.R. Specific aspects of contemporary triathlon: Implications for physiological analysis and performance. *Sports Med.* **2002**, *32*, 345–359. [CrossRef] [PubMed]
3. Smith, D.; Lee, H.; Pickard, R.; Sutton, B.; Hunter, E. Power demands of the cycle leg during elite triathlon competition. In Proceedings of the 2nd INSEP International Triathlon Congress European Symposium, Alicante, Spain, 24–26 March 2011.
4. Heiden, T.; Burnett, A. The effect of cycling on muscle activation in the running leg of an Olympic distance triathlon. *Sports Biomech.* **2003**, *2*, 35–49. [CrossRef] [PubMed]
5. Hausswirth, C.; Le Meur, Y.; Bieuzen, F.; Brisswalter, J.; Bernard, T. Pacing strategy during the initial phase of the run in triathlon: Influence on overall performance. *Eur. J. Appl. Physiol.* **2010**, *108*, 1115–1123. [CrossRef]
6. Chapman, A.; Vicenzino, B.; Hodges, R.; Dowlan, S.; Hahn, A.; Alexander, M.; Milner, T. Cycling impairs neuromuscular control during running in triathletes: Implications for performance, injury and intervention. *J. Sci. Med. Sport* **2009**, *12*, S61. [CrossRef]
7. Millet, G.P.; Vleck, V.E. Physiological and biomechanical adaptations to the cycle to run transition in Olympic triathlon: Review and practical recommendations for training. *Br. J. Sports Med.* **2000**, *34*, 384–390. [CrossRef]
8. Piacentini, M.F.; Bianchini, L.A.; Minganti, C.; Sias, M.; Di Castro, A.; Vleck, V. Is the Bike Segment of Modern Olympic Triathlon More a Transition towards Running in Males than It Is in Females? *Sports* **2019**, *7*, 76. [CrossRef]
9. Millet, G.P.; Millet, G.Y.; Candau, R.B. Duration and seriousness of running mechanics alterations after maximal cycling in triathletes. Influence of the performance level. *J. Sports Med. Phys. Fit.* **2001**, *41*, 147–153.
10. Millet, G.P.; Bentley, D.J. The physiological responses to running after cycling in elite junior and senior triathletes. *Int. J. Sports Med.* **2004**, *25*, 191–197.
11. Millet, G.P.; Millet, G.Y.; Hofmann, M.D.; Candau, R.B. Alterations in running economy and mechanics after maximal cycling in triathletes: Influence of performance level. *Int. J. Sports Med.* **2000**, *21*, 127–132. [CrossRef]
12. Le Meur, Y.; Dorel, S.; Rabita, G.; Bernard, T.; Brisswalter, J.; Hausswirth, C. Spring–mass behavior and electromyographic activity evolution during a cycle–run test to exhaustion in triathletes. *J. Electromyogr. Kinesiol.* **2012**, *22*, 835–844. [CrossRef] [PubMed]
13. Bernard, T.; Vercruyssen, F.; Grego, F.; Hausswirth, C.; Lepers, R.; Vallier, J.M.; Brisswalter, J. Effect of cycling cadence on subsequent 3 km running performance in well trained triathletes. *Br. J. Sports Med.* **2003**, *37*, 154–158. [CrossRef]
14. Millet, G.P.; Dreano, P.; Bentley, D.J. Physiological characteristics of elite short- and long-distance triathletes. *Eur. J. Appl. Physiol.* **2003**, *88*, 427–430. [CrossRef] [PubMed]

15. Chapman, A.; Vicenzino, B.; Hodges, P.; Blanch, P.; Hahn, A.; Milner, T. A protocol for measuring the direct effect of cycling on neuromuscular control of running in triathletes. *J. Sports Sci.* **2009**, *27*, 767–782. [CrossRef] [PubMed]
16. Bonacci, J.; Saunders, P.U.; Alexander, M.; Blanch, P.; Vicenzino, B. Neuromuscular control and running economy is preserved in elite international triathletes after cycling. *Sports Biomech.* **2011**, *10*, 59–71. [CrossRef] [PubMed]
17. Chapman, A.; Vicenzino, B.; Blanch, P.; Dowlan, S.; Hodges, P. Does cycling effect motor coordination of the leg during running in elite triathletes? *J. Sci. Med. Sport* **2008**, *11*, 371–380. [CrossRef]
18. Walsh, J.A.; Stamenkovic, A.; Lepers, R.; Peoples, G.; Stapley, P.J. Neuromuscular and physiological variables evolve independently when running immediately after cycling. *J. Electromyogr. Kinesiol.* **2015**, *25*, 887–893. [CrossRef] [PubMed]
19. Chapman, A.; Hodges, P.; Briggs, A.; Stapley, P.; Vicenzino, B. Neuromuscular control and exercise-related leg pain in triathletes. *Med. Sci. Sports Exerc.* **2010**, *42*, 233–243. [CrossRef]
20. Walsh, J.A.; Dawber, J.P.; Lepers, R.; Brown, M.; Stapley, P.J. Is Moderate Intensity Cycling Sufficient to Induce Cardiorespiratory and Biomechanical Modifications of Subsequent Running? *J. Strength Cond. Res.* **2017**, *31*, 1078–1086. [CrossRef]
21. Quod, M.; Martin, D.; Martin, J.; Laursen, P. The power profile predicts road cycling MMP. *Int. J. Sports Med.* **2010**, *31*, 397–401. [CrossRef] [PubMed]
22. Etxebarria, N.; Hunt, J.; Ingham, S.; Ferguson, R. Physiological assessment of isolated running does not directly replicate running capacity after triathlon-specific cycling. *J. Sports Sci.* **2014**, *32*, 229–238. [CrossRef] [PubMed]
23. Lepers, R.; Theurel, J.; Hausswirth, C.; Bernard, T. Neuromuscular fatigue following constant versus variable-intensity endurance cycling in triathletes. *J. Sci. Med. Sport* **2008**, *11*, 381–389. [CrossRef] [PubMed]
24. Hausswirth, C.; Bigard, A.X.; Berthelot, M.; Thomaidis, M.; Guezennec, C.Y. Variability in energy cost of running at the end of a triathlon and a marathon. *Int. J. Sports Med.* **1996**, *17*, 572–579. [CrossRef] [PubMed]
25. Edwards, R.H. Human muscle function and fatigue. *Hum. Muscle Fatigue Physiol. Mech.* **1981**, *82*, 1–18.
26. Fitts, R.H. Cellular mechanisms of muscle fatigue. *Physiol. Rev.* **1994**, *74*, 49–94. [CrossRef] [PubMed]
27. Edwards, R.H. Biochemical bases of fatigue in exercise performance: Catastrophe theory of muscular fatigue. *Biochem. Exerc.* **1983**, *13*, 3–28.
28. Allen, D.G.; Lamb, G.D.; Westerblad, H. Skeletal muscle fatigue: Cellular mechanisms. *Physiol. Rev.* **2008**, *88*, 287–332. [CrossRef]
29. Gruet, M.; Temesi, J.; Rupp, T.; Levy, P.; Millet, G.; Verges, S. Stimulation of the motor cortex and corticospinal tract to assess human muscle fatigue. *Neuroscience* **2013**, *231*, 384–399. [CrossRef]
30. Wan, J.-J.; Qin, Z.; Wang, P.-Y.; Sun, Y.; Liu, X. Muscle fatigue: General understanding and treatment. *Exp. Mol. Med.* **2017**, *49*, e384. [CrossRef]
31. Gandevia, S.C. Spinal and supraspinal factors in human muscle fatigue. *Physiol. Rev.* **2001**, *81*, 1725–1789. [CrossRef]
32. Davis, J.M. Central and peripheral factors in fatigue. *J. Sports Sci.* **1995**, *13*, S49–S53. [CrossRef] [PubMed]
33. Meeusen, R.; Watson, P.; Hasegawa, H.; Roelands, B.; Piacentini, M.F. Central fatigue. *Sports Med.* **2006**, *36*, 881–909. [CrossRef] [PubMed]
34. Delextrat, A.; Brisswalter, J.; Hausswirth, C.; Bernard, T.; Vallier, J.-M. Does prior 1500-m swimming affect cycling energy expenditure in well-trained triathletes? *Can. J. Appl. Physiol.* **2005**, *30*, 392–403. [CrossRef]
35. Guezennec, C.Y.; Vallier, J.M.; Bigard, A.X.; Durey, A. Increase in energy cost of running at the end of a triathlon. *Eur. J. Appl. Physiol. Occup. Physiol.* **1996**, *73*, 440–445. [CrossRef]
36. Hue, O.; Le Gallais, D.; Chollet, D.; Boussana, A.; Prefaut, C. The influence of prior cycling on biomechanical and cardiorespiratory response profiles during running in triathletes. *Eur. J. Appl. Physiol. Occup. Physiol.* **1998**, *77*, 98–105. [CrossRef] [PubMed]
37. Kreider, R.B.; Boone, T.; Thompson, W.R.; Burkes, S.; Cortes, C.W. Cardiovascular and thermal responses of triathlon performance. *Med. Sci. Sports Exerc.* **1988**, *20*, 385–390. [CrossRef] [PubMed]
38. Hausswirth, C.; Bigard, A.X.; Guezennec, C.Y. Relationships between running mechanics and energy cost of running at the end of a triathlon and a marathon. *Int. J. Sports Med.* **1997**, *18*, 330–339. [CrossRef] [PubMed]
39. Quigley, E.J.; Richards, J.G. The effects of cycling on running mechanics. *J. Appl. Biomech.* **1996**, *12*, 470–479. [CrossRef]

40. Wu, S.S.; Peiffer, J.J.; Brisswalter, J.; Nosaka, K.; Abbiss, C.R. Factors influencing pacing in triathlon. *Open Access J. Sports Med.* **2014**, *5*, 223. [CrossRef]
41. Blocken, B.; van Druenen, T.; Toparlar, Y.; Malizia, F.; Mannion, P.; Andrianne, T.; Marchal, T.; Maas, G.-J.; Diepens, J. Aerodynamic drag in cycling pelotons: New insights by CFD simulation and wind tunnel testing. *J. Wind Eng. Ind. Aerodyn.* **2018**, *179*, 319–337. [CrossRef]
42. McCole, S.; Claney, K.; Conte, J.-C.; Anderson, R.; Hagberg, J. Energy expenditure during bicycling. *J. Appl. Physiol.* **1990**, *68*, 748–753. [CrossRef]
43. Gaul, L.; Thomson, S.; Griffiths, I. Optimizing the breakaway position in cycle races using mathematical modelling. *Sports Eng.* **2018**, *21*, 297–310. [CrossRef]
44. Kyle, C.R. Reduction of wind resistance and power output of racing cyclists and runners travelling in groups. *Ergonomics* **1979**, *22*, 387–397. [CrossRef]
45. Lukes, R.; Chin, S.; Haake, S. The understanding and development of cycling aerodynamics. *Sports Eng.* **2005**, *8*, 59–74. [CrossRef]
46. Kyle, C.R.; Burke, E. Improving the racing bicycle. *Mech. Eng.* **1984**, *106*, 34–45.
47. Chapman, A.R.; Vicenzino, B.; Blanch, P.; Knox, J.J.; Dowlan, S.; Hodges, P.W. The influence of body position on leg kinematics and muscle recruitment during cycling. *J. Sci. Med. Sport* **2008**, *11*, 519–526. [CrossRef] [PubMed]
48. Fintelman, D.; Sterling, M.; Hemida, H.; Li, F.X. Effect of different aerodynamic time trial cycling positions on muscle activation and crank torque. *Scand. J. Med. Sci. Sports* **2016**, *26*, 528–534. [CrossRef] [PubMed]
49. Vleck, V.E.; Burgi, A.; Bentley, D.J. The consequences of swim, cycle, and run performance on overall result in elite olympic distance triathlon. *Int. J. Sports Med.* **2006**, *27*, 43–48. [CrossRef]
50. Hausswirth, C.; Lehénaff, D.; Dréano, P.; Savonen, K. Effects of cycling alone or in a sheltered position on subsequent running performance during a triathlon. *Med. Sci. Sports Exerc.* **1999**, *31*, 599–604. [CrossRef] [PubMed]
51. Menaspà, P.; Quod, M.; Martin, D.; Peiffer, J.; Abbiss, C. Physical demands of sprinting in professional road cycling. *Int. J. Sports Med.* **2015**, *36*, 1058–1062. [CrossRef]
52. Menaspà, P.; Abbiss, C.R.; Martin, D.T. Performance analysis of a world-class sprinter during cycling grand tours. *Int. J. Sports Physiol. Perform.* **2013**, *8*, 336–340. [CrossRef]
53. Hausswirth, C.; Brisswalter, J. Strategies for improving performance in long duration events. *Sports Med.* **2008**, *38*, 881–891. [CrossRef]
54. Gottschall, J.S.; Palmer, B.M. The acute effects of prior cycling cadence on running performance and kinematics. *Med. Sci. Sports Exerc.* **2002**, *34*, 1518–1522. [CrossRef]
55. Vercruyssen, F.; Brisswalter, J.; Hausswirth, C.; Bernard, T.; Bernard, O.; Vallier, J.-M. Influence of cycling cadence on subsequent running performance in triathletes. *Med. Sci. Sports Exerc.* **2002**, *34*, 530–536. [CrossRef] [PubMed]
56. Vercruyssen, F.; Suriano, R.; Bishop, D.; Hausswirth, C.; Brisswalter, J. Cadence selection affects metabolic responses during cycling and subsequent running time to fatigue. *Br. J. Sports Med.* **2005**, *39*, 267–272. [CrossRef]
57. Brisswalter, J.; Hausswirth, C.; Smith, D.; Vercruyssen, F.; Vallier, J.M. Energetically optimal cadence vs. freely-chosen cadence during cycling: Effect of exercise duration. *Int. J. Sports Med.* **2000**, *21*, 60–64. [CrossRef] [PubMed]
58. Vercruyssen, F.; Hausswirth, C.; Smith, D.; Brisswalter, J. Effect of exercise duration on optimal pedalling rate choice in triathletes. *Can. J. Appl. Physiol.* **2001**, *26*, 44–54. [PubMed]
59. Lepers, R.; Millet, G.; Maffiuletti, N.; Hausswirth, C.; Brisswalter, J. Effect of pedalling rates on physiological response during endurance cycling. *Eur. J. Appl. Physiol.* **2001**, *85*, 392–395. [CrossRef]
60. Le Meur, Y.; Bernard, T.; Dorel, S.; Abbiss, C.R.; Honnorat, G.; Brisswalter, J.; Hausswirth, C. Relationships between triathlon performance and pacing strategy during the run in an international competition. *Int. J. Sports Physiol. Perform.* **2011**, *6*, 183–194. [CrossRef]
61. Vleck, V.E.; Bentley, D.J.; Millet, G.P.; Bürgi, A. Pacing during an elite Olympic distance triathlon: Comparison between male and female competitors. *J. Sci. Med. Sport* **2008**, *11*, 424–432. [CrossRef]
62. Wu, S.S.X.; Peiffer, J.J.; Brisswalter, J.; Nosaka, K.; Lau, W.Y.; Abbiss, C.R. Pacing strategies during the swim, cycle and run disciplines of sprint, Olympic and half-Ironman triathlons. *Eur. J. Appl. Physiol.* **2015**, *115*, 1147–1154. [CrossRef]

63. Le Meur, Y.; Hausswirth, C.; Dorel, S.; Bignet, F.; Brisswalter, J.; Bernard, T. Influence of gender on pacing adopted by elite triathletes during a competition. *Eur. J. Appl. Physiol.* **2009**, *106*, 535–545. [CrossRef] [PubMed]
64. Peeling, P.; Bishop, D.; Landers, G. Effect of swimming intensity on subsequent cycling and overall triathlon performance. *Br. J. Sports Med.* **2005**, *39*, 960–964. [CrossRef] [PubMed]
65. Aisbett, B.; Lerossignol, P.; McConell, G.K.; Abbiss, C.R.; Snow, R. Influence of all-out and fast start on 5-min cycling time trial performance. *Med. Sci. Sports Exerc.* **2009**, *41*, 1965–1971. [CrossRef] [PubMed]
66. Bailey, S.J.; Vanhatalo, A.; Dimenna, F.J.; Wilkerson, D.P.; Jones, A.M. Fast-start strategy improves VO2 kinetics and high-intensity exercise performance. *Med. Sci. Sports Exerc.* **2011**, *43*, 457–467. [CrossRef]
67. Le Meur, Y.; Hausswirth, C.; Dorel, S.; Bignet, F.; Brisswalter, J.; Bernard, T. Erratum to: Influence of gender on pacing adopted by elite triathletes during a competition. *Eur. J. Appl. Physiol.* **2011**, *111*, 1231–1233. [CrossRef]
68. Peeling, P.; Landers, G. Swimming intensity during triathlon: A review of current research and strategies to enhance race performance. *J. Sports Sci.* **2009**, *27*, 1079–1085. [CrossRef] [PubMed]
69. Dengel, D.R.; Flynn, M.G.; Costill, D.L.; Kirwan, J.P. Determinants of success during triathalon competition. *Res. Q. Exerc. Sport* **1989**, *60*, 234–238. [CrossRef]
70. Vleck, V.E.; Bentley, D.J.; Millet, G.P.; Cochrane, T. Triathlon event distance specialization: Training and injury effects. *J. Strength Cond. Res.* **2010**, *24*, 30–36. [CrossRef]
71. Hue, O.; Valluet, A.; Blonc, S.; Hertogh, C. Effects of multicycle–run training on triathlete performance. *Res. Q. Exerc. Sport* **2002**, *73*, 289–295. [CrossRef]
72. Karniel, A.; Mussa-Ivaldi, F.A. Does the motor control system use multiple models and context switching to cope with a variable environment? *Exp. Brain Res.* **2002**, *143*, 520–524. [CrossRef] [PubMed]
73. Chapman, A.; Vicenzino, B.; Blanch, P.; Hodges, P. Do differences in muscle recruitment between novice and elite cyclists reflect different movement patterns or less skilled muscle recruitment? *J. Sci. Med. Sport* **2009**, *12*, 31–34. [CrossRef] [PubMed]
74. Etxebarria, N.; Ingham, S.A.; Ferguson, R.A.; Bentley, D.J.; Pyne, D.B. Sprinting after having sprinted: Prior high-intensity stochastic cycling impairs the winning strike for Gold. *Front. Physiol.* **2019**, *10*, 100. [CrossRef]
75. Swann, C.; Moran, A.; Piggott, D. Defining elite athletes: Issues in the study of expert performance in sport psychology. *Psychol. Sport Exerc.* **2015**, *16*, 3–14. [CrossRef]
76. Groslambert, A.; Grappe, F.; Bertucci, W.; Perrey, S. A perceptive individual time trial performed by triathletes. *J. Sports Med. Phys. Fit.* **2004**, *44*, 147–156.
77. Suriano, R.; Bishop, D. Physiological attributes of triathletes. *J. Sci. Med. Sport* **2010**, *13*, 340–347. [CrossRef]
78. Bernard, T.; Hausswirth, C.; Le Meur, Y.; Bignet, F.; Dorel, S.; Brisswalter, J. Distribution of power output during the cycling stage of a triathlon world cup. *Med. Sci. Sports Exerc.* **2009**, *41*, 1296–1302. [CrossRef] [PubMed]
79. Vleck, V.; Santos, S.; Bentley, D.; Alves, F. Influence of prior cycling on the OBLA measured during incremental running in triathletes. *Annu. Congr. Br. Assoc. Sports Exerc. Sci. Leeds J. Sports Sci.* **2005**, *23*, 93–223.
80. Díaz, V.; Peinado, A.B.; Vleck, V.E.; Alvarez-Sanchez, M.; Benito, P.J.; Alves, F.B.; Calderón, F.J.; Zapico, A.G. Longitudinal changes in response to a cycle–run field test of young male national "Talent identification" and senior elite triathlon squads. *J. Strength Cond. Res.* **2012**, *26*, 2209–2219. [CrossRef] [PubMed]
81. Bentley, D.; Delextrat, A.; Vleck, V.; Reid, A. Reliability of a sequential running-cycling-running test in trained triathletes. *Annu. Congr. Br. Assoc. Sports Exerc. Sci. J. Sports Sci.* **2005**, *23*, 93–223.
82. Vleck, V.; Alves, F.B. Triathlon Transition Tests: Overview and Recommendations for Future Research. *RICYDE Revista Internacional de Ciencias del Deporte* **2011**, *7*, I–III. [CrossRef]
83. Millet, G.Y.; Lepers, R. Alterations of neuromuscular function after prolonged running, cycling and skiing exercises. *Sports Med.* **2004**, *34*, 105–116. [CrossRef]
84. Finn, H.T.; Rouffet, D.M.; Kennedy, D.S.; Green, S.; Taylor, J.L. Motoneuron excitability of the quadriceps decreases during a fatiguing submaximal isometric contraction. *J. Appl. Physiol.* **2018**, *124*, 970–979. [CrossRef] [PubMed]
85. Temesi, J.; Rupp, T.; Martin, V.; Arnal, P.J.; Feasson, L.; Verges, S.; Millet, G.Y. Central fatigue assessed by transcranial magnetic stimulation in ultratrail running. *Med. Sci. Sports Exerc.* **2014**, *46*, 1166–1175. [CrossRef] [PubMed]

86. Burden, A.; Trew, M.; Baltzopoulos, V. Normalisation of gait EMGs: A re-examination. *J. Electromyogr. Kinesiol.* **2003**, *13*, 519–532. [CrossRef]
87. Rouffet, D.M.; Hautier, C.A. EMG normalization to study muscle activation in cycling. *J. Electromyogr. Kinesiol.* **2008**, *18*, 866–878. [CrossRef]
88. Ehrmann, F.E.; Duncan, C.S.; Sindhusake, D.; Franzsen, W.N.; Greene, D.A. GPS and injury prevention in professional soccer. *J. Strength Cond. Res.* **2016**, *30*, 360–367. [CrossRef] [PubMed]
89. Buchheit, M.; Simpson, B.M. Player-tracking technology: Half-full or half-empty glass? *Int. J. Sports Physiol. Perform.* **2017**, *12*, S2-35–S2-41. [CrossRef]
90. Gabbett, T.J.; Ullah, S. Relationship between running loads and soft-tissue injury in elite team sport athletes. *J. Strength Cond. Res.* **2012**, *26*, 953–960. [CrossRef] [PubMed]
91. Bianchi, L.; Angelini, D.; Orani, G.P.; Lacquaniti, F. Kinematic coordination in human gait: Relation to mechanical energy cost. *J. Neurophysiol.* **1998**, *79*, 2155–2170. [CrossRef] [PubMed]
92. Lacquaniti, F.; Grasso, R.; Zago, M. Motor patterns in walking. *Physiology* **1999**, *14*, 168–174. [CrossRef]
93. Hicheur, H.; Terekhov, A.V.; Berthoz, A. Intersegmental coordination during human locomotion: Does planar covariation of elevation angles reflect central constraints? *J. Neurophysiol.* **2006**, *96*, 1406–1419. [CrossRef] [PubMed]

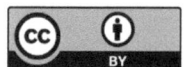

© 2019 by the author. Licensee MDPI, Basel, Switzerland. This article is an open access article distributed under the terms and conditions of the Creative Commons Attribution (CC BY) license (http://creativecommons.org/licenses/by/4.0/).

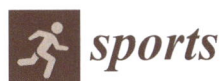 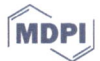

Article

Cross-Sectional Investigation of Stress Fractures in German Elite Triathletes

Pauline Neidel [1,*], Petra Wolfram [2], Thilo Hotfiel [3,4], Martin Engelhardt [4], Rainer Koch [5], Geoffrey Lee [6] and Stefan Zwingenberger [1]

1. Department of Sports Medicine at the University Center for Orthopaedics and Traumatology, University Medicine Carl Gustav Carus, Technical University Dresden, 01307 Dresden, Germany; Stefan.Zwingenberger@uniklinikum-dresden.de
2. Department for Sports Science, German Triathlon Federation, 60528 Frankfurt/Main, Germany; wolfram.petra@googlemail.com
3. Department of Orthopaedic Surgery, Friedrich-Alexander-University Erlangen-Nuremberg, 91054 Erlangen, Germany; Thilo.Hotfiel@fau.de
4. Department of Trauma and Orthopedic Surgery, Klinikum Osnabrück, 49076 Osnabrück, Germany; Martin.Engelhardt@klinikum-os.de
5. Department of Medical Statistics and Biometry, Medical Faculty Carl Gustav Carus at Technical University Dresden, 01307 Dresden, Germany; rainer.koch.01@gmx.de
6. Kennedy Institute of Rheumatology, Nuffield Department of Orthopaedics, Rheumatology, and Musculoskeletal Sciences, University of Oxford, Oxford OX3 7FY, UK; geoffrey.lee@kennedy.ox.ac.uk
* Correspondence: Pauline.neidel@t-online.de; Tel.: +49-171-566-8136

Received: 25 February 2019; Accepted: 10 April 2019; Published: 15 April 2019

Abstract: Triathlon is a popular sport for both recreational and competitive athletes. This study investigated the rates and patterns of stress fractures in the German national triathlon squad. We developed a web-based retrospective questionnaire containing questions about the frequency of stress fractures, anatomic localisation and associated risk factors. The survey was conducted as an explorative cross-sectional study. Eighty-six athletes completed the questionnaire. Twenty athletes (23%) sustained at least one stress fracture. All documented stress fractures were located in the lower extremities. Factors associated with a higher risk for stress fractures were female gender, competitive sport prior to triathlon career, Vitamin D or iron deficiency, menstrual disturbances and a high number of annual training hours. Disseminating knowledge among athletes and their professional community in order to raise awareness about early symptoms and relevant risk factors could help to improve prevention and reduce the incidence of stress fractures.

Keywords: triathlon; injury; stress fracture; risk factors; prevention

1. Introduction

Triathlon is an endurance sport that is growing in popularity. Given its multisport nature, it comprises three disciplines in one event: swimming, cycling, and running. There are numerous competitive events ranging from sprint distance (0.75 km–20 km–5 km) to long distance triathlon (3.8 km–180 km–42 km). Moreover, related formats are duathlon or relay competitions. The Olympic Games reflects the highest achievable sporting event for short distance athletes. Triathlon has been included in the Olympic Program since Sydney 2000. Among long distance triathletes, the Ironman® World Championships Hawaii, represents the most famous competition.

In Germany, triathlon is governed by the Deutsche Triathlon Union (DTU). Currently, DTU includes 58,000 members, and continues to grow [1]. An important function of the DTU is the development and promotion of young and elite athletes. These are organized in a system of different national and federal state squads [2]. In order to provide a structured training environment, DTU has set up several national training bases where most of the squad athletes are located [2].

Injuries and the consecutive loss of training and cancellation of competitions inevitably have an impact on athletes. Various studies showed that in triathlon, overuse injuries are more common than acute injuries, accounting for up to 79% [3–6]. Recent observations of DTU confirm the rising incidence of stress fractures among their squad athletes [7]. Furthermore, the latest cases of stress fractures in professional long-distance triathletes like Jan Frodeno and Ben Hoffmann, forcing them to default the World Championships in Hawaii, show the devastating consequences of this injury [8,9]. Consequently, the need to identify potential risk factors led to the conception of this study. Another aspect is that, to our knowledge, there is no investigation about the occurrence of stress fractures in triathletes. In order to improve the prevention of stress fractures and the management of risk factors, it is crucial to understand which athletes are prone to this injury. Therefore, data about the occurrence of stress fractures and their anatomic localisation, as well as relevant factors that are aetiologically associated with stress fractures, were requested. The primary aim of this study was to identify the prevalence of stress fractures among German elite-triathletes. The secondary aim was to find factors that may act as possible predictors of stress fractures such as gender, BMI, triathlon career, nutritional deficiencies, menstrual irregularities or biomechanical factors. This could lead to new hypotheses and further studies to find causal relationships.

2. Materials and Methods

This investigation was carried out as an explorative cross-sectional study using a web-based questionnaire. In November 2017, athletes of the 2017 DTU-Triathlon squad were contacted by email either directly or indirectly via their national coach. Beforehand, all national coaches were introduced to the study during a DTU Elite Sport Conference. They received both a description of the study for informed consent and an online link with access to the web-based questionnaire. Athletes were then asked to complete the questionnaire on a voluntary basis. Participants gave their informed consent by completing the questionnaire. In January 2018, the survey period was closed.

The study particularly focused on elite athletes. Therefore, a precondition for participation was the membership to a German national squad (A-, B- or C-team) or Federal State squad (D- or D/C-team). In 2017, the German national team involved 59 athletes. Distributed over the 16 state federations; the Federal State squads included 209 athletes. Consequently, 268 athletes were potentially available and contacted for this investigation.

All information was collected retrospectively using both open-ended and multiple choice questions. The questionnaire was distributed into three sections: 1. General questions about anthropometric information, e.g., age, gender or body weight; 2. Questions with regard to their training habits and health issues such as menstrual function or nutritional status; 3. Questions about the occurrence of stress fractures divided into the time before, during and after the fracture. Athletes who had not yet sustained a stress fracture were allowed to exit the questionnaire after finishing the second section. All information was gathered by laypeople.

After the survey period, all data were collated into Microsoft Excel® (Version 15.0; Microsoft Corporation, Redmond, WA, USA) and anonymised. Subsequently, data were transferred to SAS® (Version 9.4; SAS Institute, Cary, NC, USA) for statistical analysis. For the purpose of data description, the results were specified by median (Q_1; Q_3), average (±SD) and minima and maxima. The central tool for the measurement of risk was univariate Odds Ratio (OR), followed by a test for significance using Pearson's chi-square-test, Fisher's exact test (when sample size was low) or Wald-tests (for continuous variables). Univariate ORs were estimated using an SAS-Macro which was based on Wald confidence limits. For all tests, the significance level was set to 5%. The calculation of the incidence rate was performed as division of the sum of the number of stress fractures with the sum of total person-years under risk. Due to the chosen study design, that is cross-sectional investigation, and due to the high number of targeted events, ORs should not be interpreted as measurements of relative risks.

All procedures were carried out in accordance with the local ethics committee of Technical University Dresden (Protocol number: EK 399102017; Date of approval: 26 September 2017) as well as with the Declaration of Helsinki.

3. Results

3.1. All Survey Participants

A total of 136 athletes (50.7%) responded to the survey. Fifty athletes did not complete the questionnaire in its entirety. They mostly left the Online-survey in the first part (General questions) right after the beginning of the survey. Therefore, they were excluded from analysis due to incomplete data. Consequently, 86 (63.2%) athletes could be subjected to analysis. Of the 86 participants, 47 were male (55%) and 39 were female (45%) athletes. The anthropometric characteristics and training habits are shown in Table 1. On average, the athletes were 17.45 years old when they submitted the questionnaire. According to the age group definitions of DTU [10], the age group "Under 18" was the highest proportion. The distribution of athletes to the different squads is shown in Table 2 following the definitions of the German squad system until 2017 [11].

Table 1. Anthropometric characteristics, triathlon career, weekly training habits and the number of competitions of all participants, the group of athletes who sustained a stress fracture and of those who did not sustain a stress fracture are listed. All numbers refer to the 2017 season due to the retrospective nature of the survey. For all categories, average values (±SD), minima and maxima are shown.

Categories	All Participants Average (±SD)—Min/Max	Injured Participants Average (±SD)—Min/Max	Non-Injured Participants Average (±SD)—Min/Max
Anthropometric characteristics			
Age (years)	17.5 (±3.3)—12/34	18.0 (±2.7)—12/23	17.3 (±3.4)—13/34
BMI (kg/m^2)	19.9 (±1.4)—16/24	20.4 (±1.9)—16/24	19.8 (±1.2)—16/22
Triathlon career			
Experience in triathlon (years)	6.4 (±2.8)—1/14	5.9 (±2.7)—3/11	6.5 (±2.9)—1/14
Weekly training habits			
Duration/week, Total (h)	16.4 (±5.5)—7/46	19.5 (±8.0)—8/46	15.5 (±4.1)—7/25
Duration/week, Swim (h)	6.0 (±2.4)—0/20	7.2 (±3.4)—3/20	5.7 (±2.0)—0/10
Duration/week, Bike (h)	4.1 (±1.9)—0/10	5.1 (±2.1)—2/10	3.8 (±1.8)—0/8
Duration/week, Run (h)	3.9 (±1.7)—1/12	4.6 (±2.1)—3/12	3.7 (±1.6)—1/12
Duration/week, Others (h)	2.3 (±1.3)—0/6	2.7 (±1.5)—1/6	2.1 (±1.3)—0/6
Distance/week, Swim (km)	16.3 (±5.6)—1/40	19.5 (±6.4)—6/40	15.6 (±4.8)—1/25
Distance/week, Bike (km)	110.2 (±55.6)—4/241	131.6 (±57.2)—31/241	105.7 (±52.9)—0/240
Distance/week, Run (km)	34.6 (±13.6)—4/70	37.6 (±13.9)—7/70	34.2 (±13.0)—6/60
Annual competitions			
Competitions (no.)	8.4 (±3.2)—0/21	7.8 (±4.0)—0/15	8.7 (±3.0)—0/21

Table 2. The membership to either the German national squad or one of the 16 Federal State squads is shown. According to the squad system until 2017, squads are further divided into an A-, B- or C-team within the national squad and into a D/C- or D-team in the Federal State squad. For all categories, absolute and relative proportions are listed.

Categories		N (%) (n = 86)	Total (n = 86)
German national squad	A	1 (1%)	15 (17%)
	B	10 (12%)	
	C	4 (5%)	
Federal State squad	D/C	13 (15%)	71 (83%)
	D	58 (67%)	

Of all participants, 56 (65%) had competed in another sport prior to their triathlon career. The most frequent sports were swimming (36%) and track and field sports (29%). All athletes participated mainly over short distances like Super Sprint (<0.5 km, <13 km, <3.5 km) and Sprint distance (0.75 km–20 km–5 km). As shown in Table 3, some athletes suffer from biomechanical issues, nutritional deficits or, referring to the female athletes, from menstrual irregularities. Treatment of the biomechanical issues was mainly carried out by specific shoe inserts or physical therapy. Amongst the nutritional supplementation, Vitamin D and iron supplements were most frequently taken.

Table 3. Categorical variables to describe gender distribution, biomechanical issues, nutritional deficits and menstrual irregularities. The numbers refer to the group of all athletes, injured and non-injured athletes. For all categories, numbers and percentages are shown.

Categories	All Participants N (%) (n = 86)	Injured Participants N (%) (n = 20)	Non-Injured Participants N (%) (n = 66)
Gender			
Female gender	39 (45%)	12 (60%)	27 (41%)
Male gender	47 (55%)	8 (40%)	39 (59%)
Biomechanical issues			
Misalignment of feet	27 (31%)	4 (20%)	23 (35%)
Misalignment of leg axis	14 (16%)	2 (10%)	12 (18%)
Unequal leg length	10 (12%)	1 (5%)	9 (14%)
Unspecified	3 (3%)	0	3 (5%)
Treatment [1]	19 (35%)	3 (43%)	16 (24%)
Nutritional deficits			
Iron deficiency	29 (34%)	9 (45%)	20 (30%)
Vitamin D deficiency	10 (12%)	3 (15%)	7 (11%)
Nutritional supplementation	24 (28%)	9 (45%)	15 (23%)
Menstrual irregularities [2]			
Irregular menstrual cycles	12 (31%)	5 (42%)	7 (11%)
Amenorrhea	5 (13%)	5 (42%)	0

[1] Refers to those athletes who claimed a biomechanical issue. [2] Refers only to female athletes (n = 39).

3.2. Injured Participants

At the time of submission, 24 athletes had sustained a stress fracture. Yet, only 20 responses could be statistically analysed because four participants reported self-diagnosed stress fractures or different injuries. Those replies had to be sorted out due to the low validity of self-reported stress fractures [12]. Hence, 15 athletes with one stress fracture, four athletes with two stress fractures, one athlete with three stress fractures and 66 athletes with no stress fracture were transferred into the evaluation. This totaled 23%. Taking the number of occurrences per total person-years into consideration, the incidence rate was 4.8%/year (95% CI (approximate confidence interval: 3.0–6.5%). Among the group of injured athletes, 8 (40%) were male and 12 (60%) were female athletes. Their detailed description can be found in Tables 1 and 3. Seven athletes belonged to the German national squad and 13 athletes to a Federal State squad, especially to the D-Team. Fifteen athletes (75%) were active in a different competitive sport prior to their triathlon career. Common sports were swimming (N (%): 7 (47%)) and track and field sports (N (%): 7 (47%)). The number of biomechanical issues, nutritional deficiencies and menstrual irregularities can be found in Table 3.

All stress fractures were localised in the lower extremities. The main anatomic localisations were the metatarsal bones (52%). In four cases (19%), athletes sustained a fracture of the femur or femoral neck, respectively. In six cases, the lower leg was affected—2 times (10%) for each tibia, fibula and calcaneus. Athletes sustained their first reported stress fracture with an average age of 16.9 (±2.5) years. Minimum age was 12 years and maximum age was 22 years.

Prior to the occurrence of the stress fracture, 12 athletes (57%) had increased their training. This mainly (75%) referred to an increase in the distance per week, especially of the running distance. Furthermore, it seems plausible that 10 athletes (48%) had participated in a training camp for 10.45 (±3.50) days on average. However, changes of diet, body weight, equipment or technique played a minimal role. Likewise, a predominant hard surface or a specific running technique did not influence the injury occurrence.

All athletes felt pain in the particular location as initial symptom. For the most part, the pain arose in training N (%): 16 (76%)), during (N (%): 19 (90%)) or after (N (%): 16 (76%)) activity and was increasing (N (%): 16 (70%)) or was consistent (N (%): 5 (22%)) in the course of time, respectively. However, regardless of the anatomic localisation, all symptoms were assigned to running. There was only one exception, namely a hip fracture which was noticed in swimming although the specific athlete reported to have felt the pain during the pushing-off movements off the wall.

The median value from the onset of symptoms until medical consultation was seven days (Q_1: 3; Q_3: 15). Further, between the first medical consultation and the time of diagnosis passed a median of three days (Q_1: 1; Q_3: 7) with a range of 0–150 days. X-ray (N (%): 13 (62%)) and magnetic resonance tomography (MRI) (N (%): 12 (57%)) were mainly used as diagnostic tools. Computer tomography was only used in three cases (13%).

The vast majority (N (%): 17 (81%)) received conservative treatment. However, in two cases athletes had to undergo surgery: firstly, a stress fracture of the metatarsals and secondly, a stress fracture of the tibia. The median value of training downtime in terms of rehabilitation was 70 days (Q_1: 28; Q_3: 120) with a wide range of 6–180 days. The longest break (120 days; Q_1: 110; Q_3: 135) was seen in stress fractures of the femur, followed by stress fractures of the tibia (69 days; Q_1: 49; Q_3: 90) and calcaneus (60 days; Q_1: 55; Q_3: 65). In contrast, the shortest break in training was caused by stress fractures of the metatarsal bones (50 days; Q_1: 28; Q_3: 120) and fibula (55 days; Q_1: 48; Q_3: 63). While training was interrupted in the affected discipline, most of the athletes trained in alternative sports such as swimming (N (%): 14 (78%)) and biking (N (%): 11 (61%)). Taking all athletes with stress fractures into consideration, the period from symptom onset until return to training amounted to 80 days, disregarding the fact that there may have been temporal overlaps.

3.3. Risk Factors

The following table (Table 4) shows the results of the analysis of univariate Odds Ratio (OR):

Table 4. Categories with OR > 1 and OR < 1 are listed. ORs are given for each category as well as 95% confidence intervals and p-values. The calculation of the p-value was based on chi-squared tests and Wald tests with single or multiple fractures as event.

Category	OR	95% CI	p-Value
Female gender	2.2	0.8–6.0	0.1330
Competitive sport prior to triathlon	1.8	0.6–5.7	0.2898
Vitamin D deficiency	1.6	0.4–6.8	0.5612
Iron deficiency	2.2	0.7–6.6	0.1544
Nutritional supplementation	2.8	1.0–8.0	0.0517
Total amount of training [2]	1.2	1.0–1.3	0.0173
Irregular menstrual cycles [1]	1.7	0.4–7.4	0.4533
BMI [2]	1.3	0.9–1.9	0.1541
Distance/week, Run [2]	1.0	1.0–1.1	0.6080
Misalignment of feet	0.4	0.1–1.3	0.1008
Misalignment of leg axis	0.5	0.1–2.4	0.3732
Experience in triathlon/Years in triathlon [2]	0.9	0.7–1.1	0.2872
Number of competitions [2]	0.9	0.8–1.1	0.1990
Unequal leg length	0.3	0.0–2.5	0.2333

[1]: This category only applies to female athletes. [2]: For quantitative variables, an increase of OR refers to an increase by one unit of measurement.

4. Discussion

A central aim of this investigation was the identification of factors that may be associated with an increase of risk for stress fractures. This is of importance because identifying factors that place athletes at greater risk for injury can be crucial to reduce the occurrence of injuries [4]. Hence, this knowledge can help to improve prevention and knowledge about stress fractures and can also lead to new hypotheses to find causal relationships.

Taking all aspects into consideration, among German elite triathletes, athletes with the following factors were associated with sustaining a stress fracture: female gender, background in competitive sports, Vitamin D or iron deficiency, nutritional supplementation, irregular menstrual cycles and high total training amounts.

When projected on an entire year, the duration of training amounted to 853 h per year. In contrast, the national guidelines for adolescent athletes of age group "Jugend A" only recommends 700 h training per year [13]. Therefore, the participating athletes exceeded the standard requirements.

The main observations including practical implications were as follows: The majority of the recorded stress fractures arose after an increase of training which may be associated with attending a training camp. The first related sign was pain during or after running training. After one week, a physician was consulted, who could enable a prompt diagnosis with the aid of radiological imaging. Conservative treatment was the predominant course and alternative sports were trained in the 70-day training downtime.

This study is the first that has explored stress fractures exclusively in the unique population of elite triathletes. Comparative information can therefore only be determined by studies about cross and field athletes or athletes in general (i.e., Bennell et al. [14] or Changstrom et al. [15]) or studies about overuse injuries in triathlon (i.e., Collins et al. [16], Korkia et al. [3], Burns et al. [4] or Vleck et al. [6]).

The athletes surveyed were predominantly of the younger generations (average age: 17.45 years) who were restricted to starting on the shorter distances according to the regulations of DTU [10]. At this point of their career, the adolescent athletes place particular emphasis on the substantial increase of training volume in order to improve their physical stress tolerance [13,17]. However, in younger generations the full extent of training volume is not yet reached [17].

In comparison with other studies, the average age in the present study was clearly younger [3,4,6,18]. Furthermore, the participants did not include amateur athletes, but rather ambitious athletes that execute triathlon professionally and had to verify their status as squad members through performance tests or competition results [2]. In the majority of previous studies, no distinction in terms of professionalism was made.

Various studies showed that triathletes were rather prone to overuse injuries than to acute trauma [5]. A key research issue was to investigate the frequency and incidence of stress fractures among professional triathletes. In the present survey, 20 athletes (23%) already sustained a stress fracture prior to the survey period. A reason for this relatively high amount of stress fractures may be the low response rate or an over-representation due to selection bias [19,20]. The total incidence rate per year across all athletes was 4.8% (95% CI: 3.0–6.5%). In comparison with other studies that found incidence rates of 6.5–9.7% among athletes of different sports, this number is relatively low [21]. More precisely, runners and gymnasts show the highest incidence rates, whereas the lowest are found in swimming and diving [15,22,23]. These assumptions are relevant in triathlon since running training is given a high priority. Even though swim training requires a high proportion of the total training volume as well, it plays a minor role in injury aetiology [3].

In this study, as in many others, all stress fractures were located in the lower extremities [3,4,24,25]. Even further, McHardy et al. [5] showed that the lower extremities are the most affected anatomic site for all kinds of injuries in triathlon. In the context of overuse injuries specifically, the lower extremities are affected in 72–75% of cases [4]. Compared to cross and field athletes and runners, 61–78% of the stress fractures were also mainly located in the lower extremities [15,26].

Therapeutic decisions are often based on the common classification into high- and low-risk fractures depending on anatomic localisation [26,27]. Owing to the methodical approach to implement a questionnaire with laypeople, precise anatomic localisation cannot be described. For this reason, a clear classification into high- and low-fractures is needed.

Most previous studies agree that the aetiology appears multifactorial [25,26,28]. Accordingly, stress fractures evolve when different intrinsic and extrinsic components come together and frequently in combination with changes in training volume or intensity [4–6,26,29]. The multiple different risk factors are the subject of controversial discussion. However, it is the general consensus that women are at greater risk for stress fractures than men [14,15,23,30]. This corresponds to the findings of this study and to Fredericson et al. [31] who found a 1.5–3-times higher risk of females developing stress fractures.

The "Female Athlete Triad (FAT)" comprises eating disorders, menstrual disturbances and low bone density and represents an underlying pathomechanism [32]. Correspondingly, the FAT was also seen in the present study: ten out of 17 (59%) of the female athletes who suffer from menstrual disturbances also sustained a stress fracture. Moreover, of the 12 female athletes with stress fractures, only two did not show menstrual irregularities. According to Bennell et al. [33], amenorrhoeic athletes have a higher stress fracture rate and a 2–4 times greater risk than athletes with regular menses.

Further development led to a more complex definition and understanding of the FAT, namely the Relative Energy Deficiency in Sport (RED-S) [34]. RED-S describes a syndrome which influences a broad range of physiological functions (i.e., metabolic rate, menstrual function, bone health or immunity), all initially resulting from a relative energy deficiency [34]. Consequently, RED-S may lead to serious short-term and long-term effects on optimal health and performance, including an increased risk for stress fractures [34]. Besides, a major difference between FAT and RED-S is that men can be affected as well.

In sports such as running or triathlon, where athletes may benefit from a low BMI/body weight, athletes are likely to be more prone to RED-S [26]. Despite the fact that in our survey the average BMI (19.9 kg/m^2 (±1.4); Min/Max: 16/24) was within the normal range, they can still show inadequate intake of nutrients and energy. In this context, the exposed nutritional deficiencies as well as the low BMI of the athlete with three stress fractures could indicate an insufficient energy intake. Nevertheless, in previous studies a relation between BMI and the occurrence of stress fractures could not be clearly identified [35,36]. Even though body composition cannot be associated as a risk factor for stress fractures, the surveillance of BMI and its individual trend is still a helpful clinical tool to monitor health and nutritional status [33].

Nearly all studies agree that running is a major risk factor for triathlon-related injuries [3,4,6,16,24,25,33,37]. Thus, a high or increasing running mileage in preparation leads to an increased injury incidence [4,31]. Although athletes with stress fractures completed a higher distance in running training than their fellow athletes without stress fractures, an increase of OR could not be found. Nevertheless, all athletes took first notice of related symptoms during running. However, even more important in injury aetiology is less the total amount of training, but rather rapid changes in training programme without adequate time for adaptation [3,26,31]. In the present study, half of the athletes (52%) stated to have increased their training amount prior to the occurrence of the injury. Some athletes (46%) had even attended a training camp, where training mileage is typically boosted. Therefore, this seems to be a plausible pathomechanism in the study population.

In competitive sports, the prevention of injuries, along with short healing time, is by far the most important aim of sports medicine [14]. The multifactorial aetiology plays a key role in prevention work. Due to this multifactorial nature, stress fractures cannot be traced back only to training manners but likewise, they cannot be prevented only by training management. Indeed, the injury aetiology is understood as an interaction of several different individual factors. For this purpose, risk factors such as Vitamin D deficiency and menstrual disturbances should be subject to targeted monitoring and diagnostics. In the case of positive diagnostic tests, they should obviously also be targeted for treatment. At the same time, attention should be drawn towards an adequate energy intake to avoid the emergence of RED-S [34]. Whenever there is evidence for the assumption that RED-S or menstrual disturbances exist, energy intake should be increased and/or physical activity should be reduced [34].

Increases or changes in training, especially in running, i.e., in training camps, should be carried out gradually and with sufficient time for adaptation. Including low-impact sports and discharging days could be an approach to reduce physical load [36,37].

Stress fractures occur along a continuum from stress reactions to eventually stress fractures [33]. This continuous progress also includes the chance to break the cycle by identifying early symptoms such as a load-dependent pain in the lower extremities, followed by a period of reduced activity [33]. As a result, healing time and time off training may be reduced. Since athletes often underestimate the severity of symptoms, they should be made aware of the importance of early diagnosis particularly [25,38]. In the end, cooperation between sport physicians, physiotherapists, coaches and athletes is crucial to enhance prevention work.

Treatment after the occurrence of stress fractures should always be controlled by symptoms and must be continued until complete freedom of pain [26,39]. Simultaneously, risk factors need to be addressed in order to avoid further fractures [23].

The major limitations of this investigation are the limited measurement of exposure time, selection bias as a result of the voluntary participation, missing data of Non-Responders and the study design (cross-sectional study). It must be argued that cross-sectional studies cannot reveal causal relationships but only observed relationships. However, it is suitable to reveal new hypotheses and to identify potential risk factors. Furthermore, similar strategies were also adopted in other studies [3,5,15,18,28]. Carrying out a prospective cohort study with adequate power could explore causality in future studies.

The different exposure times of athletes were combined with the sum of person-years under risk in the denominator of the calculation of incidence rate. An individual approach or a differentiation to specific phases of training were not performed. In addition, due to the relatively low number of participants, there are only a few statistically significant results. Furthermore, carrying out multivariate analyses did not provide reasonable models. Thus, a sufficient statistic model could not be developed and confounder-associated estimations of risk were impossible.

The survey was based on information of medical amateurs (including nutritional deficiencies and misalignment of feet and leg axis) in spite of the limited validity of self-reported injuries [12,40]. Another limitation is that no standardised methods and definitions were applied to all studies [5,6,41]. For this reason, a comparison of study results may be problematic.

In order to enhance reliability and significance, the results need to be reexamined by studies with a larger sample size. All aspects and results need to be interpreted with consideration of the presented limitations.

5. Conclusions

Stress fractures in elite triathletes are a common injury and are highly relevant. It has been shown that running is closely linked to injury aetiology. Likewise, fracture localisations were similar to those seen in runners. Various factors could be assigned to the occurrence of stress fractures which underlines the multifactorial aetiology. In order to disseminate knowledge about relevant risk factor and typical disease progressions athletes, coaches, physiotherapists and sports physicians should be educated. By addressing potential risk factors and adjustment of training strategies especially in running, prevention may be improved and downtimes in training reduced. Future studies should be designed to identify causes of stress fractures.

Author Contributions: All authors contributed to this work. P.N., S.Z., P.W., T.H. and R.K. participated in the conceptualization, methodology, software, validation, formal analysis, investigation, resources, data curation, writing—original draft preparation, writing—review and editing, visualization. M.E. and G.L. participated in the review and editing, supervision and project administration.

Funding: We acknowledge support by the Open Access Publication Funds of the SLUB/TU Dresden.

Conflicts of Interest: The authors declare no conflict of interest.

References

1. Deutsche Triathlon Union e.V. Triathlon in Zahlen. Available online: https://www.dtu-info.de/triathlon-in-zahlen.html (accessed on 4 March 2018).
2. Deutsche Triathlon Union e.V. DTU Nominierungskriterien Kader. Available online: https://www.dtu-info.de/a/dateien/leistungssport/Nominierungskriterien/2018/DTU_Nominierungskriterien%20Kader%202017-2020.pdf (accessed on 7 July 2018).
3. Korkia, P.K.; Tunstall-Pedoe, D.S.; Maffulli, N. An epidemiological investigation of training and injury patterns in British triathletes. *Br. J. Sports Med.* **1994**, *28*, 191–196. [CrossRef] [PubMed]
4. Burns, J.; Keenan, A.-M.; Redmond, A.C. Factors associated with triathlon-related overuse injuries. *J. Orthop. Sports Phys. Ther.* **2003**, *33*, 177–184. [CrossRef] [PubMed]
5. McHardy, A.; Pollard, H.; Fernandez, M. Triathlon injuries: A review of the literature and discussion of potential injury mechanisms. *Clin. Chiropr.* **2006**, *9*, 129–138.
6. Vleck, V.E.; Bentley, D.J.; Millet, G.P.; Cochrane, T. Triathlon event distance specialization: Training and injury effects. *J. Strength Cond. Res.* **2010**, *24*, 30–36. [CrossRef] [PubMed]
7. Hotfiel, T.; Wolfram, P.; Engelhardt, M. *Unpublished Personal Communication—Steigende Anzahl von Stressfrakturen*; Deutsche Triathlon Union e.V.: Leipzig, Germany, 2017.
8. Deutsche Presse Agentur Saison-Aus wegen Stressfraktur: Frodeno verpasst Ironman-WM auf Hawaii. Available online: http://www.spiegel.de/sport/sonst/ironman-wm-auf-hawaii-jan-frodeno-muss-teilnahme-absagen-a-1227680.html (accessed on 26 November 2018).
9. Müller, S. Ironman-WM 2018. Ben Hoffman muss Hawaii-Start Absagen. Available online: http://tri-mag.de//szene/ben-hoffman-muss-hawaii-start-absagen-146365 (accessed on 26 November 2018).
10. Deutsche Triathlon Union e.V. Die Sportordnung der Deutschen Triathlon Union. Available online: https://www.dtu-info.de/a/dateien/regelwerk-ordnungen/Ordnungen/SpO_2018_V_1_2_sw.pdf (accessed on 7 July 2018).
11. Bundesministerium des Innern; Deutscher Olympischer Sportbund; Sportministerkonferenz Konzept zur. Neustrukturierung des Leistungssports und der Spitzensportförderung. Available online: https://www.bmi.bund.de/SharedDocs/downloads/DE/publikationen/themen/sport/sport-spitzensport-neustrukturierung.pdf?__blob=publicationFile&v=1 (accessed on 15 November 2018).
12. Øyen, J.; Torstveit, M.K.; Sundgot-Borgen, J. Self-reported versus diagnosed stress fractures in Norwegian female elite athletes. *J. Sports Sci. Med.* **2009**, *8*, 130.
13. Pöller, S.; Möller, T. *Rahmentrainingskonzeption Nachwuchs der Deutschen Triathlon Union*, 1st ed.; Deutsche Triathlon Union: Leipzig, Germany, 2013.
14. Bennell, K.L.; Malcolm, S.A.; Thomas, S.A.; Reid, S.J.; Brukner, P.D.; Ebeling, P.R.; Wark, J.D. Risk factors for stress fractures in track and field athletes. A twelve-month prospective study. *Am. J. Sports Med.* **1996**, *24*, 810–818. [CrossRef]
15. Changstrom, B.G.; Brou, L.; Khodaee, M.; Braund, C.; Comstock, R.D. Epidemiology of stress fracture injuries among US high school athletes, 2005–2006 through 2012–2013. *Am. J. Sports Med.* **2015**, *43*, 26–33. [CrossRef]
16. Collins, K.; Wagner, M.; Peterson, K. Overuse injuries in triathletes. *Am. J. Sports Med.* **1989**, *17*, 675–680. [CrossRef]
17. Neumann, G.; Pfützner, A.; Hottenrott, K. *Das große Buch vom Triathlon*; 2. überarb. Aufl.; Meyer & Meyer: Aachen, Germany, 2010; ISBN 978-3-89899-595-5.
18. Zwingenberger, S.; Valladares, R.D.; Walther, A.; Beck, H.; Stiehler, M.; Kirschner, S.; Engelhardt, M.; Kasten, P. An epidemiological investigation of training and injury patterns in triathletes. *J. Sports Sci.* **2014**, *32*, 583–590. [CrossRef]
19. Hernán, M.A.; Hernández-Díaz, S.; Robins, J.M. A Structural approach to selection bias. *Epidemiology* **2004**, *15*, 615–625. [CrossRef]
20. Hammer, G.P.; du Prel, J.-B.; Blettner, M. Avoiding bias in observational studies. *Dtsch. Aerzteblatt Online* **2009**, *106*, 664–668. [CrossRef]
21. Wentz, L.; Liu, P.-Y.; Haymes, E.; Ilich, J.Z. Females have a greater incidence of stress fractures than males in both military and athletic populations: A systemic review. *Mil. Med.* **2011**, *176*, 420–430. [CrossRef]

22. Brüntrup, J. Viele Läufer Bekommen Stressfrakturen. Available online: https://www.aerztezeitung.de/panorama/sport/sportmedizin/article/450731/viele-laeufer-bekommen-stressfrakturen.html (accessed on 11 September 2018).
23. Moreira, C.A.; Bilezikian, J.P. Stress fractures: Concepts and therapeutics. *J. Clin. Endocrinol. Metab.* **2016**, *102*, 525–534. [CrossRef] [PubMed]
24. Shaw, T.; Howat, P.; Trainor, M.; Maycock, B. Training patterns and sports injuries in triathletes. *J. Sci. Med. Sport* **2004**, *7*, 446–450. [CrossRef]
25. Cipriani, D.J.; Swartz, J.D.; Hodgson, C.M. Triathlon and the multisport athlete. *J. Orthop. Sports Phys. Ther.* **1998**, *27*, 42–50. [CrossRef] [PubMed]
26. Hotfiel, T.; Lutter, C.; Heiß, R. Stressreaktionen/-frakturen—Newsletter der Gesellschaft für Orthopädisch-Traumatologische Sportmedizin. *GOTS* **2018**.
27. Patel, D.S.; Roth, M.; Kapil, N. Stress fractures: Diagnosis, treatment, and prevention. *Am. Family Phys.* **2011**, *83*, 39–46.
28. Duckham, R.L.; Brooke-Wavell, K.; Summers, G.D.; Cameron, N.; Peirce, N. Stress fracture injury in female endurance athletes in the United Kingdom: A 12-month prospective study: Stress fractures in female endurance athletes. *Scand. J. Med. Sci. Sports* **2015**, *25*, 854–859. [CrossRef] [PubMed]
29. Migliorini, S. Risk factors and injury mechanism in triathlon. *J. Hum. Sport Exerc.* **2011**, *6*, 309–314. [CrossRef]
30. Rizzone, K.H.; Ackerman, K.E.; Roos, K.G.; Dompier, T.P.; Kerr, Z.Y. The epidemiology of stress fractures in collegiate student-athletes, 2004–2005 through 2013–2014 academic years. *J. Athl. Train.* **2017**, *52*, 966–975. [CrossRef] [PubMed]
31. Fredericson, M.; Jennings, F.; Beaulieu, C.; Matheson, G.O. Stress fractures in athletes. *Top. Magn. Reson. Imaging* **2006**, *17*, 309–325. [CrossRef]
32. Koenig, S.J.; Toth, A.P.; Bosco, J.A. Stress fractures and stress reactions of the diaphyseal femur in collegiate athletes: An analysis of 25 cases. *Am. J. Orthop.* **2008**, *37*, 476–480.
33. Bennell, K.; Matheson, G.; Meeuwisse, W.; Brukner, P. Risk factors for stress fractures. *Sports Med.* **1999**, *28*, 91–122. [CrossRef]
34. Mountjoy, M.; Sundgot-Borgen, J.; Burke, L.; Carter, S.; Constantini, N.; Lebrun, C.; Meyer, N.; Sherman, R.; Steffen, K.; Budgett, R.; et al. The IOC consensus statement: Beyond the female athlete triad—Relative Energy Deficiency in Sport (RED-S). *Br. J. Sports Med.* **2014**, *48*, 491–497. [CrossRef]
35. Korpelainen, R.; Orava, S.; Karpakka, J.; Siira, P.; Hulkko, A. Risk factors for recurrent stress fractures in athletes. *Am. J. Sports Med.* **2001**, *29*, 304–310. [CrossRef]
36. Field, A.; Gordon, C.; Pierce, L.; Ramappa, A.; Kocher, M. Prospective study of physical activity and risk of developing a stress fracture among preadolescent and adolescent girls. *Arch. Pediatr. Adolesc. Med.* **2011**, *165*, 723–728. [CrossRef]
37. Spiker, A.M.; Dixit, S.; Cosgarea, A.J. Triathlon: Running injuries. *Sports Med. Arthrosc. Rev.* **2012**, *20*, 206–213. [CrossRef]
38. Gosling, C.M.; Forbes, A.B.; Gabbe, B.J. Health professionals' perceptions of musculoskeletal injury and injury risk factors in Australian triathletes: A factor analysis. *Phys. Ther. Sport* **2013**, *14*, 207–212. [CrossRef]
39. Larsen, P.; Elsoe, R.; Rathleff, M.S. A case report of a completely displaced stress fracture of the femoral shaft in a middle-aged male athlete—A precursor of things to come? *Phys. Ther. Sport* **2016**, *19*, 23–27. [CrossRef]
40. Gabbe, B.J.; Finch, C.F.; Bennell, K.L.; Wajswelner, H. How valid is a self reported 12 month sports injury history? *Br. J. Sports Med.* **2003**, *37*, 545–547. [CrossRef]
41. Kienstra, C.M.; Asken, T.R.; Garcia, J.D.; Lara, V.; Best, T.M. Triathlon injuries: Transitioning from prevalence to prediction and prevention. *Curr. Sports Med. Rep.* **2017**, *16*, 397–403. [CrossRef]

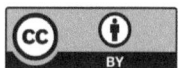 © 2019 by the authors. Licensee MDPI, Basel, Switzerland. This article is an open access article distributed under the terms and conditions of the Creative Commons Attribution (CC BY) license (http://creativecommons.org/licenses/by/4.0/).

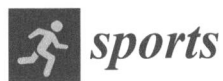

Article

Is the Bike Segment of Modern Olympic Triathlon More a Transition towards Running in Males than It Is in Females?

Maria Francesca Piacentini [1,*], Luca A Bianchini [1], Carlo Minganti [1], Marco Sias [2], Andrea Di Castro [3] and Veronica Vleck [4]

1. Department of Movement, Human and Health Sciences, University of Rome "Foro Italico", 00135 Rome, Italy; luca.bianchini.tri@gmail.com (L.A.B.); carlo.minganti@uniroma4.it (C.M.)
2. Department of Biomedical Sciences for Health, University of Milan, 20133 Milan, Italy; marco.sias92@gmail.com
3. Institute of Sports Science, 00100 Rome, Italy; dicastro.training@gmail.com
4. CIPER, Faculdade de Motricidade Humana, University of Lisbon, 1499-002 Lisbon, Portugal; vvleck@fmh.ulisboa.pt
* Correspondence: mariafrancesca.piacentini@uniroma4.it

Received: 6 March 2019; Accepted: 28 March 2019; Published: 29 March 2019

Abstract: In 2009, the International Triathlon Union created a new triathlon race format: The World Triathlon Series (WTS), for which only athletes with a top 100 world ranking are eligible. Therefore, the purpose of this study was to analyze the influence of the three disciplines on performance within all the WTS Olympic distance races within two Olympic cycles, and to determine whether their relative contribution changed over the years. Methods: For each of a total of 44 races, final race time and position as well as split times (and positions), and summed time (and position) at each point of the race were collected and included in the analysis. Athletes were divided into 4 groups according to their final race placing (G1: 1st–3rd place; G2: 4–8th place; G3: 8–16th place and G4: ≥17th place). Two-way multivariate ANOVAs were conducted to compare the main effects of years and rank groups. For females, there were significant differences in the swim and bike segment only between G4 and the other groups (p range from 0.001–0.029), whilst for the run segment each group differed significantly from each other ($p < 0.001$). For males, there were significant differences in swim only between G4 and the other groups (p range from 0.001–0.039), whilst for the running segment each group differed significantly from the others ($p < 0.001$). Although we found running to be the segment where there were significant differences between performance groups, it is apparently important for overall success that a good runner be positioned with the first cycling pack. However, bike splits were not different between either of the four male groups or between the first 3 groups of the females. At this very high level of performance, at least in the males, the bike leg seems to be a smooth transition towards running.

Keywords: endurance; elite athletes; performance

1. Introduction

Triathlon is an endurance sport consisting of sequential swimming, swimming to cycling (T1), cycling, cycling to running (T2) and running over a variety of distances [1] and has evolved considerably since it became an Olympic sport [2]. The draft legal 1.5 km swim, 40 km bike, 10 km run event debuted at the Sydney 2000 Games and since then research has focused on the effects of one discipline on the other rather than on the effects of drafting in swimming and biking (for reviews see [3,4]).

In 2009 the International Triathlon Union (ITU) changed the racing format from a single world championship race to a series of events called the World Triathlon Series (WTS) [5] during which athletes compete head to head to collect points to become world champion. WTS is restricted to the best athletes in the world (i.e., those who are ranked up to about 150 in the ITU list, according to points that can be obtained by continental, World Cup or WTS level races). The WTS doubles as an opportunity for Olympic qualification, and athletes need to perform consistently to score the points that are necessary to be eligible for selection. Points are attributed according to race performance within a cut-off time of 5% of the best male and 8% of the best female finisher (ITU regulation-www.triathlon.org), and the World Champion is the athlete that accumulates more points and thus performs more consistently throughout the season. Seventy seven percent of races are Olympic distance and the remainder are sprint distance (involving a 0.75 km swim, a 20 km draft legal bike leg and a 5 km run). The ability of an athlete to attain ranking points depends on his/her absolute performance level (both overall and within each single discipline) and on how s/he experiences residual fatigue from the previous discipline [6]. Drafting during swimming has been shown to reduce the energy cost of a subsequent cycling bout [7,8] whilst drafting during cycling can reduce energy cost by 39% with a consequent improvement in running performance [1].

Although total race time for the Olympic distance event varies between 106–110 minutes for elite males and between 119–121 minutes for elite female athletes, it is difficult to compare one race with another because there is neither any official standardization of event distance, nor any method of weighting course difficulty (in terms of topography, climate, environmental and other factors such as drafting) in place, and all of said factors may affect the overall finishing time. Elite athletes spend about 15% of their total race time swimming, 55% of total race time cycling, and 30% of time running. Males take 17, 57 to 60 and 30 minutes respectively to do so, and females 19, 63 to 67, and 35 minutes, respectively [9,10].

Another aspect that has been investigated is the impact of each discipline on overall performance. Landers et al [11] analyzed world cup races in 1999 and reported that exiting the water in the first pack of swimmers can determine the final finishing position. In fact, 90% of male and 70% of female winners were all placed within said first pack of swimmers. Vleck et al. [12] found that, when comparing the top 50% and bottom 50% finishers of an ITU World Cup, the top 50% was faster up to the first buoy of the swim, and that thereafter the two groups did not differ in swimming speed. Moreover, overall race performance was significantly correlated with both average swimming velocity and with position after the swim stage. The speed in the bike section was not different between the top and bottom 50% of finishers but was significantly higher for the second group (lower 50%), who exited the water with the task of reducing the time gap of the leaders by the start of the triathlon run. The need to play catch up impacted negatively on athletes' running speed. Cycling speed during the first section (13.4 km in this case) was inversely related to later running speed and the best runners were the best athletes overall. As the best triathletes can use less than 8 seconds to transition from one discipline to the other, it is also important for tactical reasons (such as avoiding collisions in the transition area) for an athlete to arrive in T2 at the front of the group [4]. Figueiredo et al. [10] reported that, in both sexes, cycling and running made the greatest contribution to the overall Olympic distance performance of top 50 finishers (i.e., approximately 36% and 47%, respectively) over the 1989–2014 period. Across the years, swimming contribution significantly decreased for women and men, whereas that of running only increased in men. However, this analysis did not take the introduction of draft legal cycling into account. Fröhlich et al. [13] showed, in males, that at Olympic distance World Championship level, running performance consistently makes the greatest contribution to which athlete wins. They concluded that "the swim and the cycle act as so-called feeders for the run and have to lay the foundations for the run, which decides over winning or losing more than the other two disciplines." However, they performed their analysis on only one race per year. Moreover, as separate swim, T1, bike, T2 and run times were not available for all races, they used (T1 times plus swim times), and (T2 times plus bike times) together. Millet and Vleck [4] have demonstrated, in males, that individual athlete's offset from the fastest T2 time can have an important influence on how far they eventually finish behind the race winner.

No longitudinal analyses within this genre have yet been published on all draft-legal, Olympic distance, higher level, WTS format. The purpose of the present study, therefore, was to analyze the trends in both overall and discipline specific Olympic distance triathlon performance, within the WTS only, of different performance levels of male and female triathletes, for the 2009–2016 period. The second aim was to study the differential times (i.e., the time differences to the fastest split time at that moment of the race) in T1 or out of T2. We hypothesized that swimming and cycling performance levels would level off over time and that running would be the main distinguishing factor between medalists and non-medalists. Our secondary hypothesis was that the entry into T1 would be less important than the exit from T2 in male athletes compared to female athletes. Because females seem less able than males at bridging cycle packs [6], the entry into T1 would be a determinant aspect of overall performance.

2. Materials and Methods

The data for this study were retrieved from the ITU world triathlon series website (wts.triathlon.org) and took into consideration only the WTS Olympic distance races from 2009–2016 for both sexes, including the most two recent Olympic Games (London 2012 and Rio 2016). Because the data are public and available on the internet, no formal ethics committee approval was necessary. For each race, final race time and position as well as split times (and positions) and summed time (and position) at each point of the race (S, S + T1, S + T1 + B, S + T1 + B + T2, S + T1 + B + T2 + R, where S, B and R equate to swimming, cycling and running, respectively) were retrieved and included in the analysis. In total, 44 races and 1670 male and 1706 female performances were examined (Table 1).

Table 1. Represents the number of races and athletes analyzed each year.

Year	Races	Females	Males
2009	8	239	266
2010	6	266	271
2011	6	308	286
2012	6	268	204
2013	5	151	142
2014	4	113	150
2015	4	163	156
2016	5	198	195
Total	44	1706	1670

Thereafter, for each race, participants were divided into 4 groups according to their final race placing i.e., G1: 1st–3rd place; G2: 4–8th place; G3: 8–16th place and G4: $\geq$17th place. Those athletes who did not finish the race in question were excluded from analysis. In accordance with the results of previous work that has highlighted the importance of the exit from the swim and the positioning in running to final race performance [3,6,12], the raw times were converted into differential times (offset from 1st in that leg) for T1 and T2 only.

Statistical Analysis

The statistical package IBM SPSS version 20 (IBM, Chicago, IL, USA) was used for the analysis. Values are presented as mean and standard deviations and before the analysis, the Kolmogorov–Smirnov test was applied to test the normal distribution of the data. The men's and the women's data were treated separately. Two-way multivariate ANOVAs were conducted to compare the main effects of years (i.e., from 2009–2016) and rank groups (i.e G1, G2, G3, G4) on time measures for each component of the race (i.e the swim, bike, and run). Before the analysis, the Levene's test for homogeneity of variance was performed to verify the assumption of the test. Furthermore, separate

ANOVAs were conducted to compare the effects on differential times in T1 and T2 (offset from the 1st in T1 and from the first out of T2) per year and per group. The same analysis was conducted taking only the medalists into account.

Univariate effects within MANOVAs were examined only if the overall MANOVA was significant. When significant interaction was observed (years for rank groups), follow-up tests were conducted by splitting the sample into the four rank groups and running separate ANOVAs to explore the different effect of years. When multiple comparisons were performed, post-hoc Fisher's protected least significant difference (LSD) test with Bonferroni correction was used.

The significance level for all comparisons was set at $P \leq 0.05$. In addition, effects size (ES) were calculated for all variables as partial eta-squared (η2p). Partial eta-squared values below 0.01, between 0.01–0.06, between 0.06–0.14, and above 0.14 were considered to have trivial, small, medium, and large effect sizes, respectively [14].

3. Results

For female athletes, analysis showed a multivariate effect for years (Wilks' $\lambda = 0.867$; $F_{21,1685} = 11.68$, $p < 0.001$; η2p = 0.047) and for rank groups (Wilks' $\lambda = 0.639$; $F_{9,1697} = 91.22$, $p < 0.001$; η2p = 0.139) although no interaction effect (years for rank groups) was found.

Univariate tests indicated significant effects on the three disciplines both by year (swim: $F_{7,1699} = 9.052$; $p < 0.001$; η2p = 0.036 – bike: $F_{87,1699} = 14.47$; $p < 0.001$; η2p = 0.057–run: $F_{7,1699} = 7.23$; $p < 0.001$; η2p = 0.029) and by group (swim: $F_{3,1704} = 9.84$; $p < 0.001$; η2p = 0.017–bike: $F_{3,1704} = 4.24$; $P = 0.005$; η2p = 0,008–run: $F_{3,1704} = 295.07$; $p < 0.001$; η2p = 0.346). Post-hoc for rank groups showed significant differences in the swim and bike segment only between G4 and the other groups (p range from 0.001–0.029) whilst for the run segment each group differed significantly from each other. ($p < 0.001$) (Figure 1)

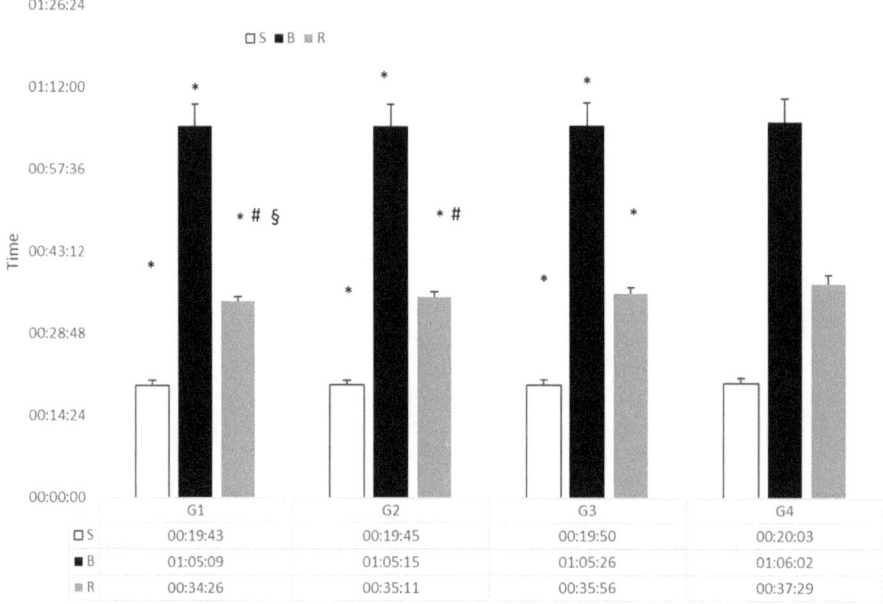

Figure 1. Split segment times for each of the female groups. S: Swim, B: bike, R: run, * different from G4, # diff from G3, § diff from G2.

The significant differences in the post-hoc by year for total time and for single legs are not reported because no trend of particular interest was noticed.

The analysis of the males showed a multivariate effect for years (Wilks' λ = 0.849; $F_{21,1649}$ = 13.17, $p < 0.001$; $\eta 2p$ = 0.053) and for group (Wilks' λ = 0.601; $F_{9,1661}$ = 102.90, $p < 0.001$; $\eta 2p$ = 0.156) while no interaction effect (year for rank groups) was found. Univariate tests indicated significant effects on the three disciplines by year (swim: $F_{7,1663}$ = 11.49; $p < 0.001$; $\eta 2p$ = 0,047–bike: $F_{7,1663}$ = 18.65; $p < 0.001$; $\eta 2p$ = 0.074–run: $F_{7,1663}$ = 7.19; $p < 0.001$; $\eta 2p$ = 0.039).

By group differences were found for swimming ($F_{3,1667}$ = 6.21; $p < 0.001$; $\eta 2p$ = 0.011) and for the run ($F_{3,1667}$ = 321.86; $p < 0.001$; $\eta 2p$ = 0.371) while no effect was found for the bike leg between groups. Post-hoc for rank groups (Figure 2) showed significant differences in swim only between G4 and the other groups (p range from 0.001–0.039), while for the running segment each group differed significantly from the others ($p < 0.001$).

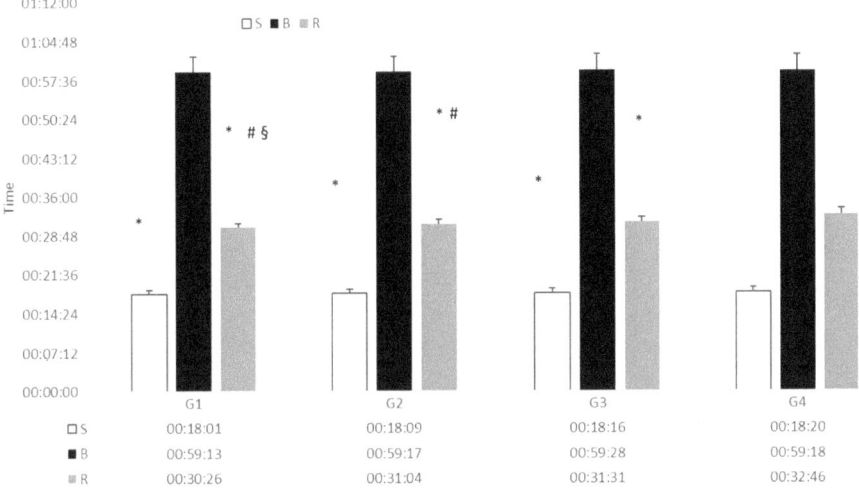

Figure 2. Split segment times for each of the male groups. S: Swim, B: bike, R: run, * different from G4, # diff from G3, § diff from G2.

Similarly to the women, the significant differences in the post-hoc by year for total time and for single legs are not reported because no trend of particular interest was noticed.

Analysis of differential times in entry in T1 and exit from T2 (offset from the 1st in that moment of the race) for women (Table 2) showed differences by rank groups in T1 ($F_{3,1703}$ = 16.38 $p < 0.001$, $\eta 2p$ = 0.040), with G1 (medalists) being significantly different from the others ($p < 0.001$). For exit from T2, all groups differed from each other ($F_{3,1703}$ = 65.69; $p < 0.001$, $\eta 2p$ = 0.142). For males (Table 3), the analysis showed a difference by rank groups both in entry in T1 ($F_{3,1663}$ = 42.01, $p < 0.001$, $\eta 2p$ = 0.091) and in exit from T2 ($F_{3,1663}$ = 45.05 $p < 0.001$, $\eta 2p$ = 0.100), with only the first group differing ($p < 0.001$) from the others in both cases.

Finally, when analyzing only G1 (medalists), no effect per year, final position or interaction years by position were found both for entry in T1 and exit in T2. Table 4 shows the position of each athlete of G1 in entry in T1 in exit of T2 and run split, for women and men respectively for the whole period (2009–2016).

Table 2. Offset time from the first in T1 and the first out of T2 for each group of female athletes.

Groups	Offset Entering T1 (sec)	Offset Existing T2 (sec)
G1	28 ± 12	12 ± 8
G2	30 ± 8 *	19 ± 15 *
G3	35 ± 7 *	35 ± 15 *#
G4	43 ± 10 *	66 ± 26 *#§

* different from G1, # diff from G2, § diff from G3 $p < 0.05$.

Table 3. Offset time from the first in T1 and the first out of T2 for each group of male athletes.

Groups	Offset Entering T1 (sec)	Offset Exiting T2 (sec)
G1	15 ± 2	21 ± 11
G2	24 ± 4 *	38 ± 10 *
G3	30 ± 5 *	54 ± 16 *
G4	35 ± 6 *	61 ± 15 *

* different from G1 $p < 0.05$.

Table 4. Position of the medalists in T1, T2 and run split over the years.

	Females			Males		
	1st	2nd	3rd	1st	2nd	3rd
T1 position	14 ± 5	16 ± 5	13 ± 4	10.2 ± 4.5	14.3 ± 4	18.2 ± 4
T2 position	8.6 ± 4	8.2 ± 4	7.4 ± 1.5	7.7 ± 4	9.6 ± 3	10.7 ± 2
Run split	2.1 ± 1	3.8 ± 1.5	5.3 ± 2.2	2.2 ± 0.8	3.8 ± 2.6	4.5 ± 1.4

4. Discussion

The purpose of the present study was to analyze the contribution of each segment of the Olympic distance triathlon to overall performance since the inception of the new WTS race format. With this new format athletes gain points that count towards the allocation of the 55 start places for the Olympic Games [9] within the WTS, within which only the best athletes in the world are allowed to compete. Our main finding was that there were differences in swim time, bike time and run time both per year and per group in the females. Within the males, such differences were observed only for swimming and running. Regarding swimming, we found no difference in segment times, in both sexes, between the first 3 groups (best 16 athletes overall)

Researchers have increasingly attempted to identify the optimal strategy for triathlon success since it became an Olympic sport, via assessment of predictors of performance, of the impact of one triathlon discipline on the other as compared to its component single disciplines, and of the best strategy to adopt during a race [2]. Although recent studies have put forward different analyses to understand the impact of the three disciplines on overall performance [9,10,13,15], the current study is the first to compare the performances over two Olympic cycles of the very top-level group of elite triathletes who competed in the WTS. Indeed, we observed smaller time differences between groups and athletes at the WTS level, i.e., every athlete which was ranked within the top 150 worldwide, than have been recorded in the literature to date. This is likely because most of said studies and some of the previously reported studies [10,13] examined performance in lower tier (albeit still elite) events, which have less restrictive criteria for athlete eligibility. Due to the strict selection process, on average only 60 athletes are allowed to start each WTS event. Various studies have previously recorded very high correlations between swimming prowess and overall performance. Landers et al. [11] showed that 90% of male winners and 70% of female winners exited in the first pack of swimmers. Ofoghi et al. [16] utilized Bayesian networks to analyze the differential time, calculated as the difference between each time in that segment of the race and the first athlete at that moment of the race, at different race points and use it to predict the likelihood of finishing on the podium. They reported that the medalists swam significantly faster than the lower placed athletes (i.e., those who finished 4–10th and above 10th place). On the other hand, Cejuela et al., [17] when analyzing the top races from 2000–2008, observed a low correlation between swimming and overall performance. Therefore, it seems that at least for the best athletes (placing up to 16th overall in the event) swimming performance levelled off from the introduction of new WTS format, and that swimming performance does not discriminate between different performance levels at the top level of professional triathlon.

Nonetheless, swimming position still seems to be a good determinant of overall success [6,11,12] because, although its contribution might be low, the strategic positioning within this segment may be critical to overall race performance. In fact, just analyzing contribution of each segment (or changes per year) does not reflect the race dynamics in relation to the race leaders in each moment of the race [10]. We therefore analyzed the offset of each athlete per group from the first athlete entering T1. We found that the men in G1 were generally 16" off from the fastest swimmer, and that this offset was higher in the other performance groups (G2: 24", G3: 29", G4: 34"). No differences were observed between the first 3 groups in the females but not only did G4 females swim significantly slower, but the G4 female group was the group with the highest offset from the fastest swimmer.

Exiting the water with a limited offset from the fastest swimmer, was shown to influence entry into the first pack(s) in the bike leg, influencing overall finishing position [6]. Depending on the individual athletes relative cycling and running ability [18], failure to enter said pack(s), and a subsequent increase in power output/effort during the bike leg in order to try to catch up to the front pack(s), may then negatively impact running performance. In accordance with the results of previous studies [6,17] we found no differences in bike splits within male different ranking groups. As regards to the women, only the first 16 athletes (G1 to G3) had similar bike splits confirming that even at this level females are divided in more groups, further apart, as compared to males.

Therefore, running seems to have the major impact on overall WTS race performance. Figuereido et al [10] showed that, over a 26-year period, the average contribution of the cycling and running stage has much more impact on overall performance of the top 50 Olympic distance finishers compared to swimming, irrespective of athlete sex. Moreover, they found that for women, swimming contribution decreased while cycling and running contribution remained unchanged. For males, running contribution significantly increased over time. Fröhlich et al [13] analyzed individual data from the world championships from 2003–2007 for all finishers as compared to the top 20, using multiple linear regression. They again highlighted the importance of running in the Olympic distance triathlon, as the discipline where performance is most related to the overall time and finishing position. Clearly, above average running performance is essential to placing well, especially in G1. Moreover, the better cyclists need to be able to keep the best runners behind them in order to have a chance to perform optimally. All the groups that were analyzed in the present study differed for running time, being G1 the fastest. We found that, over all the years and races that were analyzed, both the female and the male winners had, on average, the 2nd run split; the second finisher exhibited, on average, the 4th run split; whilst the third finisher had, on average, the 5th run split -despite there being no particular differences between the first three athletes in their position at the exit from T2 (Table 2). This appears to confirm that running is the most important determinant of overall triathlon performance [10], and that it is crucial for an athlete to arrive in the transition (T2) at the front of the group to avoid collisions or jams [4].

The second transition has been considered another important segment of the race. Because athletes often finish within seconds of each other, run times have levelled off and exiting T2 fast is important to gain precious seconds. Interestingly, male G1 was the group that over the years came closer to the exit from T2, (from 40" in 2009 to only 9" in 2016). In contrast, G3 and G4 slowed down over the years (increasing the gap from the first athlete out of T2). This could be partly because men generally arrive in larger groups in T2, as compared to female athletes, and therefore need to exit extremely quickly from T2 in order to gain precious seconds on their opponents. For the women, all the groups differed for T2 meaning that G1 was the group that was closer in time to the race leader at that moment, with no particular differences observed over the years. This supports the assertion that females may be less able to coalesce different bike packs into one [6], and that less athletes consequently enter transition zones at the same time.

Similarly, Cejuela et al [17] studied nine top level male competitions from 2000–2008. Their analysis included the lost time in each transition—calculated as the time lag between the first triathlete who started cycling or running and the rest of the athletes who arrived in the transition area with the same pack. They found a low correlation between T1 and overall performance; however, the lost time in T1 was different for each swimming pack (when 5" gaps between swimmers were taken to indicate a different pack). Even in this case, they found very low correlations between time lost and overall performance, probably because of the very flat biking routes that allowed groups to reunify. On the other hand, they confirmed that time lost in T2 is inversely related to performance. Considering the levelling off of running performance, the quicker the exit from T2 (and lower time loss) will for sure be beneficial for overall performance and final positioning.

Although, as already reported, we found running to be the segment where there were significant differences between performance groups, [17], it is apparently important for overall success that a good runner be positioned with the first cycling pack in order to have the possibility to win the race [12]. However, bike splits did not differ between male groups. At this very high level, the bike leg seems to be a smooth transition towards running, at least for the male athletes.

In conclusion, for males it appears that exiting the water close to the first athlete and exiting T2 close to the first athlete, with a fast running split, is a major determinant of success. For the women, exit from both T1 and T2 seem a major determinant of performance, as is a very fast running split. Over the years, the offset of G1 from the first athlete to exit T2 remained stable, whilst that of G2–G4 significantly worsened. The gender difference we observed in the relative influence of performance within specific sections of WTS competition to overall result can be explained by the greater number of bike packs that are seen in the women's races and their different race tactics. Because females seem less able than males at bridging cycle packs [6], their entry into T1, in contrast to males, seems to be a key aspect of overall performance.

Practical Applications

Based on the results of this analysis, we would suggest that both for males and females it is worthwhile to train the actual practice of T2 transitions. This is particularly the case in those athletes who are weaker overall, and- who will consequently (as this is a function of ranking) have their bikes placed further from the transition exit, and therefore likely have more potential to be caught up in "traffic jams." In line with the findings of Vleck et al. [6], strengthening of female biking ability to the point that athletes become better able to bridge gaps to a leading pack (through the ability to sustain short high power output bursts immediately followed by steady lower level effort, and improvement of climbing ability in the case of hilly courses) is advisable, as, depending on the athlete, it may have a significant influence on overall race placing. Run training ("brick" sessions) and performance remain of paramount and increasing importance but at present the disciplines that precede the triathlon run appear to have more impact on overall race performance in females than they do in males. The pacing characteristics of performance at this level have not as yet been established but this can clearly be the key to overall race placing, particularly in males where the performance density is better and the ability to complete a fast, sprint type, run finish can be definitive. Moreover, the data presented in this paper may prove be helpful in the selection of young talented athletes, who need to compete at a young age and not come into triathlon from one of its disciplines in isolation.

Author Contributions: Methodology, L.A.B., A.D.C. and M.S.; formal analysis, C.M.; investigation, L.A.B., M.F.P.; data curation, C.M. and L.A.B.; writing—original draft preparation, M.F.P.; writing—review and editing, V.V.; supervision, M.F.P. and V.V.

Funding: V.V. was funded by the "Fundação para a Ciência e a Tecnologia" (the Foundation for Science and Technology), Portugal (www.fct.pt): grant number SFRHBPD104394/2014.

Conflicts of Interest: The authors declare no conflict of interest.

References

1. Bentley, D.J.; Millet, G.P.; Vleck, V.E.; McNaughton, L.R. Specific aspects of contemporary triathlon: implications for physiological analysis and performance. *Sports Med.* **2002**, *32*, 345–359. [CrossRef] [PubMed]
2. Millet, G.P.; Bentley, D.J.; Vleck, V.E. The relationships between science and sport: application in triathlon. *Int. J. Sports Physiol. Perform.* **2007**, *2*, 315–322. [CrossRef] [PubMed]
3. Millet, G.P.; Vleck, V.E. *Triathlon Specificity*; Seifert, L., Chollet, D., Mujika, I., Eds.; World Book of Swimming: from Science to Performance; Nova Science Publishers, Inc.: Hauppage, NY, USA, 2010; pp. 481–495.
4. Millet, G.P.; Vleck, V.E. Physiological and biomechanical adaptations to the cycle to run transition in Olympic triathlon: review and practical recommendations for training. *Br. J. Sports Med.* **2000**, *34*, 384–390. [CrossRef] [PubMed]
5. Mujika, I. Olympic preparation of a world-class female triathlete. *Int. J. Sports Phys. Perf.* **2014**, *9*, 727–731. [CrossRef] [PubMed]
6. Vleck, V.E.; Bentley, D.J.; Millet, G.P.; Burgi, A. Pacing during an elite Olympic distance triathlon: comparison between male and female competitors. *J. Sci. Med. Sport* **2008**, *11*, 424–432. [CrossRef] [PubMed]
7. Delextrat, A.; Tricot, V.; Bernard, T.; Vercruyssen, F.; Hausswirth, C.; Brisswalter, J. Drafting during swimming improves efficiency during subsequent cycling. *Med. Sci. Sports Exerc.* **2003**, *35*, 1612–1619. [CrossRef] [PubMed]
8. Bentley, D.J.; Libicz, S.; Jougla, A.; Coste, O.; Manetta, J.; Chamari, K.; Millet, G.P. The effects of exercise intensity or drafting during swimming on subsequent cycling performance in triathletes. *J. Sci. Med. Sport* **2007**, *10*, 234–243. [CrossRef] [PubMed]
9. Rüst, C.A.; Lepers, R.; Stiefel, M.; Rosemann, T.; Knechtle, B. Performance in Olympic triathlon: changes in performance of elite female and male triathletes in the ITU World Triathlon Series from 2009 to 2012. *Springer Plus*. 2013, p. 685. Available online: http://www.springerplus.com/content/2/1/685 (accessed on 21 December 2013).
10. Figueiredo, P.; Marques, E.A.; Lepers, R. Changes in Contributions of Swimming, Cycling, and Running Performances on Overall Triathlon Performance Over a 26-Year Period. *J. Strength Cond. Res.* **2016**, *30*, 2406–2415. [CrossRef] [PubMed]
11. Landers, G.J.; Blanksby, B.A.; Ackland, T.R.; Monson, R. Swim Positioning and its Influence on Triathlon Outcome. *Int. J. Exerc. Sci.* **2008**, *1*, 96–105. [PubMed]
12. Vleck, V.E.; Burgi, A.; Bentley, D.J. The consequences of swim, cycle, and run performance on overall result in elite olympic distance triathlon. *Int. J. Sports Med.* **2006**, *27*, 43–48. [CrossRef] [PubMed]
13. Fröhlich, M.; Klein, M.; Pieter, A.; Emrich, E.; Gießing, J. Consequences of the Three Disciplines on the Overall Result in Olympic-distance Triathlon. *Int. J. Sports Sci. Eng.* **2008**, *2*, 204–210.
14. Cohen, J. *Statistical Power Analysis for the Behavioural Sciences*, 2nd ed.; Erlbaum: Hillsdale, NJ, USA, 1988; p. 283.
15. Malcata, R.M.; Hopkins, W.G.; Pearson, S.N. Tracking career performance of successful triathletes. *Med. Sci. Sports Exerc.* **2014**, *46*, 1227–1234. [CrossRef] [PubMed]
16. Ofoghi, B.; Zeleznikow, J.; Macmahon, C.; Rehula, J.; Dwyer, D.B. Performance analysis and prediction in triathlon. *J. Sports Sci.* **2016**, *34*, 607–612. [CrossRef]
17. Cejuela, R.; Cala, A.; Pérez-Turpin, J.A.; Villa, J.G.; Cortell, J.M.; Chinchilla, J.J. Temporal activity in particular segments and transitions in the Olympic triathlon. *J. Hum. Kinetics* **2013**, *36*, 87–95. [CrossRef]
18. Horne, M. The relationship of race discipline with overall performance in sprint and standard distance triathlon age-group world championships. *Int. J. Sports Sci. Coach.* **2017**, *12*, 814–822. [CrossRef]

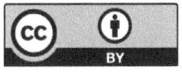

© 2019 by the authors. Licensee MDPI, Basel, Switzerland. This article is an open access article distributed under the terms and conditions of the Creative Commons Attribution (CC BY) license (http://creativecommons.org/licenses/by/4.0/).

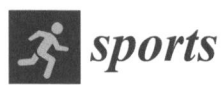 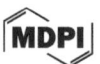

Review

The Characteristics of Endurance Events with a Variable Pacing Profile—Time to Embrace the Concept of "Intermittent Endurance Events"?

Joao Henrique Falk Neto [1,*], Martin Faulhaber [2] and Michael D. Kennedy [1]

[1] Athlete Health Lab., Faculty of Kinesiology, Sport and Recreation, University of Alberta, Edmonton, AB T6G 2R3, Canada; kennedy@ualberta.ca
[2] Department of Sport Science, University of Innsbruck, 6020 Innsbruck, Austria; martin.faulhaber@uibk.ac.at
* Correspondence: falkneto@ualberta.ca

Abstract: A variable pacing profile is common in different endurance events. In these races, several factors, such as changes in elevation or race dynamics, lead participants to perform numerous surges in intensity. These surges are so frequent that certain events, such as cross-country (XC) skiing, mountain biking (MTB), triathlon, and road cycling, have been termed "intermittent endurance events". The characteristics of these surges vary depending on the sport: MTB and triathlon require athletes to perform numerous short (<10 s) bouts; XC skiing require periods of short- and moderate- (30 s to 2 min) duration efforts, while road cycling is comprised of a mix of short-, moderate-, and long-duration (>2 min) bouts. These bouts occur at intensities above the maximal metabolic steady state (MMSS), with many efforts performed at intensities above the athletes' maximal aerobic power or speed (MAP/MAS) (i.e., supramaximal intensities). Given the factors that influence the requirement to perform surges in these events, athletes must be prepared to always engage in a race with a highly stochastic pace. The aim of this review is to characterize the variable pacing profile seen in endurance events and to discuss how the performance of multiple maximal and supramaximal surges in intensity can affect how athletes fatigue during a race and influence training strategies that can lead to success in these races.

Keywords: surges; sprints; anaerobic power reserve; extreme intensity domain; cycling; triathlon; mountain biking; cross-country skiing

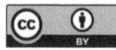

1. Introduction

The distribution of effort throughout a race is termed pacing, pacing strategy, pacing profile, or pacing pattern [1,2] and is a key factor for optimal endurance exercise performance [3]. When high-level athletes are able to pace themselves in short- (approximately 4 min) to long- (up to 2 h) distance events, the distribution of power output usually follows a J-shaped pattern [4]. The initial section of the race is performed at a higher intensity than the average race pace and represents the fast start [5]. Once this phase is completed, the athletes reduce their intensity and maintain an even pace for most of the race. This phase allows the athletes to recover from the intense effort of the fast start, maintaining an intensity that is sustainable during the race and that allows energy to be conserved for the finishing sprint [5]. This sprint, called the end-spurt, is considered a key race-defining moment [6] where multiple events are won [4,7–9].

In many endurance events, however, an even-paced phase does not occur. In these events, the athletes alternate between efforts above and below the average race intensity throughout the race, characterizing a variable pacing profile [1]. These variations in pacing can be so frequent that some endurance events resemble what occurs in team sports [10] and have been referred to as "intermittent endurance events". The term has been utilized to describe events in cross-country skiing [11], mountain biking [10,12,13], road cycling [14,15], and the cycling leg of different triathlon events [16,17]. Changes in topography, course characteristics, and race dynamics and tactics are some of the factors that ensure that athletes will have to perform several variations in intensity during the race, with the characteristics of these surges unique to each sport.

These surges are performed at intensities that are not sustainable [18], occurring above the maximal metabolic steady state (MMSS) (the intensity associated with the athlete's critical power (CP) or the 2nd ventilatory threshold (VT2)) or at supramaximal intensities (above the intensity associated with the achievement of maximal oxygen uptake (VO_2max)) during a graded exercise test, also known as maximal aerobic power (MAP) or speed (MAS). Surges at intensities equivalent to 120 to 160% of the athlete's MAP are common [10,16,19–21], with even higher values (200% to 300% MAP) reported in the literature [10]. A period of low-intensity work (approximately 40% to 60% MAP) [21,22] allows the athletes to recover from the strenuous effort and to cope with the demands of producing frequent bursts of power throughout a race.

Given the frequency, duration, and intensity of these surges, this intermittent profile can have important implications for performance. Compared to performing the same amount of work at a constant intensity, a variable profile leads to greater physiological stress and faster fatigue development and negatively influences subsequent performance [23,24]. A change in the pacing profile might also influence the determinants of performance [3,25], with success in these events related to more than just the traditional factors related to endurance performance (namely, VO_2max, the intensity associated with the athlete's lactate threshold (LT) and movement economy) [3]. The ability to perform repeated efforts at a high intensity [8,10,22] and greater anaerobic capacity and power [10,26–28] have been hypothesized to be the key to success in these events. The importance of a higher MAP and VO_2max [11,29–31] to performance has also been highlighted. Understanding the specific demands of these races may open new avenues to influence performance in these events [22].

The aim of this review is to characterize the variable pacing profile seen in endurance events and its implications to performance. This review will (1) elucidate the factors that contribute to a variable pacing profile, (2) describe the characteristics (intensity, duration, work-to-rest ratio) of the surges in intensity that occur in these events, and (3) address the consequences of these surges in intensity to endurance exercise performance.

2. Methods

This is a narrative review focused on describing the variable pacing profile that occurs in endurance events. A literature review was performed with the following search terms: "variable pacing", "intermittent pacing", "pacing pattern", "pacing strategies", "power output distribution", "power profile", and "power demands". These terms were combined with "cycling", "triathlon", "cross-country skiing", and "mountain biking", as events in these sports have been previously described as intermittent endurance events [10,11,13,15,17]. Further, papers on the "physiological demands", "physical demands", and "physiological requirements" of these sports were analyzed. Papers were included in the analysis of variable pacing profile if they provided sufficient information to describe the surges in intensity that occur during the races. Subsequently, a manual search within each identified paper was done to find further papers that provided information about the characteristics of the variable pacing profile in these events.

3. Factors That Contribute to a Variable Pacing Profile in Endurance Events

Several factors are implicated in the variable pacing profile that is seen in endurance events. While the course's characteristics provide the most obvious reason for changes in intensity to occur, race dynamics, tactics, and even the influence of governing bodies can contribute to a variable pacing profile.

3.1. Out with Old, in with the New—New Race Formats and Changes in Regulations Influenced the Races' Pacing Profiles

Numerous endurance events have recently been created or modified across different sports to make races more spectacular and spectator friendly [10,17]. Cross-country skiing, for example, had eight out of 12 Olympic events in Sochi 2014 that were different from the 1994 Winter Olympics. Shorter events, such as sprint skiing, and an increase in the number of races with a mass start (10 of the 12 Olympic races now involve mass starts) [32] have increased the demands of surges in intensity and the requirement of sprinting ability in the sport [9,27].

Mountain biking and triathlon have also evolved in their race formats. In Olympic XC MTB (XCO), race duration and lap length were reduced, while the requirement for technical sections in the course increased. Current regulations require races to last between 80 and 100 min, with a lap length of 4–6 km, over a variety of terrains [10,21]. Short track XC MTB (XCC), a new race format introduced in 2018, is performed in loops of no more than 2 km and maximum race times of 20 min [33]. The cycling leg of Olympic and sprint distance triathlons is also performed in shorter loops (3.5 to 5 km) [30], and new race formats, such as super sprints and the team mixed-relay event [34], can be performed in even shorter courses.

The shorter courses have increased the number of tight turns and sharp corners in these events, increasing the number of repetitive, high-intensity accelerations that are performed [10,17,20]. In sprint and Olympics distance triathlon, for example, the number of dangerous curves performed per kilometer has a strong correlation with the variability index (a measure of the variations in power output during a race) and to the number of supramaximal efforts performed [30]. These changes to race formats ensure that several variations in intensity will occur during a race, regardless of the influence of other factors on the races' pacing profile.

3.2. Uphill, Downhill, and Technical Demands—How the Course's Characteristics Influence Pacing Profile

The technical demands of sports, such as MTB, also contribute to the number of surges that are performed. MTB courses present the athletes with numerous jumps, climbs, descents, and other technical features [13,21]. Navigating these challenges requires the performance of multiple short (8 to 15 s) efforts during the race [12,35]. The fact that the number of surges performed per lap in MTB is not significantly reduced when athletes break into smaller packs corroborates that many of these surges occur as a product of the course's characteristics [13]. Similar influence of the terrain and technical features have also been reported in cyclocross [36] and off-road triathlon [37].

Further, changes in elevation provide their own challenge in different sports. In cross-country skiing, for example, races must have an equal distribution of flat, uphill, and downhill terrain [32]. The time spent in uphill sections, thus, varies based on the event, with shorter efforts (20 to 40 s) reported in sprint skiing [28,38] and longer efforts (up to 4 min) during longer distance races [39,40]. Likewise, in road cycling, mountainous stages require longer efforts (6 to 10 min) at intensities just above that associated with the maximal metabolic steady state (MMSS), while semi-mountainous stages require shorter (30 s to 2 min), more intense efforts [15].

3.3. Breaking Away—The Influence of Race Dynamics to a Variable Pacing Profile

The number and characteristics of the surges might also vary according to the race's dynamics. Riding in a group leads to a higher number of surges performed as the athletes try to stay within or break away from the pack [14,20]. For example, the four athletes competing as a team in the mixed-relay triathlon performed 17, 11, 8, and 12 surges (>600 W) in intensity during the cycling leg of the race (approximately 11 min) [34]. The athlete who only performed 8 surges was described as chasing a pack, while the others were riding within a group.

The tactics of the chase group might also influence the surges in intensity. In road cycling, it is possible that the group will allow the breakaway to occur earlier in the race, leading to a surge that is less intense [14]. Later in the race, the power output of the surge is higher, and the intensity remains elevated for a further 30 s to 5 min to try to ensure the success of the action [7,14]. As the race nears its end, multiple 5 to 15 s sprints are performed in the 20 min prior to the end-spurt, as the competitors gradually attempt to break away from the pack or position themselves for a successful sprint to the finish line [7,8,41].

Race tactics and dynamics also play an important role in races where position within the packs is important (for example, single-track races where opportunities to pass a competitor are limited), such as MTB [21] and mass-start cross-country skiing [9]. In these events, a longer sprint (around 20 to 30 s) is performed at the beginning of the race as the athletes try to position themselves for the subsequent laps. Athletes might also perform more surges (skiing) or surges that are more intense (MTB) during the initial lap [9,21] to ensure optimal tactical positioning for the remainder of the race. Despite the negative influence that these intense efforts can have on performance, the benefits of competing within the front pack offset the greater metabolic demands of the increased intensity [9,12].

A summary of the factors contributing to surges in intensity and their consequences on the characteristics of the surges is presented in Table 1. A brief analysis of these factors shows that these are intrinsic to the sport (e.g., course characteristics), reflect changes made by governing bodies to make races more spectator friendly, or cannot be predicted (e.g., race dynamics, competitors' tactics). Even increased media exposure can lead an athlete to attempt a breakaway from the group [14]. As such, athletes must be prepared to engage in a highly stochastic race, with the characteristics of these efforts and their importance for overall performance varying according to the sport and the event.

Table 1. Summary of factors that contribute to a variable pacing pattern in intermittent endurance events and how it affects the characteristics of the surges.

Factors Contributing to Surges	Effect on Variable Pacing Pattern	Influence on Characteristics of Surges	Sports Influenced by It
Changes in elevation/topography	Variations in intensity according to the duration and length of the climb	Performance of short- (<15 s) (MTB), moderate- (30 s to 2 min), and long- (>2 min) (XC skiing, road cycling) efforts during the race	MTB, XC skiing, Road cycling
Course's characteristics	Repetitive accelerations, tight turns, dangerous curves, technical sections	Performance of multiple short (<15 s) efforts	Triathlon, MTB
Race format	Mass start races, competing in shorter loops	Performance of multiple short (<15 s) efforts, end-spurt determines winner	MTB, XC skiing, Road cycling
Race tactics/dynamics	Tactical positioning, breakaways, pack riding	Longer and more intense surges in first lap (tactical positioning), less intense and shorter surges earlier in the race (breakaway), higher number of surges prior to finishing sprint, need to sustain higher intensity following surge later in the race	MTB, XC skiing, Road Cycling, Triathlon

4. Characteristics of Surges in Intensity in Variable Pacing Endurance Events

The characteristics of the surges in intensity that occur during a race vary depending on the sport. The variable pacing profile of events in XC skiing, MTB, road cycling, and the cycling leg of different triathlon races, events referred to as "intermittent endurance events" is described below. An overview of the characteristics of the surges in intensity in these sports is presented in Table 2.

Table 2. Characteristics of variable pacing profile in different sports.

Study	Participants and Competition Level	Race Characteristics		Characteristics of Surges			Recovery Duration/Work to Rest Ratio	Time Spent/Work Done in Each Intensity Zone
		Distance/Average Duration	Average Intensity	Number	Duration	Intensity		
Triathlon								
Mixed Relay (MR)								
Sharma & Périard [34]	4 elite (2 males, 2 females) World Championships	Males: 10.5 min Females: 11.5 min	NR	11 and 12 (males) 17 and 8 (females)	NR	>650 W >400 W (8 W/kg)	NR	48% and 62% above 85% 4MMAP (males) 58% and 64% above 85% 4MMAP (females)
Sprint (SD) and Olympic Distance (OD)								
Bernard et al. [16]	10 Elite triathletes (5 males, 5 females) World Cup	40 km 72 min females 63 min males	66.0 ± 7.1% MAP L1-L2 60.7 ± 9.1% MAP L3-L4 52.7 ± 7.5% MAP L5-L6	44 13 13	7 s 15 s 7 s	>100% MAP >100% MAP >60% MAnP	NR	Z1: 51 ± 9% Z2: 17 ± 6% Z3: 15 ± 3% Z4: 17 ± 6%
Etxebarria et al. [20]	5 elite male triathletes (12 race profiles from 7 ITU international races)	40 km	252 ± 33 W (3.9 ± 0.5 W/kg)	34 ± 14 *	NR	>600 W	NR	NR
Cejuela et al. [30]	4 male triathletes 13 WTS races (6 SD, 8OD) Tokyo 2021 Olympic Games (OD)	Approx. 40 km (average of 8.86 laps per race) for OD Approx. 20 km (average of 5.4 laps per race) for SD	58.3% MAP (mean power) 65% MAP (normalized power) Athlete's mean MAP across study: 450 W	Average of 13.9 ± 3.6 peaks (surges) per km	NR	Peaks reported as efforts above MAP Power profile during races— 5 s MMP: 795 ± 102 W (approx. 176% MAP) 30 s MMP: 499 ± 62 W (approx. 110% MAP) 60 s MMP: 411 ± 48 W (approx. 91% MAP)	NR	Time Z1: 51.9 ± 6.5% Z2: 17.3 ± 3.9% Z3: 13.3 ± 2.6% Z4: 17.4 ± 5.0 Work done Z1: 22.0 ± 5.8% Z2: 20.4 ± 4.0% Z3: 20.0 ± 3.5% Z4: 37.5 ± 10%

Table 2. Cont.

Study	Participants and Competition Level	Race Characteristics		Characteristics of Surges			Recovery Duration/Work to Rest Ratio	Time Spent/Work Done in Each Intensity Zone
		Distance/Average Duration	Average Intensity	Number	Duration	Intensity		
Smith et al. [42]	3 elite triathletes (1 male, 2 females) ITU World Cup	40 km (6 laps)	Male: 238.3 ± 167.4 W Female 1: 229 ± 111 W Female 2: 225 ± 124 W	Male: 8 (a single lap) Females: Numerous per lap (NR)	NR	Male: 600 W (threshold power estimated to be 320–350 W) Females: >500 W	NR	NR
Mountain Biking								
Granier et al. [10]	8 male (5 U23, 3 elite) 13 international races	5 to 8 laps 28.15 ± 5.41 km 90 ± 9 min	283 ± 22 W 68 ± 5% MAP	18 ± 4 (per lap)	10 s $	559 ± 46 W	Every 40 ± 14 s	Z1: 25 ± 5% Z2: 21 ± 4% Z3: 13 ± 3% Z4: 16 ± 3% Z5: 26 ± 5%
Naess et al. [13]	5 male, 2 females (23.4 years, 68.5 kg), National Standard	3.8 km Loop 19 km for females (5 laps) 23 km for males (6 laps) 96 ± 7 min (lap time: 16 ± 2 min)	249 ± 63 W 3.6 ± 0.7 W 180 ± 4 bpm 63 ± 4% MAP 76 ± 9% CP	Approx. 90 per lap (above CP, not supra-maximal) Starting loop had 17 ± 3	8 s (5.2–11.6)	1.18 to 1.41 (Fraction of CP) SL: 1.41 ± 0.07 Remainder of race has an average of 1.2	NR	Zero PO: 27% ± 3% Time > CP: 40 ± 8% Time > MAP: 26 ± 8%
Hays et al. [21]	16 male juniors or U23 (national or international level) Simulated race in official racetrack	3 laps (5.1 km) Simulated: 64 ± 1.5 min Competition: 66 ± 2 min	NR	22.1 11.8 5.7 3.1 1.8	1–5 s 5–10 s 11–15 s 16–20 s >20 s	>MAP (specific intensity not reported)	NR	L1, L2, L3, respectively: NP: 18.8 ± 4.3%, 18.9 ± 4.6%, 19.8 ± 6.0% Z1: 27.0 ± 8.1%, 31.2 ± 9.8%, 33.5 ± 10.2% Z2: 11.9 ± 4.9%, 12.3 ± 5.2%, 13.6 ± 5.0% Z3: 9.5 ± 5.1%, 9.7 ± 4.3%, 9.1 ± 4.5% Z4: 32.8 ± 8.2%, 27.9 ± 7.9%, 24.0 ± 8.2%

213

Table 2. Cont.

Study	Participants and Competition Level	Race Characteristics		Characteristics of Surges				Recovery Duration/Work to Rest Ratio	Time Spent/Work Done in Each Intensity Zone
		Distance/Average Duration	Average Intensity	Number	Duration	Intensity			
				Road Cycling					
Peiffer et al. [8]	7 professional female cyclists	31 races where the rider of interest finished in the top-5. Average race time of 179.4 ± 33.4 min	167 ± 24 W	68 efforts above 80% of the maximal final sprint (numerous 5-, 15-, 30-, 60-, 240-, and 600-second efforts above 80% MMP80 also occurred)	15 s	>80% of MSP 80 (80% of the PO of the final sprint) Other sprints were above 80% of mean maximal power for specific duration.		NR	NR
				XC Skiing #					
				Sprint Skiing					
Sandbaak et al. [28]	12 elite male XC skiers (3 WCs)	240 ± 5 s (234–248); 1820 m.	NR	3 (S3, S4, S7)	S3: 18.8 ± 0.5 s S4: 51.4 ± 2.3 s S7: 15.0 ± 0.7 s Total of 85.2 ± 3.1 s	160% VO$_2$max (476 ± 42 W) for S4 Not reported for S3 and S7.		NR (S5 + S6, approx. 50 s-1:1)	NR 36% Uphill (>MAP) 27% Flat 30% Downhill 7% Curved
Ihalainen et al. [38]	11 female XC skiers (Scandinavian Cup)	250.4 ± 5.8 s	NR	3 (S2, S5, S7)	S3: 21.1 ± 0.9 s S5: 22.1 ± 0.9 s S7: 38.2 ± 2.0 s	NR		NR S3 + S4: approx. 41.5 s S6: 14.1 s	NR

Table 2. Cont.

Study	Participants and Competition Level	Race Characteristics		Characteristics of Surges			Recovery Duration/Work to Rest Ratio	Time Spent/Work Done in Each Intensity Zone
		Distance/Average Duration	Average Intensity	Number	Duration	Intensity		
Distance Skiing								
Sandbaak et al. [39]	10 elite females (highest ranked in the world to top-15 Norway) VO₂max = 68.0 ± 4.8 mL/kg/min	10 km (2 × 5-km laps) Total of 56% uphill (483 ± 31 s), 16% flat (193 + 10 s), 28% downhill (218 ± 8 s) Total of 894 s	NR	5 (per lap)	S3: 42 ± 2 s S5: 41 ± 3 s S7: 162 ± 10 s S9: 152 ± 11 s S14: 85 ± 4 s Total of 483 ± 31 s	NR	S4 = 25 s (downhill) S6: 46 s (downhill) S8: 31 s (downhill) S10–S13: 128 s (downhill and flat)	NR 56% uphill (>CP/MAP) 16% flat 28% downhill
Staunton et al. [40]	19 (9 female, 10 male) tier 3 athletes, FIS-sanctioned	Approx. 4900 m per lap Men: 3 laps (14,678 m) Women: 2 laps (9743 m) Total of 165 m of climbing Total Time Women: 28 min 44 ± 58 s Men: 38 min 37 ± 57 s	NR	4 (per lap) S1, S3, S5, S7	Women S1: 226 ± 10 s S3: 67 ± 3 s S5: 243 ± 11 s S7: 61 ± 3 s Men S1: 194 ± 5 s S3: 56 ± 2 s S5: 210 ± 10 s S7: 52 ± 2 s	NR	Women S2: 102 ± 2 s S4: 36 ± 1 s S6: 55 ± 1 s S8 + S9: 86 s Men S2: 94 ± 3 S4: 33 ± 1 s S6: 51 ± 1 S8 + S9: 78 s	NR

4MMAP: 4-min maximal aerobic power (surrogate of maximal aerobic power(MAP)); NR: not reported; SL: starting lap; L1—LN: lap number; CP: critical power; S1—SN: section number; MMP: maximal mean power over different durations; MSP: maximal sprinting power of the finishing sprint; Z1 to Z5: intensity zones; #: surges reported in XC skiing represent duration of uphill sections in different events; *: average; ±: standard deviation of the races reported in the study; $: value reported via personal communication with the author.

4.1. Cross-Country Skiing

Changes in elevation are a key factor in the surges in intensity reported in XC skiing. In sprint skiing races (0.8 to 1.8 km, approximately 3 min in duration) [43], the time spent in individual uphill sections was reported to range between 15 and 50 s, with two different studies [28,38] reporting uphill times of approximately 15, 18, 21, 22, 38, and 51 s. In shorter climbs, intensities of 140–160% of the athletes' VO_2max have been reported [28], with only a short period (20 to 40 s) spent in flat and/or downhill sections prior to the next uphill section [28,38]. As the race distance increases, so does the length of the uphill sections. In events ranging from 10 km to 15 km, male and female skiers withstand uphill sections lasting between 40 and 226 s [39,40]. Despite the duration, these efforts are still performed at intensities above the athletes' VO_2max but vary based on the length of the section (approximately 115% VO_2max for longer climbs and 140–160% VO_2max during shorter ones) [22]. The work-to-rest ratio is similar to that of shorter races. For example, between two uphill sections (42 and 41 s in duration, respectively), athletes competing in a 10 km race spent approximately 25 s in the subsequent downhill section [39]. A short period on a flat or downhill section after a long climb has also been reported in longer races (21.8 km) [9], with a flat and downhill section occurring back to back only twice during the race (14 segments). XC skiing races, thus, are a sequence of uphill–downhill or flat–uphill, with work-to-rest ratios of 2:1, 1:1, and 1:2 reported between climbs [9,28,38–40].

In addition to the challenges imposed by the terrain, the increased number of mass start races also influenced the pacing profile in the sport. In these races, narrow tracks often limit the ability to advance in the field. Further, an accordion effect (when competitors in front reduce their speed, but soon accelerate, with the fluctuation in speed propagating backwards) has recently been reported [9]. The accordion effect can lead to additional accelerations and decelerations and also to more incidents during the race for those skiers not in the leading pack [9]. Positional advantage is, therefore, important, and athletes perform the initial lap of the race at an intensity that is higher than that of the subsequent laps, with the higher intensity potentially due to a greater number or intensity of surges performed [9]. Lastly, mass start races are won in the finishing sprint, with several competitors performing an all-out sprint to the finish line. In a 21.8 km race, a group of 10 athletes sprinted over the last 1.2 km of the race, with only 2.4 s separating the top five skiers and a photo finish required to determine the winner [9].

Given its characteristics, success in the sport requires the ability to withstand high intensities (110–160% VO_2max) during uphill sections and to recovery quickly from these efforts in the downhill sections (40–60% VO_2max) [11,22,32,44]. These demands are magnified in mass start races where further surges are required to attain a better position in the field. Navigating these demands while retaining the ability to sprint to the finish line is essential for success in these events.

4.2. Mountain Biking

The changes to the regulations (reduction in race duration and increase in technical constraints) have altered the demands of the sport. XC MTB races last 80–100 min and are comprised of an explosive start followed by a pattern of intermittent bursts throughout the race [12,21]. The initial burst has been shown to last approximately 68.5 ± 5.5 s, and to occur at an intensity of 481 ± 122 W (6.63 ± 1.34 W/kg, equivalent to approximately 118% of the athletes' MAP) [12,45]. It must be noted, however, that this data is from prior to the regulation changes. Recent studies have yet to describe the initial surge but have highlighted that the initial lap of the race is performed at a higher intensity than other laps [21,45], due to the performance of numerous surges in intensity that can range between 200 and 300% of the athlete's MAP, reflecting that athletes need to optimally position themselves early in the race. The benefit of positional advantage for the single-track sections of the race compensates for the negative effects of the intense effort earlier in the race, even if the intensity of some surges approaches the athletes' maximal anaerobic power (MAnP) [10].

Analyzing the surges in intensity in relation to the athletes' CP, Naess et al. [13] reported an average of 90 surges in intensity above CP per lap (3.8 km, 16 ± 2 min). These surges had an average duration of approximately 8 s and ranged in intensity from 120% to 140% of the athlete's CP. Granier et al. [10] described the supramaximal (>MAP) surges over 13 international races (90 ± 9 min) and reported an average of 18 bursts of intensity each lap (laps varied between 3.5 and 5.6 km, with races ranging between 5 and 8 laps). These surges had an average duration of 10 s and were performed at an intensity of approximately 559 W ± 46 W (equivalent to 136% of the athletes' MAP). Throughout the race, the number of surges performed per lap either remains constant [10] or is reduced [13], while the intensity of the surges is gradually reduced [10,13]. It is not clear if the change in intensity is a result of athletes trying to avoid fatiguing before the end of the race or a result of athletes separating into smaller packs [13].

Combined, these studies indicate that XC MTB requires multiple short (8 to 10 s) efforts above CP and MAP. These occur approximately every 30 to 50 s [13], leading to a work-to-rest ratio of approximately 1:4 or 1:5. Between surges, intensity is reduced to 40% to 60% of the athletes' MAP, and periods of even lower intensity (no power produced or less than 10% MAP), typically a downhill section, are common [21]. This pattern leads athletes to spend a significant portion of race time (25 to 40%) below their first ventilatory threshold (VT1) or above their MAP (25% to 30% of the race) [10,13,21]. This has led authors to emphasize that the ability to perform numerous surges in intensity above MAP should be a key training goal [10,21]. In addition, the numerous supramaximal surges in the sport have also altered athletes' profiles, with the MAnP of MTB athletes increasing by 15% over a 10-year period [10,26]. Given the numerous variations in intensity, high-intensity repeatability (i.e., the ability to perform multiple surges in intensity) [46] has been highlighted as the strongest predictor of performance in a group of elite XCO athletes, along with maximal pedaling rate and relative maximal aerobic power [21].

4.3. Road Cycling

Road cycling is characterized by prolonged periods of low- and high-intensity exercise and numerous short, high-intensity surges throughout the race [14]. These surges can be as frequent as in other intermittent sports, despite many races in road cycling lasting several hours [8]. The changes in intensity occur when athletes have to overcome varying conditions (uphill sections or headwinds, for example), attempt a breakaway, or have to respond to attacks from other competitors [14]. The characteristics of these surges differ depending on the reason for their occurrence. For example, the variations in intensity that occur due to changes in elevation depend on the race profile. One-day, single-stage, flat races require a higher number of short-duration efforts, with the ability to produce high power outputs in durations ranging from 5 to 30 s being a key factor for performance [15]. Semi-mountainous stages require the ability to perform slightly longer efforts (30 s to 2 min), while time trials and mountainous stages require longer duration (>10 min), sustained, maximal power outputs [15]. The influence of the course's characteristics is also seen in criterium races, with a greater number of short (6 to 10 s) surges above MAP compared to hilly and flat races (70, 40, and 20 sprints above MAP, respectively) due to the numerous accelerations out of corners in these shorter loop races [47].

The surges in intensity that occur due to race dynamics vary in their characteristics depending on when they occur in the race. Earlier in the race, the surges are performed at a lower intensity since the larger group might allow the breakaway to occur. Later in the race, however, power output remains elevated for a subsequent 30 s to 5 min following an attempted breakaway, to ensure the success of the action [14]. Throughout the race, the characteristics of the surges might also change. In women's races, the athletes performed 68 efforts of at least 15 s that exceeded 80% of the average power of the final sprint to the finish line, with these being more prevalent during the second (25%), third (26%), and fifth (31%) quintiles of the race [8]. The later stages of the race are particularly challenging. Abbis et al. [14] reported that in the 10 min prior to establishing a breakaway numerous 5–15 s efforts, at a very high intensity (700 to 1000 W, approx. 9.5–14.0 W/kg) are performed. A difference in the amount of time spent at high intensities (>6.6 W/kg) for short efforts (<3.8 s) was also reported between the penultimate and the final 5 min of the race, highlighting the importance of being able to perform multiple short, high-intensity efforts at the end of the race [7,41]. Menaspa et al. [7] also reported that the final 5 min of the race had twice as many surges in intensity when compared to the previous 5 min. The increase in the number of surges in intensity contributes to the last 60 min of the race being, on average, 15% more intense than the other sections of the race [7]. The need to perform multiple short (3 to 10 s efforts) bursts of intensity likely explains why a top-5 or top-10 finish for males and females is largely determined by shorter duration (5 and 10 s) absolute and relative maximal mean power (MMP), even in races with different characteristics (flat vs. mountainous, for example) [48,49].

Particularly in the later moments of the race, team dynamics also play an important role. As a team attempts to win the race with their designated sprinter, the cyclist's teammates might provide drafting and tactical assistance [50], potentially influencing the demands experienced by the athlete. In the last 60 s preceding the finishing sprint, the position of the cyclist within the bunch (closer to the front of the pack) and the number of teammates in front of the athlete are related to the chances of a successful sprint [51,52]. These last moments of the race include numerous surges in intensity and a higher overall intensity [7,51,52], with the demands likely different between athletes within the same team. It is important to notice that the athlete's specialization (e.g., climber or sprinter) is another factor to be considered. Compared to climbers and flat specialists, sprinters might possess higher power outputs in short (5 to 30 s) durations, while climbers might be better suited to sustain longer efforts (5 to 60 min) [53,54]. An analysis of the demands of the Tour de France, for example, has shown that sprinters endure a greater load during mountainous stages [55]. In this context, sprinters with good climbing ability might be better positioned to win as other competitors (e.g., flat-terrain sprinters) might be dropped before the finish line [51].

The ability to perform numerous surges in intensity and stay within the leading pack allows the athletes the chance to win the race, by sprinting to the finish line. In women's races, the average sprint finish required an effort of approximately 20 s in duration, with a peak power output of 886 W (SD 91, range 716–1088, 13.9 W/kg) and an average power output of 679 W (SD 101) or 10.6 (1.5) W/kg [8]. For males, the finishing sprint lasted approximately 13.2 s (ranging between 9 and 17 s), with a peak power output of 1248 W (SD 122) and an average power output of 1020 W (SD 77, range 865–1140) or 14.2 (SD 1.1, 12.2–15.8) W/kg [7,41].

These studies demonstrate that success in road cycling requires several efforts of different durations that vary in their demands according to the race's characteristics (e.g., flat vs. mountainous) and where they might occur during the race (early in the race vs. in the 5 min preceding the finishing sprint, for example). In addition, a winning performance requires one final sprint to the finish line, performed for an average of 13 to 20 s (for males and females, respectively), and reaching an average intensity that is more than 200% of the athlete's MAP.

4.4. Triathlon

The cycling leg of a super sprint (such as the mixed-relay, MR), sprint (SD), and Olympic (OD) distance triathlons is essential for overall race performance. Positioning at the end of the cycling leg is significantly correlated with race performance [30], and athletes who complete the 2nd transition in the leading pack have a higher probability of winning a medal [56]. This leg is characterized by high variability in power output and cadence, and many short intensity bursts alternated with moderate intensity periods [16,17,20]. However, different methods of classifying these surges lead to large variations in the numbers reported in the literature. Etxebarria et al. [20] found that athletes competing in OD races completed an average of 34 (±14) surges per race, with a surge identified as any 1 s period where the intensity surpassed 600 W (more than 200% of the average race intensity of 252 ± 33 W). The number varied significantly between (ranging from 11 to 55) and within the races, with three athletes in the same event completing 35, 40, and 54 surges. A recent study [30] shows even higher numbers in OD and SD races, with an average of 13.9 peaks of power output above MAP per kilometer. Bernard et al. [16] also reported the duration of surges above the athletes' MAP, showing that the athletes completed 57 surges of seven seconds and 13 efforts of 15 s throughout the race. In addition, 13 periods of seven consecutive seconds, with intensities above 60% of the athletes' ManP, were also recorded. Race dynamics also significantly influence the number of surges performed during a race. During the cycling leg of the mixed-relay triathlon (300 m swim, 7 km bike, 2 km run), for example, the athletes perform anywhere between 8 and 17 sprints (depending on their position within the team, which might affect if they are riding with a group or chasing a pack) [34]. The male athletes in the event performed 11 and 12 peaks above 650 W during approximately 10.5 min of the race, while the female athletes performed 8 and 17 bursts of intensity above 400 W, with the difference between the two female athletes due to one athlete being chasing a group while the other was riding with a pack [34]. The fact that athletes perform several efforts even when not racing with a group highlights the influence of the course's characteristics in the number of surges performed.

The influence of changes in elevation to the variable pacing profile seen in the different triathlon events requires further investigation. Along with a technical course, changes in elevation are responsible for an increased variability in power output in off-road triathlons, with the races resembling what is found in XCO mountain biking [37]. For road events, however, no correlation was found between the athletes' power profile and the presence of uphill sections [30]. A further factor to be considered is how the athlete's characteristics and performance on the other legs might influence their race. A strong swimmer might create a gap to the chase pack, leading to a bike leg with little influence from other competitors. The athlete's locomotor profile [6] might also dictate that some athletes will excel with a variable pacing profile, while others will perform better following a constant pacing effort. Corroborating this assertion, a recent investigation [57] highlighted the importance of determining the order of the athletes within a mixed-team relay to ensure that the athletes that excel in specific circumstances (i.e., racing in a group or in a non-drafting situation) can match the requirements of the race.

The duration of the races and the number of surges reported indicate that the cycling leg of a triathlon event might require athletes to perform a 7 to 15 s effort per minute [16,30,34], with these efforts exceeding the athletes' MAP [16,34]. In this context, work-to-rest ratios of 1:4 to 1:6 can be expected. Between surges, the intensity is low (approximately 60% MAP) [20,23]. This pattern leads athletes to spend a significant amount of time in intensity zones close to or above their MAP. In the MR and OD races, athletes spent approximately 18% of their race time above MAP [16,20,30], with the amount of work completed in this intensity (as a percentage of total work done in the race) reported to be even higher (37.5%, on average) [30]. Shorter races, such as the MR, might have even higher demands. In the same team, male athletes (positions 2 and 4) were reported to spend 48% and 62% of race time at intensities above 85% of their MAP, while the female athletes (positions 1 and 3) spent 58% and 64% of the race time above this threshold [34].

Further analysis of the surges in intensity during the cycling leg of a triathlon is required as studies have reported peaks of power output above the athletes' MAP [16,30] or above an arbitrary power output [20,34]. The variations in the characteristics of the surges (duration, frequency, intensity) per lap are also not well established in the literature. For example, the final moments of the cycling leg have been described to occur at a higher intensity than the previous laps, as athletes attempt to position themselves for the start of the running leg [58]. It is possible that this could lead to greater variations in intensity in the final moments of the cycling leg. In turn, this might influence the athlete's performance during the running leg of the event [17,59].

5. Intermittent Endurance Events: Potential Implications for Performance

The completion of numerous surges in intensity has important implications for performance in these events. Two key areas related to performance are highlighted: the development of fatigue during the races and the importance of different determinants of endurance performance to success in these events.

5.1. Fatigue Development during the Race

The surges that occur during races are performed at intensities that range from above the MMSS (a surge in intensity at 110% of the athlete's critical power in XC MTB, for example) [13] to supramaximal intensities, with values up to 300% of the athletes' MAP reported in the literature [10]. These intensities encompass two different intensity domains: the severe (intensities from the MMSS to approximately 136% of the athlete's MAP) and the extreme (intensities above 136% of the athlete's MAP) domains [18,60]. The increased reliance on anaerobic energy production in these domains leads to an accumulation of H^+, inorganic phosphate (Pi), and blood lactate, along with a drop in phosphocreatine concentrations (PCr) and pH within the muscle [18,61,62]. These factors are implicated in the development of central and peripheral fatigue [61,62].

The magnitude of central and peripheral fatigue is determined by the duration and intensity of the exercise. In self-paced trials, central fatigue is greater following longer duration efforts [63]. Similarly, during repeated supramaximal efforts, peripheral fatigue develops earlier, with central fatigue presenting a later onset [64]. Further, the magnitude of central and peripheral fatigue is dependent on the intensity domain in which the exercise is performed. At task failure, central fatigue is similar following exercise in the moderate, heavy, and severe intensity domains, while it is absent in the extreme intensity domain. Conversely, peripheral fatigue is greater following exercise performed in the severe or extreme intensity domains [61]. Endurance events with an intermittent pacing profile might then present a particular scenario in which the supramaximal surges in intensity will lead to a larger magnitude of peripheral fatigue, while the duration of the exercise (and the continuous demands of subsequent sprints) will also increase the degree of central fatigue. This combination of central and peripheral fatigue is likely to increase the physiological demands of the race and potentially hinder performance.

When compared to performing the same amount of work at a constant intensity, a variable pacing consisting of multiple maximal and supramaximal surges leads to higher levels of blood lactate, heart rate, ventilation, oxygen consumption, and perceived exertion [24,59]. Subsequent performance is also impaired to a greater extent [23,24]. Figure 1 provides an overview of reported surges during different events and the intensity they represent.

Further, once exercise intensity exceeds the MMSS, only a limited amount of work, the athletes' W', can be performed [18]. The W' represents a finite work capacity above CP and is related to the accumulation of metabolites related to fatigue, such as inorganic phosphate (Pi), adenosine diphosphate, and hydrogen ions (H^+) [18,65,66]. A strong relationship between full depletion of W' and task failure in the severe and extreme intensity domains has been observed [61,65,67]. Importantly, the rate of utilization and the size of W' might vary based on the intensity of the efforts. The more intense, the faster the depletion, with the W' for efforts in the extreme intensity domain potentially smaller than for efforts in the severe intensity domain [68]. This anaerobic capacity is attributed to three different energy sources—local oxygen stores (aerobic contribution), high energy phosphates (alactic contribution), and anaerobic glycolysis (lactic contribution) [13,66,69]. During exhaustive exercise, the contribution of these sources is 5–10%, 20–30%, and 60–70%, respectively [11]. While the recovery of local O_2 stores and PCr is quick (20 s halftime), the recovery of the lactic component of W' is much slower [65,70]. Efforts that lead to substantial accumulation of blood lactate might also delay the recovery of PCr and impact movement economy [71]. It is best for the athletes, then, that the supramaximal efforts performed are not as intense or prolonged to fully deplete their W' or to significantly impair their ability to recover from the efforts, hastening their fatigue development.

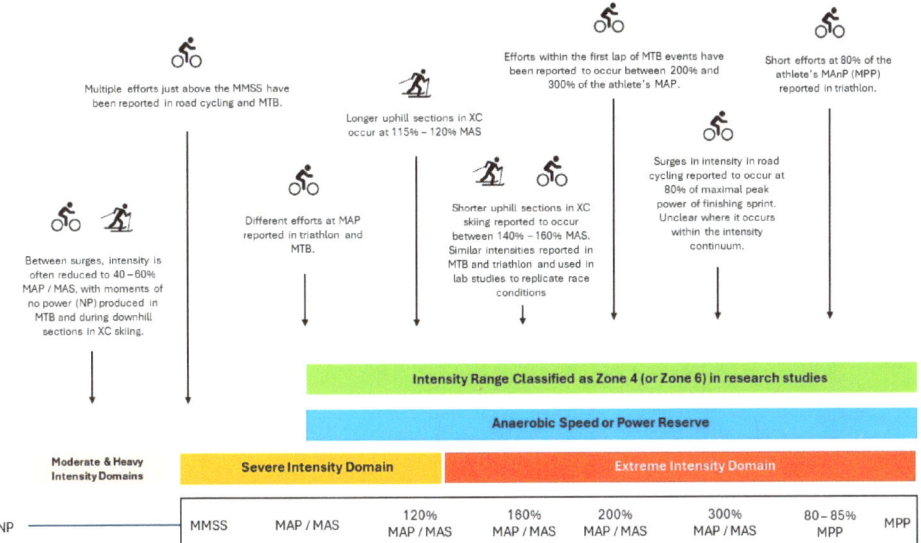

Figure 1. The range of intensities of the surges reported in the literature and their relation to intensity domains and the athletes' anaerobic power reserve (APR). The image illustrates the numerous surges in the severe and extreme intensity domains and how classifying these as a single intensity zone (green bar) does not accurately represent their physiological demands. NP: no power, MMSS: maximal metabolic steady state, MAP: maximal aerobic power, MAS: maximal aerobic speed, MPP: maximal peak power.

The level of W' depletion reported in the literature supports this assertion. In MTB, most of the surges in intensity deplete only a fraction (less than 10%) of the athletes' W', and very few efforts reach 50% of their W' [13]. While the duration of the efforts in the sport remains constant, the intensity is reduced (with a reported W' depletion of 11% per surge in the initial lap vs. 3–5% throughout the remainder of the race) [13]. A similar pattern occurs in XC skiing, where the magnitude of the depletion of the athlete's anaerobic capacity (assessed through the maximal accumulated oxygen debt (MAOD)) in each surge is considered small (approximately 50% or less) in relation to the athlete's total anaerobic capacity [11,22]. The accumulated depletion of anaerobic sources during a race, however, is much greater than the athletes' capacity. Athletes can expend up to 3.8 times their anaerobic capacity during a XC skiing race [11], with similar levels of expenditure and replenishment of the W' also reported in MTB [13] and off-road triathlon races [37].

This greater level of anaerobic capacity expenditure is possible because the intense efforts are interspersed with periods at low intensity. This pattern of intense surges and low-intensity efforts leads athletes to spend a significant amount of race time at intensities above the MMSS and their MAP/MAS, along with long periods at intensities below the first ventilatory threshold (in the moderate-intensity domain) (Figure 2). At these lower intensities, athletes can recover their W' and minimize the increases in muscle activity and oxygen consumption [65,66]. W' reconstitution occurs in a biexponential way, with a faster initial recovery (e.g., a 30% reconstitution in the first 30 s after exercise to exhaustion), followed by a slower recovery of the remaining portion [70]. Recovery of fatigue-related substrates (e.g., resynthesis of PCr) and clearance of fatigue-related metabolites from muscle (e.g., H^+) also occur [65,66,69,70], allowing the athletes to avoid the attainment of a limiting intramuscular environment. The reduction in the intensity of the surges throughout the races has been hypothesized to occur so that athletes avoid achieving this level of metabolic stress [13]. In this context, the ability to minimize the metabolic disturbances due to repeated efforts above the MMSS and at supramaximal intensities is essential to performance in these events.

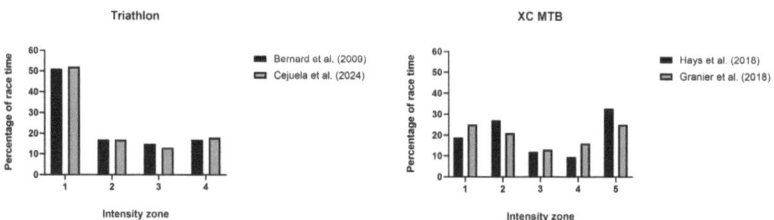

Figure 2. Time spent at different intensity zones during intermittent endurance events in triathlon (top) and mountain biking (bottom). Data for triathlon from Bernard et al. [16] and Cejuela et al. [30]; data for mountain biking from Granier et al. [10] and Hays et al. [21]. Training zones in triathlon correspond to: Z1: below VT1, Z2: between VT1 and VT2, Z3: between VT2 and MAP, Z4: above MAP. In MTB: Z1: no power or 10% below MAP, Z2: 10% MAP to below VT1, Z3: VT1 to VT2, Z4: VT2 to MAP, Z5: above MAP.

5.2. Impact of a Variable Pacing Profile on Determinants of Endurance Performance

A change in the distribution of power output during an endurance event alters the contribution of different factors that determine performance [3,25]. In endurance events with a variable pacing profile, the athletes' MAP/MAS and VO_2max might have an increased importance to performance. A higher MAP and VO_2max improves recovery following repeated sprints [72–74] and contributes to faster recovery of W' [69,70], while also allowing athletes to minimize the number of supramaximal efforts they complete. As time to fatigue in supramaximal efforts is related to the percentage of the APR at which the efforts are completed [6,75], a higher MAP might lead to efforts performed at a lower % of the athlete's APR. Unpublished data from our lab show that performing sprints at a higher supramaximal intensity leads to greater physiological stress and hinders subsequent performance. In the study, 15 well-trained (tier 2) [76] male endurance athletes completed a protocol simulating the work-to-rest ratio reported in some intermittent endurance events [10,16]. The participants were asked to complete fifteen 10 s sprints, interspersed with 50 s of low-intensity cycling (60% MAP). The protocol was performed under three different conditions, depending on the intensity of the sprints, either at the intensity associated with the athletes' MAP or at 25% or 50% of their APR. Blood lactate concentrations showed a significant difference between conditions (Figure 3). Efforts at MAP were well-tolerated by all participants, but supramaximal intensities showed significantly higher blood lactate levels. Subsequent performance in a 30 s all-out effort was also significantly impaired following supramaximal efforts (Figure 4). Current recommendations to training in intermittent endurance sports corroborate these results. For MTB athletes, the performance of high-intensity interval training to enhance MAP has been recently emphasized [10,21], and similar recommendations have been made in triathlon [30] and XC skiing, where a higher VO_2max is also highlighted [28,77].

Further, the increased reliance on anaerobic energy is reflected in the changes to performance determinants over the years. Anaerobic power (MAnP) and maximal velocity (V_{max}) have been identified as important determinants of performance in MTB and XC skiing [19,29], respectively. For MTB athletes, MAnP has increased by 15% over a 10-year period [10,13]. Increasing an athlete's MAnP also raises the upper boundary of the APR, potentially leading athletes to perform supramaximal efforts at a lower percentage of their APR. The performance of intense efforts relying on anaerobic energy also increased the importance of anaerobic capacity to performance in these two sports [26–28,32].

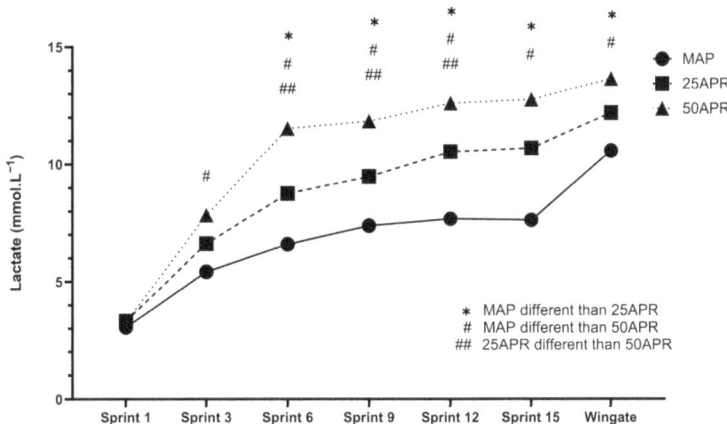

Figure 3. Blood lactate concentrations during a repeated sprint protocol performed, consisting of fifteen 10 s sprints at three different intensities. MAP: maximal aerobic power, 25APR: intensity associated with 25% of the participant's APR; 50APR: intensity associated with 25% of the participant's APR.

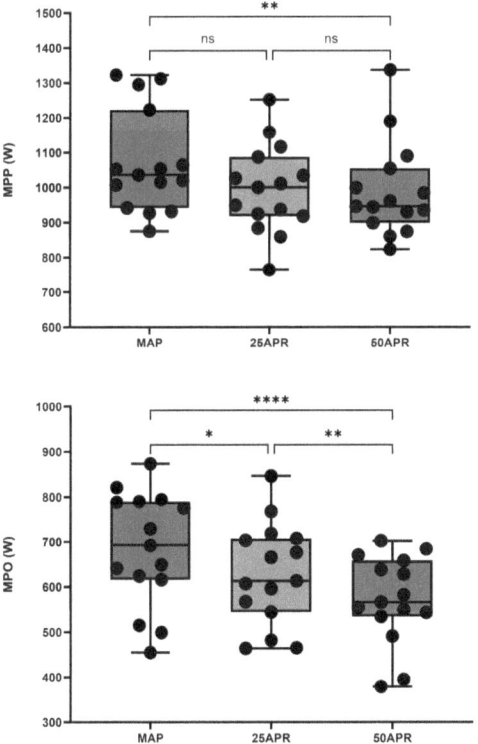

Figure 4. Performance during a 30 s Wingate, following the completion of the repeated sprint protocol. Each circle represents a data point. (**Top panel**) maximal peak power (MPP); (**bottom panel**) mean power during the 30 s effort. * $p < 0.05$, ** $p < 0.01$, **** $p < 0.001$, ns = non significant.

The ability to perform repeated efforts at intensities above CP and MAP is also essential to performance in these events. The development of repeated sprint ability (RSA) can benefit athletes involved in road cycling [8,14], MTB [10,21], XC skiing [11,19,22], and triathlon [17,30]. RSA training could improve the factors that limit the performance of multiple surges during a race (e.g., oxidative capacity, H^+ buffering) and neural factors such as muscle activation and recruitment strategies [78]. Different strategies such as short- and long-duration high-intensity interval training [79,80] and resistance training [80,81] can be utilized to improve these factors.

Lastly, the ability to tolerate the intense demands of the race without a significant decrement in performance is key to success. This trait, called physiological resilience [82] or durability [46], has been proposed as the fourth determinant of endurance performance [82]. This resiliency is related to the degree of change or decoupling in physiological responses (e.g., heart rate, blood lactate) to the same exercise intensity as work is accumulated during a race [46]. To date, only a few studies have highlighted how these responses change during endurance exercise, with results showing a shift in the athlete's physiological responses at the first [83] and second [59] thresholds as work is accumulated. When compared to exercise performed at a constant intensity, Etxebarria et al. [59] demonstrated that the magnitude of the shift in MMSS is greater after a variable intensity exercise bout with multiple supramaximal surges in performance, even when both protocols are matched for total workload. A recent study with road cyclists showed similar results, with greater decrements in high-intensity performance following variable work [84]. Indeed, it has been hypothesized that while the absolute intensity of the surges is reduced throughout a race in MTB [13], it is possible that the efforts still represent the same relative intensity, as the intensity associated with the athlete's MMSS might have changed due to the work already performed. The ability to perform and recover from numerous surges in intensity and its relationship with durability and performance warrants further investigation.

6. Practical Applications and Future Directions

6.1. Summary of Different Intensity Zones to Performance

A variable pacing profile is common in many endurance events. In these races, multiple surges in intensity are performed, with the characteristics (intensity, duration, frequency, work-to-rest ratio) of these surges varying depending on several factors (e.g., race dynamics, course profile). As such, athletes must be prepared to always engage in a highly stochastic race. These surges can occur so often that the pacing profile of certain events resembles what is seem in team sports, leading to these sport being characterized as "intermittent endurance events" [10,11].

The physiological demands of these intermittent endurance events, however, are not yet fully understood. Of the studies that compared the responses between constant and variable intensity endurance exercise, only a few [23,24,59] utilized protocols that replicate the variations in intensity seen in these events. While challenging [14], future studies should aim to replicate the duration, intensity, and work-to-rest ratio of these races. Further, the performance of supramaximal efforts is common in these events. These efforts occur within the athletes' APR. This range of intensities (from MAP to MPP) encompasses two different exercise domains (the severe and the extreme intensity domains). The factors that limit exercise within these domains are distinct in nature, and as such so are the fatigue mechanisms associated with them [61]. Distinct intensity zones might even exist within the extreme intensity domain [85]. In addition, the intensity that demarcates the severe and the extreme intensity domain is not clear, with recent studies showing that this threshold can occur at a lower percentage (120 to 130%) of the athlete's MAP [61,85] than previously thought (approximately 136% MAP) [60]. Nevertheless, current studies report the amount of time spent at supramaximal intensities as a single intensity zone (zone 4 or zone 6, in either a 3- or 5-zone model, respectively) (Figure 1) [10,13,16,21,30]. The intensity of these efforts has also been arbitrarily classified in different studies. For example, Peiffer et al. [8] classified some of the supramaximal efforts in road cycling based on a percentage of the power output of the finishing sprint in the race. In triathlon, intense efforts have been described as surpassing a certain threshold (400 W or 600 W) [20,34] or as a percentage of the athletes' MAnP [16]. Classifying these efforts according to a percentage of the athletes' APR might provide a method to standardize the intensity of the efforts, while elucidating the expected physiological demands of these surges [6].

6.2. Potential Aids for Performance Improvement and Environmental Considerations

Understanding the demands of intermittent endurance events might open new avenues for interventions that can influence performance. For example, creatine supplementation, long considered to not have an important effect on endurance performance, can enhance performance in events where multiple surges in intensity are performed [86,87]. Given their intermittent profile, training interventions that can improve performance in team sports, such as repeated sprints with blood flow restriction or in hypoxia [88,89], can also become valuable tools to enhance performance in intermittent endurance events. Lastly, heat and altitude have both been demonstrated to reduce performance during repeated sprint efforts [90,91]. Further research should investigate the influence of these environmental factors during intermittent endurance events, with particular focus on how they might influence the ability to perform multiple surges in intensity and their effect on subsequent performance.

6.3. Limitations

This review aimed to describe the variable pacing profile that occurs in different endurance events, with a particular focus on events described as "intermittent endurance events". Some limitations within the literature must be acknowledged. First, the research in this topic has been done with athletes that ranged from trained to elite or world class [76]. It is unclear if races performed at lower levels of the sport present a similar pacing profile. As such, caution is advised when translating this information to recreational- or developmental-level athletes. Second, it is important to consider the limitations of a narrative review in relation to methodological rigor and the selection of articles for inclusion. Nevertheless, we are confident that our review addresses best practices in writing a narrative review [92] and that it provides a key contribution to deepening the understanding of this topic [93]. Future studies in each individual sport presented here (and others in the literature) are necessary for a better understanding of the specific demands of endurance events with a variable pacing profile.

Author Contributions: Conceptualization, J.H.F.N. and M.D.K.; methodology, J.H.F.N. and M.D.K.; data interpretation: J.H.F.N., M.F. and M.D.K.; writing—original draft preparation, J.H.F.N.; writing—review and editing, M.D.K. and M.F.; supervision, M.D.K.; All authors have read and agreed to the published version of the manuscript.

Funding: This research was funded by a MITACS Accelerate grant (IT14510—Kennedy World Triathlon Series Edmonton) in partnership with World Triathlon Edmonton.

Conflicts of Interest: The authors declare no conflicts of interest.

References

1. Abbiss, C.R.; Laursen, P.B. Describing and understanding pacing strategies during athletic competition. *Sports Med.* **2008**, *38*, 239–252. [CrossRef]
2. Skorski, S.; Abbiss, C.R. The Manipulation of Pace within Endurance Sport. *Front. Physiol.* **2017**, *8*, 102. [CrossRef]
3. Joyner, M.J.; Coyle, E.F. Endurance exercise performance: The physiology of champions. *J. Physiol.* **2008**, *586*, 35–44. [CrossRef]
4. Hettinga, F.J.; Edwards, A.M.; Hanley, B. The Science Behind Competition and Winning in Athletics: Using World-Level Competition Data to Explore Pacing and Tactics. *Front. Sports Act. Living* **2019**, *1*, 11. [CrossRef]
5. Azevedo, R.A.; Cruz, R.; Couto, P.; Silva-Cavalcante, M.D.; Boari, D.; Lima-Silva, A.E.; Millet, G.Y.; Bertuzzi, R. Characterization of performance fatigability during a self-paced exercise. *J. Appl. Physiol. (1985)* **2019**, *127*, 838–846. [CrossRef]
6. Sandford, G.N.; Laursen, P.B.; Buchheit, M. Anaerobic Speed/Power Reserve and Sport Performance: Scientific Basis, Current Applications and Future Directions. *Sports Med.* **2021**, *51*, 2017–2028. [CrossRef]

7. Menaspà, P.; Quod, M.; Martin, D.T.; Peiffer, J.J.; Abbiss, C.R. Physical Demands of Sprinting in Professional Road Cycling. *Int. J. Sports Med.* **2015**, *36*, 1058–1062. [CrossRef]
8. Peiffer, J.J.; Abbiss, C.R.; Haakonssen, E.C.; Menaspà, P. Sprinting for the Win: Distribution of Power Output in Women's Professional Cycling. *Int. J. Sports Physiol. Perform.* **2018**, *13*, 1237–1242. [CrossRef]
9. Seeberg, T.M.; Kocbach, J.; Wolf, H.; Talsnes, R.K.; Sandbakk, Ø.B. Race development and performance-determining factors in a mass-start cross-country skiing competition. *Front. Sports Act. Living* **2022**, *4*, 1094254. [CrossRef]
10. Granier, C.; Abbiss, C.R.; Aubry, A.; Vauchez, Y.; Dorel, S.; Hausswirth, C.; Le Meur, Y. Power Output and Pacing During International Cross-Country Mountain Bike Cycling. *Int. J. Sports Physiol. Perform.* **2018**, *13*, 1243–1249. [CrossRef]
11. Gløersen, Ø.; Gilgien, M.; Dysthe, D.K.; Malthe-Sørenssen, A.; Losnegard, T. Oxygen Demand, Uptake, and Deficits in Elite Cross-Country Skiers during a 15-km Race. *Med. Sci. Sports Exerc.* **2020**, *52*, 983–992. [CrossRef]
12. Macdermid, P.W.; Stannard, S. Mechanical work and physiological responses to simulated cross country mountain bike racing. *J. Sports Sci.* **2012**, *30*, 1491–1501. [CrossRef]
13. Næss, S.; Sollie, O.; Gløersen, Ø.N.; Losnegard, T. Exercise Intensity and Pacing Pattern During a Cross-Country Olympic Mountain Bike Race. *Front. Physiol.* **2021**, *12*, 702415. [CrossRef]
14. Abbiss, C.R.; Menaspà, P.; Villerius, V.; Martin, D.T. Distribution of power output when establishing a breakaway in cycling. *Int. J. Sports Physiol. Perform.* **2013**, *8*, 452–455. [CrossRef]
15. Sanders, D.; Heijboer, M. Physical demands and power profile of different stage types within a cycling grand tour. *Eur. J. Sport. Sci.* **2019**, *19*, 736–744. [CrossRef]
16. Bernard, T.; Hausswirth, C.; Le Meur, Y.; Bignet, F.; Dorel, S.; Brisswalter, J. Distribution of power output during the cycling stage of a Triathlon World Cup. *Med. Sci. Sports Exerc.* **2009**, *41*, 1296–1302. [CrossRef]
17. Walsh, J.A. The Rise of Elite Short-Course Triathlon Re-Emphasises the Necessity to Transition Efficiently from Cycling to Running. *Sports* **2019**, *7*, 99. [CrossRef]
18. Burnley, M.; Jones, A.M. Power-duration relationship: Physiology, fatigue, and the limits of human performance. *Eur. J. Sport. Sci.* **2018**, *18*, 1–12. [CrossRef]
19. Andersson, E.; Holmberg, H.C.; Ørtenblad, N.; Björklund, G. Metabolic Responses and Pacing Strategies during Successive Sprint Skiing Time Trials. *Med. Sci. Sports Exerc.* **2016**, *48*, 2544–2554. [CrossRef]
20. Etxebarria, N.; D'Auria, S.; Anson, J.M.; Pyne, D.B.; Ferguson, R.A. Variability in power output during cycling in international Olympic-distance triathlon. *Int. J. Sports Physiol. Perform.* **2014**, *9*, 732–734. [CrossRef]
21. Hays, A.; Devys, S.; Bertin, D.; Marquet, L.A.; Brisswalter, J. Understanding the Physiological Requirements of the Mountain Bike Cross-Country Olympic Race Format. *Front. Physiol.* **2018**, *9*, 1062. [CrossRef]
22. Karlsson, Ø.; Gilgien, M.; Gløersen, Ø.N.; Rud, B.; Losnegard, T. Exercise Intensity During Cross-Country Skiing Described by Oxygen Demands in Flat and Uphill Terrain. *Front. Physiol.* **2018**, *9*, 846. [CrossRef]
23. Etxebarria, N.; Ingham, S.A.; Ferguson, R.A.; Bentley, D.J.; Pyne, D.B. Sprinting After Having Sprinted: Prior High-Intensity Stochastic Cycling Impairs the Winning Strike for Gold. *Front. Physiol.* **2019**, *10*. [CrossRef]
24. Theurel, J.; Lepers, R. Neuromuscular fatigue is greater following highly variable versus constant intensity endurance cycling. *Eur. J. Appl. Physiol.* **2008**, *103*, 461–468. [CrossRef]
25. Bellinger, P.; Derave, W.; Lievens, E.; Kennedy, B.; Arnold, B.; Rice, H.; Minahan, C. Determinants of last lap speed in paced and maximal 1500-m time trials. *Eur. J. Appl. Physiol.* **2021**, *121*, 525–537. [CrossRef]
26. Inoue, A.; AS, S.F.; Mello, F.C.; Santos, T.M. Relationship between anaerobic cycling tests and mountain bike cross-country performance. *J. Strength. Cond. Res.* **2012**, *26*, 1589–1593. [CrossRef]
27. Losnegard, T.; Hallén, J. Physiological differences between sprint- and distance-specialized cross-country skiers. *Int. J. Sports Physiol. Perform.* **2014**, *9*, 25–31. [CrossRef]
28. Sandbakk, O.; Ettema, G.; Leirdal, S.; Jakobsen, V.; Holmberg, H.C. Analysis of a sprint ski race and associated laboratory determinants of world-class performance. *Eur. J. Appl. Physiol.* **2011**, *111*, 947–957. [CrossRef]
29. Andersson, E.; Supej, M.; Sandbakk, Ø.; Sperlich, B.; Stöggl, T.; Holmberg, H.C. Analysis of sprint cross-country skiing using a differential global navigation satellite system. *Eur. J. Appl. Physiol.* **2010**, *110*, 585–595. [CrossRef]
30. Cejuela, R.; Arévalo, H.; Sellés, S. Power Profile during Cycling in World Triathlon Series and Olympic Games. *J. Sports Sci. Med.* **2024**, *23*, 25. [CrossRef]
31. Smekal, G.; von Duvillard, S.P.; Hörmandinger, M.; Moll, R.; Heller, M.; Pokan, R.; Bacharach, D.W.; LeMura, L.M.; Arciero, P. Physiological Demands of Simulated Off-Road Cycling Competition. *J. Sports Sci. Med.* **2015**, *14*, 799–810.
32. Sandbakk, Ø.; Holmberg, H.C. A reappraisal of success factors for Olympic cross-country skiing. *Int. J. Sports Physiol. Perform.* **2014**, *9*, 117–121. [CrossRef]
33. Arriel, R.A.; Meireles, A.; Souza, H.L.R.; Leite, R.C.d.M.; Marocolo, M. Mechanical demands and pacing profile adopted by elite mountain bikers during different cross-country events. *J. Phys. Educ.* **2023**, *34*, e3287. [CrossRef]
34. Sharma, A.P.; Périard, J.D. Physiological Requirements of the Different Distances of Triathlon. In *Triathlon Medicine*; Migliorini, S., Ed.; Springer International Publishing: Berlin/Heidelberg, Germany, 2020; pp. 5–17.
35. Impellizzeri, F.M.; Marcora, S.M. The physiology of mountain biking. *Sports Med.* **2007**, *37*, 59–71. [CrossRef]
36. Bossi, A.H.; O'Grady, C.; Ebreo, R.; Passfield, L.; Hopker, J.G. Pacing Strategy and Tactical Positioning During Cyclo-Cross Races. *Int. J. Sports Physiol. Perform.* **2018**, *13*, 452–458. [CrossRef]

37. Harnish, C.R.; Ferguson, H.A.; Swinand, G.P. Racing Demands of Off-Road Triathlon: A Case Study of a National Champion Masters Triathlete. *Sports* **2021**, *9*, 136. [CrossRef]
38. Ihalainen, S.; Colyer, S.; Andersson, E.; McGawley, K. Performance and Micro-Pacing Strategies in a Classic Cross-Country Skiing Sprint Race. *Front. Sports Act. Living* **2020**, *2*, 77. [CrossRef]
39. Sandbakk, Ø.; Losnegard, T.; Skattebo, Ø.; Hegge, A.M.; Tønnessen, E.; Kocbach, J. Analysis of Classical Time-Trial Performance and Technique-Specific Physiological Determinants in Elite Female Cross-Country Skiers. *Front. Physiol.* **2016**, *7*, 326. [CrossRef]
40. Staunton, C.A.; Colyer, S.L.; Karlsson, Ø.; Swarén, M.; Ihalainen, S.; McGawley, K. Performance and Micro-Pacing Strategies in a Freestyle Cross-Country Skiing Distance Race. *Front. Sports Act. Living* **2022**, *4*, 834474. [CrossRef]
41. Menaspà, P.; Quod, M.; Martin, D.; Victor, J.; Abbiss, C. Physiological demands of road sprinting in professional and U23 cycling. A pilot study. *J. Sci. Cycl.* **2013**, *2*, 35.
42. Smith, D.; Lee, H.; Pickard, R.; Sutton, B.; Hunter, E. Power demands of the cycle leg during elite triathlon competition. *Cah. De L'insep* **1999**, *24*, 224–230. [CrossRef]
43. Hébert-Losier, K.; Zinner, C.; Platt, S.; Stöggl, T.; Holmberg, H.C. Factors that Influence the Performance of Elite Sprint Cross-Country Skiers. *Sports Med.* **2017**, *47*, 319–342. [CrossRef]
44. Losnegard, T. Energy system contribution during competitive cross-country skiing. *Eur. J. Appl. Physiol.* **2019**, *119*, 1675–1690. [CrossRef]
45. Viana, B.F.; Pires, F.O.; Inoue, A.; Santos, T.M. Pacing Strategy During Simulated Mountain Bike Racing. *Int. J. Sports Physiol. Perform.* **2018**, *13*, 208–213. [CrossRef]
46. Maunder, E.; Seiler, S.; Mildenhall, M.J.; Kilding, A.E.; Plews, D.J. The Importance of 'Durability' in the Physiological Profiling of Endurance Athletes. *Sports Med.* **2021**, *51*, 1619–1628. [CrossRef]
47. Ebert, T.R.; Martin, D.T.; Stephens, B.; Withers, R.T. Power output during a professional men's road-cycling tour. *Int. J. Sports Physiol. Perform.* **2006**, *1*, 324–335. [CrossRef]
48. van Erp, T.; Lamberts, R.P. Performance Characteristics of TOP5 Versus NOT-TOP5 Races in Female Professional Cycling. *Int. J. Sports Physiol. Perform.* **2022**, *17*, 1070–1076. [CrossRef]
49. Van Erp, T.; Sanders, D. Demands of professional cycling races: Influence of race category and result. *Eur. J. Sport. Sci.* **2021**, *21*, 666–677. [CrossRef]
50. Phillips, K.E.; Hopkins, W.G. Determinants of Cycling Performance: A Review of the Dimensions and Features Regulating Performance in Elite Cycling Competitions. *Sports Med.—Open* **2020**, *6*, 23. [CrossRef]
51. Menaspà, P.; Abbiss, C.R.; Martin, D.T. Performance analysis of a world-class sprinter during cycling grand tours. *Int. J. Sports Physiol. Perform.* **2013**, *8*, 336–340. [CrossRef]
52. van Erp, T.; Kittel, M.; Lamberts, R.P. Sprint Tactics in the Tour de France: A Case Study of a World-Class Sprinter (Part II). *Int. J. Sports Physiol. Perform.* **2021**, *16*, 1371–1377. [CrossRef] [PubMed]
53. Pinot, J.; Grappe, F. The record power profile to assess performance in elite cyclists. *Int. J. Sports Med.* **2011**, *32*, 839–844. [CrossRef] [PubMed]
54. Valenzuela, P.L.; Muriel, X.; van Erp, T.; Mateo-March, M.; Gandia-Soriano, A.; Zabala, M.; Lamberts, R.P.; Lucia, A.; Barranco-Gil, D.; Pallarés, J.G. The Record Power Profile of Male Professional Cyclists: Normative Values Obtained From a Large Database. *Int. J. Sports Physiol. Perform.* **2022**, *17*, 701–710. [CrossRef] [PubMed]
55. van Erp, T.; Kittel, M.; Lamberts, R.P. Demands of the Tour de France: A Case Study of a World-Class Sprinter (Part I). *Int. J. Sports Physiol. Perform.* **2021**, *16*, 1363–1370. [CrossRef]
56. Piacentini, M.F.; Bianchini, L.A.; Minganti, C.; Sias, M.; Di Castro, A.; Vleck, V. Is the Bike Segment of Modern Olympic Triathlon More a Transition towards Running in Males than It Is in Females? *Sports* **2019**, *7*, 76. [CrossRef]
57. Quagliarotti, C.; Gaiola, D.; Bianchini, L.; Vleck, V.; Piacentini, M.F. How to Form a Successful Team for the Novel Olympic Triathlon Discipline: The Mixed-Team-Relay. *J. Funct. Morphol. Kinesiol.* **2022**, *7*, 46. [CrossRef] [PubMed]
58. Bernard, T.; Vercruyssen, F.; Mazure, C.; Gorce, P.; Hausswirth, C.; Brisswalter, J. Constant versus variable-intensity during cycling: Effects on subsequent running performance. *Eur. J. Appl. Physiol.* **2007**, *99*, 103–111. [CrossRef] [PubMed]
59. Etxebarria, N.; Hunt, J.; Ingham, S.; Ferguson, R. Physiological assessment of isolated running does not directly replicate running capacity after triathlon-specific cycling. *J. Sports Sci.* **2014**, *32*, 229–238. [CrossRef] [PubMed]
60. Hill, D.W.; Poole, D.C.; Smith, J.C. The relationship between power and the time to achieve VO(2max). *Med. Sci. Sports Exerc.* **2002**, *34*, 709–714. [CrossRef]
61. Iannetta, D.; Zhang, J.; Murias, J.M.; Aboodarda, S.J. Neuromuscular and perceptual mechanisms of fatigue accompanying task failure in response to moderate-, heavy-, severe-, and extreme-intensity cycling. *J. Appl. Physiol. (1985)* **2022**, *133*, 323–334. [CrossRef]
62. Venancio-Dallan, L.P.; Santos-Mariano, A.C.; Cristina-Souza, G.; Schamne, J.C.; Coelho, D.B.; Bertuzzi, R.; Okuno, N.M.; Lima-Silva, A.E. The effect of constant load cycling at extreme- and severe-intensity domains on performance fatigability and its determinants in young female. *Sci. Sports* **2023**, *38*, 312.e511. [CrossRef]
63. Thomas, K.; Goodall, S.; Stone, M.; Howatson, G.; Gibson, A.S.C.; Ansley, L. Central and Peripheral Fatigue in Male Cyclists after 4-, 20-, and 40-km Time Trials. *Med. Sci. Sports Exerc.* **2015**, *47*, 537–546. [CrossRef]
64. Collins, B.W.; Pearcey, G.E.P.; Buckle, N.C.M.; Power, K.E.; Button, D.C. Neuromuscular fatigue during repeated sprint exercise: Underlying physiology and methodological considerations. *Appl. Physiol. Nutr. Metab.* **2018**, *43*, 1166–1175. [CrossRef]

65. Chidnok, W.; Dimenna, F.J.; Bailey, S.J.; Vanhatalo, A.; Morton, R.H.; Wilkerson, D.P.; Jones, A.M. Exercise tolerance in intermittent cycling: Application of the critical power concept. *Med. Sci. Sports Exerc.* **2012**, *44*, 966–976. [CrossRef]
66. Chidnok, W.; DiMenna, F.J.; Fulford, J.; Bailey, S.J.; Skiba, P.F.; Vanhatalo, A.; Jones, A.M. Muscle metabolic responses during high-intensity intermittent exercise measured by (31)P-MRS: Relationship to the critical power concept. *Am. J. Physiol. Regul. Integr. Comp. Physiol.* **2013**, *305*, R1085–R1092. [CrossRef]
67. Chidnok, W.; Dimenna, F.J.; Bailey, S.J.; Wilkerson, D.P.; Vanhatalo, A.; Jones, A.M. Effects of Pacing Strategy on Work Done above Critical Power during High-Intensity Exercise. *Med. Sci. Sports Exerc.* **2013**, *45*, 1377–1385. [CrossRef]
68. Alexander, A.M.; Didier, K.D.; Hammer, S.M.; Dzewaltowski, A.C.; Kriss, K.N.; Lovoy, G.M.; Hammer, J.L.; Smith, J.R.; Ade, C.J.; Broxterman, R.M.; et al. Exercise tolerance through severe and extreme intensity domains. *Physiol. Rep.* **2019**, *7*, e14014. [CrossRef]
69. Chorley, A.; Bott, R.P.; Marwood, S.; Lamb, K.L. Physiological and anthropometric determinants of critical power, W′ and the reconstitution of W′ in trained and untrained male cyclists. *Eur. J. Appl. Physiol.* **2020**, *120*, 2349–2359. [CrossRef]
70. Caen, K.; Bourgois, G.; Dauwe, C.; Blancquaert, L.; Vermeire, K.; Lievens, E.; JO, V.A.N.D.; Derave, W.; Bourgois, J.G.; Pringels, L.; et al. W′ recovery Kinetics after Exhaustion: A Two-Phase Exponential Process Influenced by Aerobic Fitness. *Med. Sci. Sports Exerc.* **2021**, *53*, 1911–1921. [CrossRef]
71. Hoff, J.; Støren, Ø.; Finstad, A.; Wang, E.; Helgerud, J. Increased Blood Lactate Level Deteriorates Running Economy in World Class Endurance Athletes. *J. Strength. Cond. Res.* **2016**, *30*, 1373–1378. [CrossRef]
72. Bishop, D.; Girard, O.; Mendez-Villanueva, A. Repeated-sprint ability—Part II: Recommendations for training. *Sports Med.* **2011**, *41*, 741–756. [CrossRef]
73. Buchheit, M.; Hader, K.; Mendez-Villanueva, A. Tolerance to high-intensity intermittent running exercise: Do oxygen uptake kinetics really matter? *Front. Physiol.* **2012**, *3*, 406. [CrossRef]
74. Buchheit, M. Repeated-sprint performance in team sport players: Associations with measures of aerobic fitness, metabolic control and locomotor function. *Int. J. Sports Med.* **2012**, *33*, 230–239. [CrossRef]
75. Blondel, N.; Berthoin, S.; Billat, V.; Lensel, G. Relationship between run times to exhaustion at 90, 100, 120, and 140% of vVO2max and velocity expressed relatively to critical velocity and maximal velocity. *Int. J. Sports Med.* **2001**, *22*, 27–33. [CrossRef]
76. McKay, A.K.A.; Stellingwerff, T.; Smith, E.S.; Martin, D.T.; Mujika, I.; Goosey-Tolfrey, V.L.; Sheppard, J.; Burke, L.M. Defining Training and Performance Caliber: A Participant Classification Framework. *Int. J. Sports Physiol. Perform.* **2022**, *17*, 317–331. [CrossRef]
77. Seeberg, T.M.; Kocbach, J.; Danielsen, J.; Noordhof, D.A.; Skovereng, K.; Haugnes, P.; Tjønnås, J.; Sandbakk, Ø. Physiological and Biomechanical Determinants of Sprint Ability Following Variable Intensity Exercise When Roller Ski Skating. *Front. Physiol.* **2021**, *12*, 638499. [CrossRef]
78. Girard, O.; Mendez-Villanueva, A.; Bishop, D. Repeated-sprint ability—Part I: Factors contributing to fatigue. *Sports Med.* **2011**, *41*, 673–694. [CrossRef]
79. Etxebarria, N.; Anson, J.M.; Pyne, D.B.; Ferguson, R.A. High-intensity cycle interval training improves cycling and running performance in triathletes. *Eur. J. Sport. Sci.* **2014**, *14*, 521–529. [CrossRef]
80. Kristoffersen, M.; Sandbakk, Ø.; Rønnestad, B.R.; Gundersen, H. Comparison of Short-Sprint and Heavy Strength Training on Cycling Performance. *Front. Physiol.* **2019**, *10*, 1132. [CrossRef]
81. Edge, J.; Hill-Haas, S.; Goodman, C.; Bishop, D. Effects of Resistance Training on H+ Regulation, Buffer Capacity, and Repeated Sprints. *Med. Sci. Sports Exerc.* **2006**, *38*, 2004–2011. [CrossRef]
82. Jones, A.M. The fourth dimension: Physiological resilience as an independent determinant of endurance exercise performance. *J. Physiol.* **2023**. [CrossRef] [PubMed]
83. Gallo, G.; Faelli, E.L.; Ruggeri, P.; Filipas, L.; Codella, R.; Plews, D.J.; Maunder, E. Power output at the moderate-to-heavy intensity transition decreases in a non-linear fashion during prolonged exercise. *Eur. J. Appl. Physiol.* **2024**. [CrossRef] [PubMed]
84. Spragg, J.; Leo, P.; Giorgi, A.; Gonzalez, B.M.; Swart, J. The intensity rather than the quantity of prior work determines the subsequent downward shift in the power duration relationship in professional cyclists. *Eur. J. Sport Sci.* **2024**, *24*, 449–457. [CrossRef]
85. Ozkaya, O.; Jones, A.M.; Burnley, M.; As, H.; Balci, G.A. Different categories of VO2 kinetics in the 'extreme' exercise intensity domain. *J. Sports Sci.* **2023**, *41*, 2144–2152. [CrossRef] [PubMed]
86. Forbes, S.C.; Candow, D.G.; Neto, J.H.F.; Kennedy, M.D.; Forbes, J.L.; Machado, M.; Bustillo, E.; Gomez-Lopez, J.; Zapata, A.; Antonio, J. Creatine supplementation and endurance performance: Surges and sprints to win the race. *J. Int. Soc. Sports Nutr.* **2023**, *20*, 2204071. [CrossRef] [PubMed]
87. Tomcik, K.A.; Camera, D.M.; Bone, J.L.; Ross, M.L.; Jeacocke, N.A.; Tachtsis, B.; Senden, J.; LJC, V.A.N.L.; Hawley, J.A.; Burke, L.M. Effects of Creatine and Carbohydrate Loading on Cycling Time Trial Performance. *Med. Sci. Sports Exerc.* **2018**, *50*, 141–150. [CrossRef] [PubMed]
88. Hamlin, M.J.; Olsen, P.D.; Marshall, H.C.; Lizamore, C.A.; Elliot, C.A. Hypoxic Repeat Sprint Training Improves Rugby Player's Repeated Sprint but Not Endurance Performance. *Front. Physiol.* **2017**, *8*, 24. [CrossRef] [PubMed]
89. Mckee, J.R.; Girard, O.; Peiffer, J.J.; Scott, B.R. Repeated-Sprint Training With Blood Flow Restriction: A Novel Approach to Improve Repeated-Sprint Ability? *Strength Cond. J.* **2023**, *45*, 598–607. [CrossRef]

90. Girard, O.; Brocherie, F.; Bishop, D.J. Sprint performance under heat stress: A review. *Scand. J. Med. Sci. Sports* **2015**, *25* (Suppl. 1), 79–89. [CrossRef]
91. Girard, O.; Brocherie, F.; Millet, G.P. Effects of Altitude/Hypoxia on Single- and Multiple-Sprint Performance: A Comprehensive Review. *Sports Med.* **2017**, *47*, 1931–1949. [CrossRef]
92. Furley, P.; Goldschmied, N. Systematic vs. Narrative Reviews in Sport and Exercise Psychology: Is Either Approach Superior to the Other? *Front. Psychol.* **2021**, *12*, 685082. [CrossRef] [PubMed]
93. Greenhalgh, T.; Thorne, S.; Malterud, K. Time to challenge the spurious hierarchy of systematic over narrative reviews? *Eur. J. Clin. Investig.* **2018**, *48*, e12931. [CrossRef] [PubMed]

Disclaimer/Publisher's Note: The statements, opinions and data contained in all publications are solely those of the individual author(s) and contributor(s) and not of MDPI and/or the editor(s). MDPI and/or the editor(s) disclaim responsibility for any injury to people or property resulting from any ideas, methods, instructions or products referred to in the content.

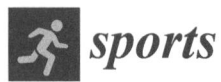

Review

Accelerating Recovery from Exercise-Induced Muscle Injuries in Triathletes: Considerations for Olympic Distance Races

Thilo Hotfiel [1,2,3,*], Isabel Mayer [3], Moritz Huettel [3], Matthias Wilhelm Hoppe [1,4], Martin Engelhardt [1,2], Christoph Lutter [5,6], Klaus Pöttgen [7], Rafael Heiss [8], Tom Kastner [2,9,10] and Casper Grim [1,2]

1. Department of Orthopedic, Trauma, Hand and Neuro Surgery, Klinikum Osnabrück GmbH, Osnabrück 49076, Germany; matthias.hoppe@klinikum-os.de (M.W.H.); martin.engelhardt@klinikum-os.de (M.E.); casper.grim@klinikum-os.de (C.G.)
2. Deutsche Triathlon Union (DTU), Frankfurt 60528, Germany; tom.kastner@iat.uni-leipzig.de
3. Department of Orthopedic Surgery, Friedrich-Alexander-University Erlangen-Nuremberg, Erlangen 91054, Germany; isabel.mayer@gmx.de (I.M.); moritz.huettel@gmx.de (M.H.)
4. Department of Movement and Training Science, University of Wuppertal, Wuppertal 42119, Germany
5. Department of Orthopedics, Rostock University Medical Center, Rostock 18057, Germany; christoph.lutter@googlemail.com
6. Department of Sports Orthopedics, Sports Medicine, Sports Traumatology, Klinikum Bamberg, Bamberg 96049, Germany
7. B·A·D Group, Darmstadt 64295, Germany; klaus@drpoettgen.de
8. Department of Radiology, University Hospital Erlangen, Erlangen 91054, Germany; rafael.heiss@klinikum-os.de
9. Department of Sport Medicine Humboldt University and Charité University Medicine, Berlin 10117, Germany
10. Institute for Applied Training Science Leipzig (IAT), Leipzig 04109, Germany
* Correspondence: thilo.hotfiel@klinikum-os.de; Tel.: +49-541-450-6245; Fax: +49-541-4562

Received: 2 May 2019; Accepted: 4 June 2019; Published: 13 June 2019

Abstract: The triathlon is one of the fastest developing sports in the world due to expanding participation and media attention. The fundamental change in Olympic triathlon races from a single to a multistart event is highly demanding in terms of recovery from and prevention of exercise-induced muscle injures. In elite and competitive sports, ultrastructural muscle injuries, including delayed onset muscle soreness (DOMS), are responsible for impaired muscle performance capacities. Prevention and treatment of these conditions have become key in regaining muscular performance levels and to guarantee performance and economy of motion in swimming, cycling and running. The aim of this review is to provide an overview of the current findings on the pathophysiology, as well as treatment and prevention of, these conditions in compliance with clinical implications for elite triathletes. In the context of DOMS, the majority of recovery interventions have focused on different protocols of compression, cold or heat therapy, active regeneration, nutritional interventions, or sleep. The authors agree that there is a compelling need for further studies, including high-quality randomized trials, to completely evaluate the effectiveness of existing therapeutic approaches, particularly in triathletes. The given recommendations must be updated and adjusted, as further evidence emerges.

Keywords: DOMS; EIMD; recovery; regeneration; muscle injuries; CWI; compression; endurance

1. Introduction

The triathlon is a multisport endurance sport in which athletes race sequentially in swimming, cycling, and running over various race distances. Due to an ever-expanding participation base and increased media interest, the triathlon is considered to be one of the fastest growing sports globally [1–3]. There are numerous event formats for both competitive and recreational events, ranging from super-sprint to long-distance triathlon, over which the International Triathlon Union (ITU) presides. In addition to the standard distance (Olympic distance) and sprint distance races, the ITU is the Governing Body overseeing the Mixed Team Relay (MTR) [4]; an innovative racing format where athletes complete a super-sprint triathlon, comprising of a 300 m swim, 6.6 km cycle and 1 km run before handing over to a teammate in the given order of female-male-female-male. The Mixed Relay is commonly held within 2–3 days of the individual race embedded within the same event. Having recently been included in the Olympic program, the Mixed Relay will make its debut at the Tokyo 2020 Olympic Games [4]. As well as being an exciting addition for spectators, it alters the demands placed upon the athletes, requiring them to work at higher intensity and greater speed throughout.

Historically, events such as the World Triathlon Series (WTS) or Olympic Games consisted of one intense and exhausting race for each athlete. Subsequently, athletes were able to recover in the days following competition until the resumption of full training or further competition; a second race start during the same competition was usually not performed. The fundamental change in triathlons from a single to multi-start event increases the demands placed upon the athlete in terms of recovery and prevention of exercise-induced muscle damages, which in turn has created a demand for research into optimizing recovery and regeneration. According to previous studies, particularly carbohydrate depletion, dehydration, hypoglycemia, electrolyte imbalance and ultrastructural muscle damage have been estimated to have a key function affecting muscle force output in triathletes [5,6]. As triathlon was established as a traditional endurance sport, common recovery practices focus mainly on the metabolic aspects (i.e., energy and carbohydrate storage, fluid intake, natrium balance [7,8]) and triathletes seem well informed about the necessity of rehydration after exercise [6]. Several studies demonstrated the presence of exercise-induced muscle injuries in triathletes [6,9,10], which is a relevant factor that impairs muscle function in triathlons, and which is known to mainly result from the running leg [6]. It was demonstrated in a recent study that post-exercise myoglobin and creatine kinase levels as indirect markers of muscle damage correlated with countermovement jumps height loss after the race [5,6]. The authors concluded that muscle fiber damage is one of the key factors for muscle fatigue in triathlons and strategies to lessen muscle fatigue during triathlon events should comprise a reduction in muscle damage [6]. However, those strategies have not been developed for triathletes up to now. Due to the adapted Olympic program, there is now a greater demand on athletes to regain high-intensity muscular activity and a high biomechanical output in order to deliver maximum performance for the MTR race [11] (Figure 1).

Understanding the benefits of each intervention requires knowledge of the underlying muscle damaging and exhausting mechanisms, pathophysiological processes and treatment interventions [12]. The design of an "ideal" recovery regime is a topic receiving a lot of attention within current elite sports research [13–16]. Therefore, the aim of this narrative review is to provide an overview of the current literature on the pathophysiology as well as treatment and prevention of muscle soreness and suggesting the clinical implications for elite triathletes.

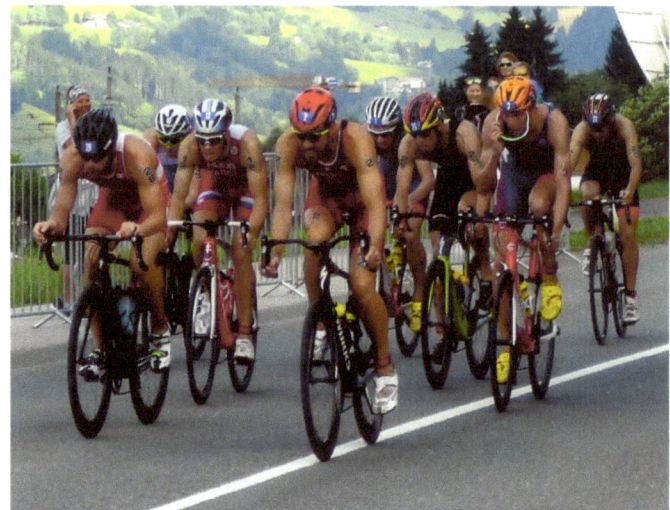

Figure 1. Scuffles for positions during cycling. High muscular demands are required. Elite triathletes need to perform i.e., over 1000 watts 3s peak power.

2. Materials and Methods

This narrative review focusses on the prevention and treatment of exercise-induced muscle injuries in relation to elite level triathletes. The existing literature on the pathogenesis, treatment, and prevention of exercise-induced muscle injuries, including original research reports, systematic and non-systematic reviews, book chapters and case reports was reviewed independently from their level of evidence. No systematic literature search was conducted. The aim of the present work was (1) to update the information about the current findings in pathogenesis of exercise-induced muscle injuries; (2) to apply current evidence for the treatment and prevention of exercise-induced muscle injuries in general; and (3) to discuss and evaluate the current findings by considering clinical and practical implications for triathlon races and competitions. For the purpose of this manuscript, the work done by an interdisciplinary authorship, consisting of biomechanists, sports scientists and sports physicians from the German Olympic Federation (DOSB) and the German Triathlon Union (DTU, Deutsche Triathlon Union), as well as scientists specializing in the field of exercise-induced muscle injuries is highlighted.

3. Results and Discussion

3.1. Mechanisms and Pathogenesis of Exercise-Induced Muscle Injures

3.1.1. Differentiation between Muscle Soreness, Exercise-Induced Muscle Damage (EIMD) and Delayed Onset Muscle Soreness (DOMS)

The clinical progression and manifestation of exercise-induced muscle damage, also known as DOMS, commonly begins 6–12 h post exercise, increasing progressively until peak pain occurs at 48–72hrs and thereafter decreasing until completely imperceptible 5–7 days post exercise [17,18]. DOMS is often accompanied by impaired muscle contraction and reduced force capacity [17,19,20], whilst a local or even global area of increased muscle tone is commonly observed [21–24]. DOMS is associated with local muscle soreness, reduced range of motion and altered biomechanical function of the adjacent joints [17,19,20,25,26]. Although the precise underlying causes of DOMS remain unknown [27], it is commonly accepted that the main mechanisms are related to ultrastructural damage of skeletal muscle integrity (exercise-induced muscle damage, EIMD) caused by intense and exhausting exercise and/or unfamiliar sporting activity [28–30] (Figure 2, Figure 3); for elite triathletes, the first scenario being the most relevant.

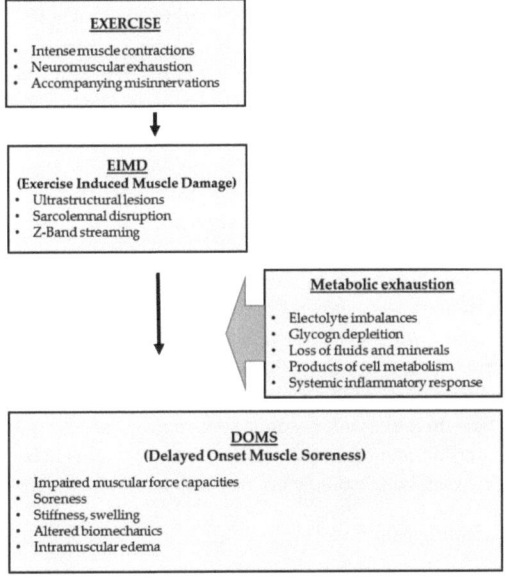

Figure 2. Illustrating the pathophysiological pathway of exercises, Exercise-induced Muscle Damage (EIMD), Delayed Onset Muscle Soreness (DOMS) and accompanying metabolic exhaustion; adapted from Heiss et al. [12].

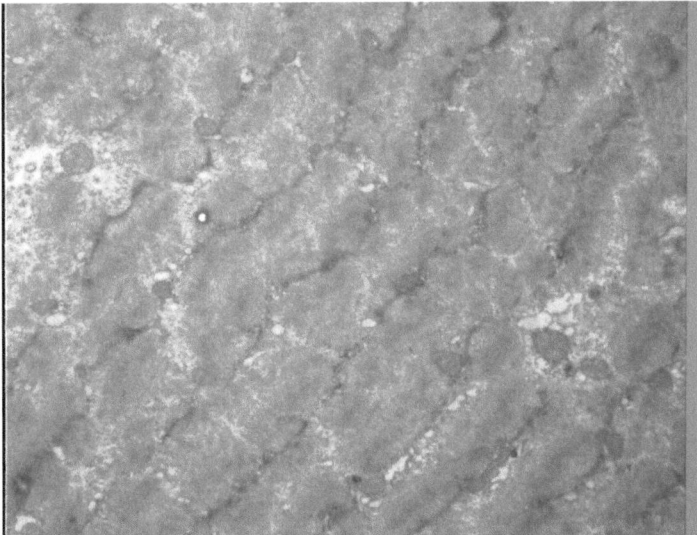

Figure 3. Z-disk disintegration and myofilament disarrangement as sign of ultrastructural damage was evaluated by electron microscopy of biopsies of human vastus lateralis 24 h after strenuous resistance exercise for 70 s under tension leading to DOMS (With kind permission, Prof. W. Bloch, German Sport University Cologne, Germany).

In the past, eccentric contractions in particular were suspected to play a key role in the development of ultrastructural muscle injuries. In this condition, external loads are greater than the force generated by the muscles fibres under concentric conditions [12,28,31]. The higher muscular force is caused by an increase in recruitment of active cross-bridges [32] and in particular, by "passive-elastic" factors (i.e., Ca^{2+} triggered increased stiffness of titin and its winding on actin [12,33]), as described in the three-filament model and winding filament by Herzog et al. [34]. However, this hypothesis is not entirely relevant to triathletes, as eccentric contractions may occur solely during running, particularly on inclined surfaces. Several studies demonstrated the presence of exercise-induced muscle injuries in triathletes [6,9,10]. However, the exact cause of muscle damage in endurance sports, in particular in triathletes in triathletes has yet to be elucidated. In triathlons, there are no isolated eccentric contractions that induce a "pure eccentric overload" as applied in several DOMS models. Instead, the disciplines of swimming, cycling, and running are associated with changes of direction and positioning and eccentric contractions are shorter and part of the entire stretch-shortening cycle [35,36]. Swimming and cycling are considered to produce minor muscle damage in the involved muscles. Running however, as weight bearing activity includes concentric and eccentric actions in the lower extremity muscles [6]. During high-intensity races, central neuromuscular exhaustion and accompanying misinnervations can be discussed to reinforce the development of ultrastructural muscle injuries in these conditions. Hence, weariness induced alterations in intra- and intermuscular coordination between the muscle fibres with associated overstressing and damaging single muscle fibers should also be considered a factor [23]. Furthermore, it is unclear if metabolic exhaustion may also reinforce the development of DOMS.

3.1.2. Inflammatory and Healing Responses

Electrolyte imbalances, leukocyte accumulation and infiltration in the exercised muscle, as well as an upregulation of circulating pro-inflammatory cytokines have been found in the context of DOMS as well as after exhausting endurance trials [27–29,37]. The released cytokines lead to a higher vascular permeability and microcirculation disturbances as they act as inflammatory mediators [38]. The presence of interstitial fluid associated with intramuscular edema and compartment swelling (Figure 4) as well as the presence of diverse inflammatory substances are described to be responsible for nociceptor activation and pain sensation [39,40]. In response to the loss of sarcolemmal integrity and permeability of the plasma membrane, DOMS is associated with increased creatine kinase (CK) activity levels, which are one of the leading indirect markers of muscle damage [19,38,41,42]. Several further markers such as Interleukin 6 (IL-6), C-reactive protein (CRP) [43], PTX-3 or LDH are upregulated during inflammation within damaged tissues [44]. However, the assessment of these parameters has been studied primarily in a scientific setting, as it is not methodological feasible in the context of triathlon competitions; therefore, generalizability is limited.

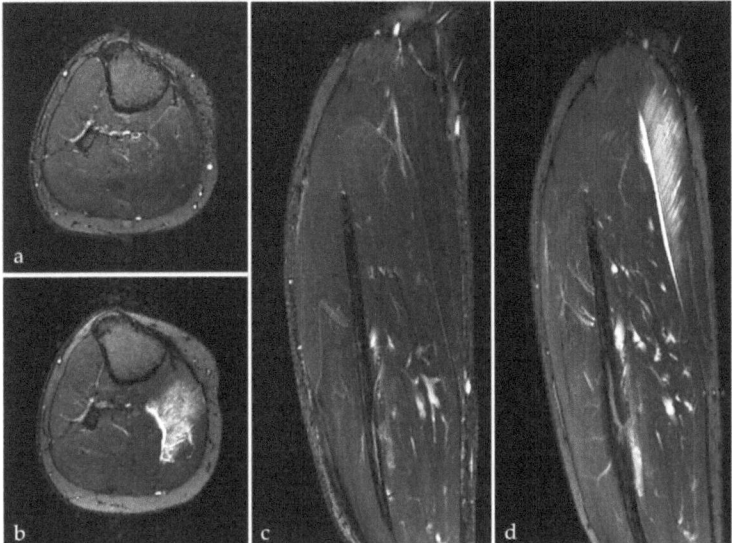

Figure 4. Axial (**a,b**) and coronal (**c,d**) T2-weighted fat-suppressed MRI images of the lower leg before (**a,c**) and 60 h after eccentric exercise (**b,d**) in the same participant. The increased signal intensity (**b,d**) reflects a rising fluid content in the gastrocnemius medialis muscle as equivalent of DOMS.

4. Treatments and Strategies to Target Exercise-Induced Muscle Injuries

It is desirable to prevent athletes from experiencing DOMS, particularly in the context of multi-start events. Based on pathophysiological factors, recovery strategies should focus on various aspects, including (1), the primary prevention of ultrastructural lesions during exercise (prevention of EIMD), (2), the treatment of inflammatory responses leading to DOMS, and (3) – in case of failure of point (1) and (2) the treatment and recovery strategies of reduce signs of DOMS [12]. A range of interventions aiming to either prevent or relieve the symptoms of DOMS, thereby accelerating the recovery process from this performance-limiting condition, have been reported.

4.1. The Role of Sleep

A reduction in total regeneration time at major sporting events containing multiple starts increases the awareness of sleep as a crucial component of the recovery process. Disturbance of sleep can be caused by early morning training, increases in training load, travel departure times, jet lag and altitude [45,46]. Sleep deprivation is associated with lower physical and mental performance [47], whilst optimal levels of sleep (in both quantity and quality) have been linked to increased performance and reduced risk of injury [48]. The greater the demand for speed, tactical awareness and technical skill within a sport, the more sensitive it is to sleep duration manipulation. Further to this, longer-term sleep manipulation is more likely to affect athletic performance than acute sleep manipulation [49]. Some studies showed a positive effect of sleep extension on subsequent performance [50,51]. A promising option in the case of an insufficient night's sleep could be the introduction of power naps, provided that the recommendation of a 30-min maximum duration is not exceeded [52,53]. For practical suggestions, refer to Table 1.

Table 1. Recommendations for improving sleep in athletes (Data adapted from Simpson et al. [54]).

Obtain adequate total sleep duration	Strategy 1: Track sleep for 2 weeks using a self-report sleep diary. Gradually increase sleep duration by 15 min every few nights, until athlete feels well rested and alert during the day. Consider increasing nighttime sleep by 30–60 min/night; this is particularly important if average sleep duration is <7 h/night	Strategy 2: Consider implementing regular naps, beginning on weekends or off-days if needed. Allow adequate time to return to full alertness after daytime naps
Maintain healthy sleep habits	Strategy 1: Develop a good sleep environment: the ideal room is cool, dark, and comfortable. Avoid having/using electronics or personal devices in bedroom	Strategy 2: Avoid alerting factors in the evening. Reduce ambient light exposure in late evening hours if possible, limit electronic device use at least 1 hr prior to bedtime, allow for a 30–60 min relaxing wind-down period before bed. Ideally, consume no caffeine after lunch; limit alcohol use in late evening
Minimizing impact of travel	Strategy 1: Factor-in time needed to adjust to new time zone; as a rule of thumb, the body can adjust to 1 h of time zone difference each day. Consider starting to shift body clock prior to departure or during flight; personalized travel planners (available online) may be helpful	Strategy 2: Reduce impact of non-jet lag travel effects: dehydration, acoustic stress, low physical activity, changes in food/drinking patterns

4.2. Compression Therapy

In recent years, there has been increasing interest in the efficacy of compression garments for post-exercise treatment in various disciplines. Existing systematic reviews have concluded that compression garments are effective in enhancing recovery from exercise-induced muscle damage [55,56], whilst the majority of previous studies failed to support a performance-enhancing effect of wearing compression garments during exercise. Results are not uniformly accepted. Inconsistent findings may be caused by heterogeneous conditions [55,57] and no consensus for optimal application time, applied pressure, composition as well as shape and design [57] could be provided thus far. Overall there is limited evidence to suggest that compression garments impact athletic performance [58–60], but there may be legitimation for its use in terms of recovery [55,57,61,62].

4.2.1. Compression Therapy during Exercise

Bringard et al. suggest that wearing compression garments during exercise may enhance muscle perfusion and decrease muscle oscillation which thereby promotes a lower energy expenditure and an improvement or maintenance in submaximal running speed [63]. Moreover, it is reported that compression garments lead to increased comfort [12,57,64] and support the underlying tissue resulting in reduced microtrauma and muscular damage [62,65]. In contrast, a systematic review by Beliard et al. reported that nine from ten studies did not show any performance enhancing effects [57], nor significant changes in objective physiological variables such as increased oxygen uptake or plasma level related changes of lactate or CK [12,63,64,66]. Only Kemmler et al. could demonstrate a significant performance effect (time under load, total work) for calf compression in male runners [66]. In summary, wearing compression garments during exercise (triathlon) might lead to marginal improvements in performance; however, evidence is inconclusive.

4.2.2. Compression Therapy Post Exercise

For post exercise compression therapy, heterogeneous modalities are discussed. For the prevention of DOMS, several studies have shown positive effects on recovery, function and strength of the treated muscle groups [12,55,57,67]. The decrease of CK levels shown in two studies [15,55,57] and the reduction of lactate level [67,68] could be seen as valid markers for improved regeneration. This could be attributed to an attenuation in the release of CK into the bloodstream, improved clearance from the circulation and enhanced repair of the damaged muscle tissue [12,57]. This theory could however not be confirmed by MRI based investigations which showed no reduction in edema or DOMS in the calf muscles [24]. In the same study, the only parameter shown to be significant was a faster normalization of muscle stiffness.

4.2.3. Intermittent Compression Therapy

A further available treatment strategy is intermittent compression therapy. The NormaTec Pulse Massage Pattern (The NormaTec PULSE recovery Systems, NormaTec, Watertown, Massachusetts, USA) works with a pulsating, dynamic, upwards moving compression with the goal of mobilizing fluids and supporting the outflow out of the extremities [12]. This method is poorly investigated with only one study exists showing local hyperermia [69]. Pneumatic compression pants did not alter the rate of muscle glycogen resynthesis, blood lactate, or blood glucose and insulin concentrations associated with a post-exercise oral glucose load [70]. Further, Haun et al. reported a decrease in DOMS and potential reduction in muscle proteolysis as well as oxidative stress [71]. There is a need for further research related to mechanistic changes.

Practical implications: Based on the evidence reviewed, there is no generalized recommendation for use of compression garments during exercise, but if the athlete reports subjective benefits, then it may have a positive impact. There is evidence suggesting that compression can play a role in enhanced post-exercise recovery, whilst evidence for dynamic compression is inconclusive.

4.3. Thermal Therapy

4.3.1. Cold Water Immersion Therapy (CWI)

Systemic cooling for post-exercise recovery and regeneration has become more widespread in elite sport. Specifically, CWI has established itself as an effective therapy to cope with EIMD and alleviate physiological and functional deficits [72]. There is high level evidence for its clinical effectiveness in regard to an enhanced regeneration [12]. Hohenauer et al. emphasized, that cooling is superior in comparison to passive recovery strategies with CWI achieving the best results in reducing the symptoms of DOMS [73]. This was confirmed by Leeder et al., especially up to 96 hrs post exercise [74]. Various aspects promoting a faster regeneration are suggested, for example, a facilitated removal of metabolites [75]; limitation of inflammation and cell damage [76]; analgesic effects through activation of M8 cation channels (TRPM8), located in a and c fibres [77]; compression through increased hydrostatic pressure [75] and especially a decreased tissue temperature, blood flow and cardiovascular strain [74,76,78]. Referring to the water temperature, the best results were found to be between 11 and 15 °C for 11–15 min. [72]. Also, the efficacy of CWI seems to be depended of the previous type of exercise. CWI is thought to be most effective in attenuating EIMD induced by whole body prolonged endurance-based exercise [79]. Inflammatory processes may be limited through a coldness dependent down regulation of intramuscular metabolism [80]; however, associated adverse effects with regards to glycogen resynthesis or lactate metabolism cannot be assumed and have to be investigated further.

Practical implications: Taking into account the different practical aspects, CWI seems to be an appropriate short-term recovery modality of exercise-induced muscle injuries in triathletes, especially within the new framework that includes mixed relay competition. Beside positive muscle injury related effects, CWI should be viewed critically in regard to glycogen and energy metabolism. The application of CWI should be adjusted to suit the environmental conditions such as climate, local equipment, conditions and, not least, the athlete's individual preference in order to be most effective.

4.3.2. Heat Therapy

The application of heat therapy is still controversially discussed, and studies have to be regarded cautiously in the examined context. Study protocols vary from experimental designs in isolated mouse soleus muscle to gain information about glycogen and energy metabolism [81], to studies focusing mainly on clinical outcomes like maximal range of movement (ROM) [82] or voluntary contraction and muscle steadiness after sauna [83]. In regards to the acute inflammatory response leading to DOMS (between 48–72hrs), whole-body heat therapy has to be regarded critically [28]. In contrast, after the outlined peak, heat therapy can support soft tissue repair, tissue nutrition and circulation [84,85]. Studies show a positive effect in gaining muscle strength associated with hypertrophy (10 weeks heat therapy without strength training) through provoked gene expression for growth and differentiation [12,86] enhanced recovery after eccentric resistance training with an acceleration of angiogenic factors in human knee extensor muscle [87] and an acceleration of muscle contractility properties and decreased muscle steadiness after whole-body heat therapy by sauna [83]. In contrast Frier et al. emphasizes pre-exercise heat stress may inhibit increases in muscle mass, potentially caused by accumulation of heat shock proteins in lower limbs of rats [88].

Practical implications: For the application of heat therapy in triathlons, no general recommendation can be made at this point. Especially for acute injuries in the first inflammation phase, cooling is the preferred strategy. After the inflammatory response or recovery without muscle injury, heat therapy can support regeneration and improved tissue healing. Unfortunately, there are no available studies with an endurance-based protocol, specifically relating to long-term muscle load such as the duration of a triathlon event.

4.4. Active Regeneration

Conventional strategies such as low intensity exercise and stretching have a long tradition in sports [89], whilst there has been a surge in innovative techniques recently which are yet to be fully investigated. Low intensity training is suggested after eccentric or high-intensity training sessions inducing DOMS, which is associated with muscle pain and tenderness [90], as well as compromised performance and swelling [28]. It has been proposed that the short-term alleviation of pain during exercise is due to the breakup of adhesions in the sore muscles, an increased removal of noxious waste products via an increased blood flow or an increased endorphin release [90]. There are two studies inducing DOMS with an eccentric exercise protocol in upper arm [91] and wrist extensor muscles [92] followed by 8–10 min ergometry; neither was unable to show any clinical advantage [90]. In contrast Hasson et al. reported a significant decrease in DOMS 48 hrs after a high velocity concentric isokinetic exercise of the knee extensors and flexors by performing a stepping exercise 24 hrs after the initial training [90,93]. In summary, study results related to recovery from DOMS are heterogenous, without any clear conclusion.

Furthermore, in regard to fatigue inducing exercise, Vanderthommen et al. were unable to show any superior effect in performance or pain of active compared to passive regeneration after isometric muscle contraction [94]. The same recovery modality of pedaling on a bicycle ergometer with a moderate load had however demonstrated an improvement in the recovery process [94]. These studies showed a superior blood lactate removal following active recovery [95,96] compared to passive recovery. In a randomized controlled trial from 2018 no positive effects of dynamic contract-relax stretching in either strength or in ROM or pain threshold could be confirmed [97]. Moreover, stretching after eccentric exercises failed to prove its efficacy [90], therefore it was concluded that there is insufficient data for stretching as a strategy to enhance recovery [98].A new form of active regeneration is foam rolling, as a method of self-myofascial release, which has become popular in recovery [12] with ubiquitous use through all performance levels. Several studies have examined the effect of post muscle damaging exercise foam rolling. All studies reported a significant reduction of pain, whilst two also showed objective benefits in sprint and jump performance and in ROM [17,99], which was, however, contradicted by the findings of Jay et al. [100]. As another clinical outcome Fleckenstein et al. observed a significant effect of foam rolling on neuromuscular exhaustion as maximal isometric voluntary force of the knee extensors and pain [101]. The only study observing the rate of blood lactate clearance was conducted after a 100 m water-rescue in life guards which was also found to be significant [102]. In conclusion, foam rolling seems to be effective in pain reduction, but further benefits have yet to be conclusively reported. The underlying physiological principles and potential risks also remain unclear [103,104].

Practical implications: As an active recovery strategy, low intensity training in form of 15 min of pedaling directly after exercise might have a recovery enhancing effect, however, there is little evidence of performance enhancement or objective support for muscle healing [12].

4.5. Nutrition

The importance of post-exercise nutrition as a critical component of recovery is widely accepted. However, evidence-based dietary recommendations specifically related to elite triathletes are still lacking. There are many studies evaluating the effects of nutritional expression of DOMS after EIMD. The importance of protein supplementation for endurance triathletes is increasingly accepted. Post-exercise protein supplementation enhances muscle protein synthesis and satellite cell activity for muscle repair, furthermore facilitates muscle glycogen resynthesis [105]. Beside this, branched-chain amino acids (BCAAs) which are mainly metabolized in skeletal muscle [106], are thought to have further positive effects on exercise-related cytokine production in cases of structural and metabolic processes due to exercise damage [12,107]. A review analyzing the effects of branched-chain amino acids (BCAAs) in endurance sports concluded that supplementation with BCAAs lowers the degree of pain and muscle damage, perceived exertion and mental fatigue, but stimulates the anabolic response in recovery and improves the immune response. There was no consensus about the dose and timing, but it seems to be most effective if there is 2–3/1 1g relationship between leucine/ isoleucine and valine amino acids [108]. Doering et al. suggest that masters athletes may have slower recovery rates due to impaired muscle remodeling mechanism, compared to younger, equally trained athletes, after muscle-damaging endurance exercise. Given this fact, masters athletes could benefit from higher doses of post exercise dietary protein intake, especially with leucine [105]. A systematic review showed that a high daily BCAA supplementation (>200 mg kg $^{-1}$ day $^{-1}$) for a long period (>10 days) was particularly effective when the extent of muscle damage was low-to-moderate and consumed pre-exercise [12,40,109]. Another important nutritional component targeting a fast and ideal recovery are the omega-3-fatty acids. By limitation of anti-inflammatory responses and oxidative stress, omega-3-fatty acids significantly reduce the DOMS sensations. Therefore, it is recommended to ingest 1.8–3 g of omega-3-fatty acids after exercise [110,111].

5. Conclusions

The present work provides an overview of the pathophysiological pathway, as well as the various treatment strategies in the field of exercise-induced muscle injuries, and evaluates their effectiveness with respect to the existing scientific evidence and practical expertise (Table 2). As a limitation of this review, there are only a few studies dealing with specific interventions in elite triathletes. Most existing investigations focusing on the pathogenesis or interventions in exercise-induced muscle injuries consist of a wide spectrum of athletes and different accompanying metabolic demands. Further, when interpreting triathlon specific data, different metabolic demands in short and long-distance athletes have to be considered, and it is unclear if given general recommendations can be completely transferred to Olympic triathletes. The authors agree that there is a compelling need for further studies, including high-quality randomized trials, to completely evaluate the effectiveness of existing therapeutic approaches. The given recommendations must be updated and adjusted as further evidence emerges.

Table 2. Overview of discussed interventions in treatment and prevention of exercise-induced muscle damages.

	Intervention	Practical Implications
Compression	• Compression therapy during exercise • Compression therapy post exercise • Intermittent compression therapy	• Overall there is evidence to suggest that compression garments are effective in the treatment of exercise-induced muscle damages (i.e., 6 h use in post-exercise set-up) • Inconsistent data exists in terms of accelerating performance • No recommendations can be made in regard to pressure level or design. • Athlete's Individual preference and comfort should be considered
Thermal therapy	• Cold water immersion therapy (CWI) • Whole body cryotherapy • Heat therapy	• CWI seems to be an appropriate short-term recovery modality of exercise-induced muscle injuries in triathletes • Besides positive muscle injury related effects, the effects of CWI on glycogen and energy metabolism should be considered critically. • The application of CWI should be adjusted to suit the environmental conditions such as climate, local equipment, conditions and not least the athlete's individual preference in order to be most effective.
Active regeneration	• Low intensity exercise • Stretching • Foam rolling	• As an active recovery strategy, low intensity training in form of 15 min of pedaling directly after exercise might have a recovery enhancing effect, however, there is little evidence of performance enhancement or objective support for muscle healing • No clear recommendations can be made on stretching or foam rolling
Oral medications and nutrition	• Protein supplementation, use of branched-chain amino acids (BCAAs)	• Post-exercise protein supplementation enhances muscle protein synthesis and satellite cell activity for muscle repair, furthermore facilitates muscle glycogen resynthesis • Branched-chain amino acids (BCAAs) are thought to have further positive effects on exercise-related cytokine production in cases of structural and metabolic processes due to exercise damage
Improving sleep	• Adequate total sleep duration • Healthy sleep habits • Minimizing impact on travel	• Please refer to Table 1

Author Contributions: T.H., M.W.H., C.G. and M.E. designed the manuscript. T.H. and R.H. have made major contributions in section "Results". I.M., M.H., C.L., K.P. and T.K. have made major contributions in drafting and writing the section "Discussion". All authors read and approved the final manuscript.

Funding: This research received no external funding.

Acknowledgments: The English language support of Annika Wing is gratefully acknowledged.

Conflicts of Interest: The authors declare no conflict of interest.

References

1. Kienstra, C.M.; Asken, T.R.; Garcia, J.D.; Lara, V.; Best, T.M. Triathlon Injuries: Transitioning from Prevalence to Prediction and Prevention. *Curr. Sports Med. Rep.* **2017**, *16*, 397–403. [CrossRef] [PubMed]
2. Olcina, G.; Timon, R.; Brazo-Sayavera, J.; Martinez-Guardado, I.; Marcos-Serrano, M.; Crespo, C. Changes in physiological and performance variables in non-professional triathletes after taking part in an Olympic distance triathlon. *Res. Sports Med. (Print)* **2018**, *26*, 323–331. [CrossRef] [PubMed]
3. Neidel, P.; Wolfram, P.; Hotfiel, T.; Engelhardt, M.; Koch, R.; Lee, G.; Zwingenberger, S. Cross-Sectional Investigation of Stress Fractures in German Elite Triathletes. *Sports* **2019**, *7*, 88. [CrossRef] [PubMed]
4. International Triathlon Union. Available online: https://www.triathlon.org/ (accessed on 1 May 2019).
5. Jeukendrup, A.E.; Jentjens, R.L.; Moseley, L. Nutritional considerations in triathlon. *Sports Med. (Auckl. NZ)* **2005**, *35*, 163–181. [CrossRef] [PubMed]
6. Del Coso, J.; Gonzalez-Millan, C.; Salinero, J.J.; Abian-Vicen, J.; Soriano, L.; Garde, S.; Perez-Gonzalez, B. Muscle damage and its relationship with muscle fatigue during a half-iron triathlon. *PLoS ONE* **2012**, *7*, e43280. [CrossRef]
7. Hiller, W.D. Dehydration and hyponatremia during triathlons. *Med. Sci. Sports Exerc.* **1989**, *21*, S219–S221.
8. Speedy, D.B.; Noakes, T.D.; Kimber, N.E.; Rogers, I.R.; Thompson, J.M.; Boswell, D.R.; Ross, J.J.; Campbell, R.G.; Gallagher, P.G.; Kuttner, J.A. Fluid balance during and after an ironman triathlon. *Clin. J. Sport Med.* **2001**, *11*, 44–50. [CrossRef]
9. Margaritis, I.; Tessier, F.; Verdera, F.; Bermon, S.; Marconnet, P. Muscle enzyme release does not predict muscle function impairment after triathlon. *J. Sports Med. Phys. Fit.* **1999**, *39*, 133–139.
10. Galan, B.S.; Carvalho, F.G.; Santos, P.C.; Gobbi, R.B.; Kalva-Filho, C.A.; Papoti, M.; da Silva, A.S.; Freitas, E.C. Effects of taurine on markers of muscle damage, inflammatory response and physical performance in triathletes. *J. Sports Med. Phys. Fit.* **2018**, *58*, 1318–1324. [CrossRef]
11. Fernandez-Revelles, A.B. Infographic. Correlation between phases and final result in Men's triathlon competition at the Olympic Games in Sydney 2000. *Br. J. Sports Med.* **2018**. [CrossRef]
12. Heiss, R.; Freiwald, J.; Hoppe, M.W.; Lutter, C.; Forst, R.; Grim, C.; Poettgen, K.; Bloch, W.; Huttel, M.; Hotfiel, T. Advances in Delayed-Onset Muscle Soreness (DOMS): Part II: Treatment and Prevention. *Sportverletz. Sportschaden* **2019**, *33*, 1–9. [CrossRef] [PubMed]
13. Crowther, F.; Sealey, R.; Crowe, M.; Edwards, A.; Halson, S. Influence of recovery strategies upon performance and perceptions following fatiguing exercise: A randomized controlled trial. *BMC Sports Sci. Med. Rehabil.* **2017**, *9*, 25. [CrossRef] [PubMed]
14. Hausswirth, C.; Mujika, I. *Recovery for Performance in Sport*; Human Kinetics: Champaign, IL, USA, 2013.
15. Meyer, T.; Ferrauti, A.; Kellmann, M.; Pfeiffer, M. *Regenerationsmanagement im Spitzensport. REGman-Ergebnisse und Handlungsempfehlungen*; Sportverlag Strauß: Hellenthal, Germany, 2016.
16. Hotfiel, T.; Seil, R.; Bily, W.; Bloch, W.; Gokeler, A.; Krifter, R.M.; Mayer, F.; Ueblacker, P.; Weisskopf, L.; Engelhardt, M. Nonoperative treatment of muscle injuries–recommendations from the GOTS expert meeting. *J. Exp. Orthop.* **2018**, *5*, 24. [CrossRef] [PubMed]
17. Pearcey, G.E.; Bradbury-Squires, D.J.; Kawamoto, J.E.; Drinkwater, E.J.; Behm, D.G.; Button, D.C. Foam rolling for delayed-onset muscle soreness and recovery of dynamic performance measures. *J. Athl. Train.* **2015**, *50*, 5–13. [CrossRef] [PubMed]
18. Valle, X.; Til, L.; Drobnic, F.; Turmo, A.; Montoro, J.B.; Valero, O.; Artells, R. Compression garments to prevent delayed onset muscle soreness in soccer players. *Muscles Ligaments Tendons J.* **2013**, *3*, 295–302. [CrossRef]
19. Kim, S.K.; Kim, M.C. The affect on delayed onset muscle soreness recovery for ultrasound with bee venom. *J. Phys. Ther. Sci.* **2014**, *26*, 1419–1421. [CrossRef] [PubMed]

20. Mizuno, S.; Morii, I.; Tsuchiya, Y.; Goto, K. Wearing Compression Garment after Endurance Exercise Promotes Recovery of Exercise Performance. *Int. J. Sports Med.* **2016**, *37*, 870–877. [CrossRef]
21. Hotfiel, T.; Kellermann, M.; Swoboda, B.; Wildner, D.; Golditz, T.; Grim, C.; Raithel, M.; Uder, M.; Heiss, R. Application of Acoustic Radiation Force Impulse (ARFI) Elastography in Imaging of Delayed Onset Muscle Soreness (DOMS): A Comparative Analysis With 3T MRI. *J. Sport Rehabil.* **2017**, 1–29. [CrossRef]
22. Pollock, N.; James, S.L.J.; Lee, J.C.; Chakraverty, R. British athletics muscle injury classification: A new grading system. *Br. J. Sports Med.* **2014**, *48*. [CrossRef]
23. Mueller-Wohlfahrt, H.W.; Haensel, L.; Mithoefer, K.; Ekstrand, J.; English, B.; McNally, S.; Orchard, J.; van Dijk, C.N.; Kerkhoffs, G.M.; Schamasch, P.; et al. Terminology and classification of muscle injuries in sport: The Munich consensus statement. *Br. J. Sports Med.* **2013**, *47*, 342–350. [CrossRef]
24. Heiss, R.; Kellermann, M.; Swoboda, B.; Grim, C.; Lutter, C.; May, M.S.; Wuest, W.; Uder, M.; Nagel, A.M.; Hotfiel, T. Effect of Compression Garments on the Development of Delayed-Onset Muscle Soreness: A Multimodal Approach Using Contrast-Enhanced Ultrasound and Acoustic Radiation Force Impulse Elastography. *J. Orthop. Sports Phys. Ther.* **2018**, *48*, 887–894. [CrossRef] [PubMed]
25. Yu, J.Y.; Jeong, J.G.; Lee, B.H. Evaluation of muscle damage using ultrasound imaging. *J. Phys. Ther. Sci.* **2015**, *27*, 531–534. [CrossRef] [PubMed]
26. Kellermann, M.H.M.; Swoboda, B.; Gelse, K.; Freiwald, J.; Grim, C.; Nagel, A.; Uder, M.; Wildner, D.; Hotfiel, T. Intramuscular perfusion response in delayed onset muscle soreness (DOMS): A quantitative analysis with contrast-enhanced ultrasound (CEUS). *Int. J. Sports Med.* **2017**, *38*, 833–841. [CrossRef] [PubMed]
27. Paulsen, G.; Mikkelsen, U.R.; Raastad, T.; Peake, J.M. Leucocytes, cytokines and satellite cells: What role do they play in muscle damage and regeneration following eccentric exercise? *Exerc. Immunol. Rev.* **2012**, *18*, 42–97. [PubMed]
28. Hotfiel, T.; Freiwald, J.; Hoppe, M.W.; Lutter, C.; Forst, R.; Grim, C.; Bloch, W.; Huttel, M.; Heiss, R. Advances in Delayed-Onset Muscle Soreness (DOMS): Part I: Pathogenesis and Diagnostics. *Sportverletz. Sportschaden* **2018**, *32*, 243–250. [CrossRef] [PubMed]
29. Peake, J.; Nosaka, K.; Suzuki, K. Characterization of inflammatory responses to eccentric exercise in humans. *Exerc. Immunol. Rev.* **2005**, *11*, 64–85. [PubMed]
30. Lewis, P.B.; Ruby, D.; Bush-Joseph, C.A. Muscle soreness and delayed-onset muscle soreness. *Clin. Sports Med.* **2012**, *31*, 255–262. [CrossRef]
31. Douglas, J.; Pearson, S.; Ross, A.; McGuigan, M. Eccentric Exercise: Physiological Characteristics and Acute Responses. *Sports Med. (Auckl. NZ)* **2017**, *47*, 663–675. [CrossRef]
32. Linari, M.; Lucii, L.; Reconditi, M.; Casoni, M.E.; Amenitsch, H.; Bernstorff, S.; Piazzesi, G.; Lombardi, V. A combined mechanical and X-ray diffraction study of stretch potentiation in single frog muscle fibres. *J. Physiol.* **2000**, *526 Pt 3*, 589–596. [CrossRef]
33. Nishikawa, K.C.; Monroy, J.A.; Uyeno, T.E.; Yeo, S.H.; Pai, D.K.; Lindstedt, S.L. Is titin a 'winding filament'? A new twist on muscle contraction. *Proc. Biol. Sci.* **2012**, *279*, 981–990. [CrossRef]
34. Herzog, W. Mechanisms of enhanced force production in lengthening (eccentric) muscle contractions. *J. Appl. Physiol. (Bethesda MD 1985)* **2014**, *116*, 1407–1417. [CrossRef] [PubMed]
35. Nicol, C.; Avela, J.; Komi, P.V. The stretch-shortening cycle: A model to study naturally occurring neuromuscular fatigue. *Sports Med. (Auckl. NZ)* **2006**, *36*, 977–999. [CrossRef] [PubMed]
36. Tesch, P.A.; Fernandez-Gonzalo, R.; Lundberg, T.R. Clinical Applications of Iso-Inertial, Eccentric-Overload (YoYo) Resistance Exercise. *Front. Physiol.* **2017**, *8*, 241. [CrossRef] [PubMed]
37. Pinho, R.A.; Silva, L.A.; Pinho, C.A.; Scheffer, D.L.; Souza, C.T.; Benetti, M.; Carvalho, T.; Dal-Pizzol, F. Oxidative stress and inflammatory parameters after an Ironman race. *Clin. J. Sport Med.* **2010**, *20*, 306–311. [CrossRef] [PubMed]
38. Yanagisawa, O.; Sakuma, J.; Kawakami, Y.; Suzuki, K.; Fukubayashi, T. Effect of exercise-induced muscle damage on muscle hardness evaluated by ultrasound real-time tissue elastography. *Springerplus* **2015**, *4*, 308. [CrossRef] [PubMed]
39. Nie, H.; Madeleine, P.; Arendt-Nielsen, L.; Graven-Nielsen, T. Temporal summation of pressure pain during muscle hyperalgesia evoked by nerve growth factor and eccentric contractions. *Eur. J. Pain* **2009**, *13*, 704–710. [CrossRef] [PubMed]
40. Kim, J.; Lee, J. A review of nutritional intervention on delayed onset muscle soreness. Part I. *J. Exerc. Rehabil.* **2014**, *10*, 349–356. [CrossRef] [PubMed]

41. Kraemer, W.J.; Bush, J.A.; Wickham, R.B.; Denegar, C.R.; Gomez, A.L.; Gotshalk, L.A.; Duncan, N.D.; Volek, J.S.; Putukian, M.; Sebastianelli, W.J. Influence of compression therapy on symptoms following soft tissue injury from maximal eccentric exercise. *J. Orthop. Sports Phys. Ther.* **2001**, *31*, 282–290. [CrossRef]
42. Ulbricht, A.; Gehlert, S.; Leciejewski, B.; Schiffer, T.; Bloch, W.; Hohfeld, J. Induction and adaptation of chaperone-assisted selective autophagy CASA in response to resistance exercise in human skeletal muscle. *Autophagy* **2015**, *11*, 538–546. [CrossRef]
43. Deme, D.; Telekes, A. Prognostic importance of lactate dehydrogenase (LDH) in oncology. *Orv. Hetil.* **2017**, *158*, 1977–1988. [CrossRef]
44. Del Giudice, M.; Gangestad, S.W. Rethinking IL-6 and CRP: Why They Are More Than Inflammatory Biomarkers, and Why It Matters. *Brain Behav. Immun.* **2018**. [CrossRef] [PubMed]
45. Roberts, S.S.H.; Teo, W.P.; Warmington, S.A. Effects of training and competition on the sleep of elite athletes: A systematic review and meta-analysis. *Br. J. Sports Med.* **2018**. [CrossRef] [PubMed]
46. Hausswirth, C.; Louis, J.; Aubry, A.; Bonnet, G.; Duffield, R.; Le Meur, Y. Evidence of disturbed sleep and increased illness in overreached endurance athletes. *Med. Sci. Sports Exerc.* **2014**, *46*, 1036–1045. [CrossRef] [PubMed]
47. Halson, S.L. Sleep in elite athletes and nutritional interventions to enhance sleep. *Sports Med. (Auckl. NZ)* **2014**, *44* (Suppl. 1), S13–S23. [CrossRef] [PubMed]
48. Watson, A.M. Sleep and Athletic Performance. *Curr. Sports Med. Rep.* **2017**, *16*, 413–418. [CrossRef] [PubMed]
49. Kirschen, G.W.; Jones, J.J.; Hale, L. The Impact of Sleep Duration on Performance Among Competitive Athletes: A Systematic Literature Review. *Clin. J. Sport Med.* **2018**. [CrossRef] [PubMed]
50. Bonnar, D.; Bartel, K.; Kakoschke, N.; Lang, C. Sleep Interventions Designed to Improve Athletic Performance and Recovery: A Systematic Review of Current Approaches. *Sports Med. (Auckl. NZ)* **2018**, *48*, 683–703. [CrossRef]
51. Thun, E.; Bjorvatn, B.; Flo, E.; Harris, A.; Pallesen, S. Sleep, circadian rhythms, and athletic performance. *Sleep Med. Rev.* **2015**, *23*, 1–9. [CrossRef]
52. Milner, C.E.; Cote, K.A. Benefits of napping in healthy adults: Impact of nap length, time of day, age, and experience with napping. *J. Sleep Res.* **2009**, *18*, 272–281. [CrossRef]
53. Waterhouse, J.; Atkinson, G.; Edwards, B.; Reilly, T. The role of a short post-lunch nap in improving cognitive, motor, and sprint performance in participants with partial sleep deprivation. *J. Sports Sci.* **2007**, *25*, 1557–1566. [CrossRef]
54. Simpson, N.S.; Gibbs, E.L.; Matheson, G.O. Optimizing sleep to maximize performance: Implications and recommendations for elite athletes. *Scand. J. Med. Sci. Sports* **2017**, *27*, 266–274. [CrossRef] [PubMed]
55. Hill, J.; Howatson, G.; van Someren, K.; Leeder, J.; Pedlar, C. Compression garments and recovery from exercise-induced muscle damage: A meta-analysis. *Br. J. Sports Med.* **2014**, *48*, 1340–1346. [CrossRef] [PubMed]
56. Marques-Jimenez, D.; Calleja-Gonzalez, J.; Arratibel, I.; Delextrat, A.; Terrados, N. Are compression garments effective for the recovery of exercise-induced muscle damage? A systematic review with meta-analysis. *Physiol. Behav.* **2016**, *153*, 133–148. [CrossRef] [PubMed]
57. Beliard, S.; Chauveau, M.; Moscatiello, T.; Cros, F.; Ecarnot, F.; Becker, F. Compression garments and exercise: No influence of pressure applied. *J. Sports Sci. Med.* **2015**, *14*, 75. [PubMed]
58. da Silva, C.A.; Helal, L.; da Silva, R.P.; Belli, K.C.; Umpierre, D.; Stein, R. Association of Lower Limb Compression Garments During High-Intensity Exercise with Performance and Physiological Responses: A Systematic Review and Meta-analysis. *Sports Med.* **2018**, *48*, 1859–1873. [CrossRef] [PubMed]
59. Venckunas, T.; Trinkunas, E.; Kamandulis, S.; Poderys, J.; Grunovas, A.; Brazaitis, M. Effect of lower body compression garments on hemodynamics in response to running session. *Sci. World J.* **2014**, *2014*, 353040. [CrossRef] [PubMed]
60. Duffield, R.; Portus, M. Comparison of three types of full-body compression garments on throwing and repeat-sprint performance in cricket players. *Br. J. Sports Med.* **2007**, *41*, 409–414; discussion 414. [CrossRef]
61. Kim, J.; Kim, J.; Lee, J. Effect of compression garments on delayed-onset muscle soreness and blood inflammatory markers after eccentric exercise: A randomized controlled trial. *J. Exerc. Rehabil.* **2017**, *13*, 541–545. [CrossRef]
62. Trenell, M.I.; Rooney, K.B.; Sue, C.M.; Thomspon, C.H. Compression Garments and Recovery from Eccentric Exercise: A (31)P-MRS Study. *J. Sports Sci. Med.* **2006**, *5*, 106–114.

63. Bringard, A.; Perrey, S.; Belluye, N. Aerobic energy cost and sensation responses during submaximal running exercise–positive effects of wearing compression tights. *Int. J. Sports Med.* **2006**, *27*, 373–378. [CrossRef]
64. Ali, A.; Caine, M.P.; Snow, B.G. Graduated compression stockings: Physiological and perceptual responses during and after exercise. *J. Sports Sci.* **2007**, *25*, 413–419. [CrossRef] [PubMed]
65. Sperlich, B.; Born, D.-P.; Kaskinoro, K.; Kalliokoski, K.K.; Laaksonen, M.S. Squeezing the muscle: Compression clothing and muscle metabolism during recovery from high intensity exercise. *PLoS ONE* **2013**, *8*, e60923. [CrossRef] [PubMed]
66. Kemmler, W.; von Stengel, S.; Kockritz, C.; Mayhew, J.; Wassermann, A.; Zapf, J. Effect of compression stockings on running performance in men runners. *J. Strength Cond. Res.* **2009**, *23*, 101–105. [CrossRef] [PubMed]
67. Hamlin, M.J.; Mitchell, C.J.; Ward, F.D.; Draper, N.; Shearman, J.P.; Kimber, N.E. Effect of compression garments on short-term recovery of repeated sprint and 3-km running performance in rugby union players. *J. Strength Cond. Res.* **2012**, *26*, 2975–2982. [CrossRef]
68. Chatard, J.C.; Atlaoui, D.; Farjanel, J.; Louisy, F.; Rastel, D.; Guezennec, C.Y. Elastic stockings, performance and leg pain recovery in 63-year-old sportsmen. *Eur. J. Appl. Physiol.* **2004**, *93*, 347–352. [CrossRef] [PubMed]
69. Martin, J.S.; Borges, A.R.; Beck, D.T. Peripheral conduit and resistance artery function are improved following a single, 1-h bout of peristaltic pulse external pneumatic compression. *Eur. J. Appl. Physiol.* **2015**, *115*, 2019–2029. [CrossRef] [PubMed]
70. Keck, N.A.; Cuddy, J.S.; Hailes, W.S.; Dumke, C.L.; Ruby, B.C. Effects of commercially available pneumatic compression on muscle glycogen recovery after exercise. *J. Strength Cond. Res.* **2015**, *29*, 379–385. [CrossRef]
71. Haun, C.T.; Roberts, M.D.; Romero, M.A.; Osburn, S.C.; Mobley, C.B.; Anderson, R.G.; Goodlett, M.D.; Pascoe, D.D.; Martin, J.S. Does external pneumatic compression treatment between bouts of overreaching resistance training sessions exert differential effects on molecular signaling and performance-related variables compared to passive recovery? An exploratory study. *PLoS ONE* **2017**, *12*, e0180429. [CrossRef]
72. Machado, A.F.; Ferreira, P.H.; Micheletti, J.K.; de Almeida, A.C.; Lemes, I.R.; Vanderlei, F.M.; Netto Junior, J.; Pastre, C.M. Can Water Temperature and Immersion Time Influence the Effect of Cold Water Immersion on Muscle Soreness? A Systematic Review and Meta-Analysis. *Sports Med. (Auckl. NZ)* **2016**, *46*, 503–514. [CrossRef]
73. Hohenauer, E.; Taeymans, J.; Baeyens, J.P.; Clarys, P.; Clijsen, R. The Effect of Post-Exercise Cryotherapy on Recovery Characteristics: A Systematic Review and Meta-Analysis. *PLoS ONE* **2015**, *10*, e0139028. [CrossRef]
74. Leeder, J.; Gissane, C.; van Someren, K.; Gregson, W.; Howatson, G. Cold water immersion and recovery from strenuous exercise: A meta-analysis. *Br. J. Sports Med.* **2012**, *46*, 233–240. [CrossRef] [PubMed]
75. Stocks, J.M.; Patterson, M.J.; Hyde, D.E.; Jenkins, A.B.; Mittleman, K.D.; Taylor, N.A. Effects of immersion water temperature on whole-body fluid distribution in humans. *Acta Physiol. Scand.* **2004**, *182*, 3–10. [CrossRef] [PubMed]
76. Wilcock, I.M.; Cronin, J.B.; Hing, W.A. Physiological response to water immersion: A method for sport recovery? *Sports Med.* **2006**, *36*, 747–765. [CrossRef] [PubMed]
77. Proudfoot, C.J.; Garry, E.M.; Cottrell, D.F.; Rosie, R.; Anderson, H.; Robertson, D.C.; Fleetwood-Walker, S.M.; Mitchell, R. Analgesia mediated by the TRPM8 cold receptor in chronic neuropathic pain. *Curr. Biol.* **2006**, *16*, 1591–1605. [CrossRef] [PubMed]
78. Swenson, C.; Sward, L.; Karlsson, J. Cryotherapy in sports medicine. *Scand. J. Med. Sci. Sports* **1996**, *6*, 193–200. [CrossRef] [PubMed]
79. Ihsan, M.; Watson, G.; Abbiss, C.R. What are the physiological mechanisms for post-exercise cold water immersion in the recovery from prolonged endurance and intermittent exercise? *Sports Med.* **2016**, *46*, 1095–1109. [CrossRef] [PubMed]
80. Merrick, M.A.; Rankin, J.M.; Andres, F.A.; Hinman, C.L. A preliminary examination of cryotherapy and secondary injury in skeletal muscle. *Med. Sci. Sports Exerc.* **1999**, *31*, 1516–1521. [CrossRef] [PubMed]
81. Blackwood, S.J.; Hanya, E.; Katz, A. Effect of post-exercise temperature elevation on post-exercise glycogen metabolism of isolated mouse soleus muscle. *J. Appl. Physiol. (1985)* **2019**. [CrossRef] [PubMed]
82. Saga, N.; Katamoto, S.; Naito, H. Effect of heat preconditioning by microwave hyperthermia on human skeletal muscle after eccentric exercise. *J. Sports Sci. Med.* **2008**, *7*, 176–183. [PubMed]

83. Cernych, M.; Baranauskiene, N.; Vitkauskiene, A.; Satas, A.; Brazaitis, M. Accelerated muscle contractility and decreased muscle steadiness following sauna recovery do not induce greater neuromuscular fatigability during sustained submaximal contractions. *Hum. Mov. Sci.* **2019**, *63*, 10–19. [CrossRef] [PubMed]
84. Halvorson, G.A. Therapeutic Heat and Cold for Athletic Injuries. *Phys. Sportsmed.* **1990**, *18*, 87–94. [CrossRef]
85. Lohman, E.B., 3rd; Bains, G.S.; Lohman, T.; DeLeon, M.; Petrofsky, J.S. A comparison of the effect of a variety of thermal and vibratory modalities on skin temperature and blood flow in healthy volunteers. *Med. Sci. Monit.* **2011**, *17*, MT72–81. [CrossRef] [PubMed]
86. Goto, K.; Oda, H.; Kondo, H.; Igaki, M.; Suzuki, A.; Tsuchiya, S.; Murase, T.; Hase, T.; Fujiya, H.; Matsumoto, I.; et al. Responses of muscle mass, strength and gene transcripts to long-term heat stress in healthy human subjects. *Eur. J. Appl. Physiol.* **2011**, *111*, 17–27. [CrossRef]
87. Kim, K.; Kuang, S.; Song, Q.; Gavin, T.P.; Roseguini, B.T. Impact of heat therapy on recovery following eccentric exercise in humans. *J. Appl. Physiol. (1985)* **2019**. [CrossRef]
88. Frier, B.C.; Locke, M. Heat stress inhibits skeletal muscle hypertrophy. *Cell Stress Chaperones* **2007**, *12*, 132–141. [CrossRef] [PubMed]
89. Freiwald, J. *Optimales Dehnen: Sport-Prävention-Rehabilitation*; Spitta Verlag: Balingen, Germany, 2013.
90. Cheung, K.; Hume, P.A.; Maxwell, L. Delayed Onset Muscle Soreness. *Sports Med.* **2003**, *33*, 145–164. [CrossRef]
91. Weber, M.D.; Servedio, F.J.; Woodall, W.R. The effects of three modalities on delayed onset muscle soreness. *J. Orthop. Sports Phys. Ther.* **1994**, *20*, 236–242. [CrossRef] [PubMed]
92. Gulick, D.T.; Kimura, I.F.; Sitler, M.; Paolone, A.; Kelly IV, J.D. Various treatment techniques on signs and symptoms of delayed onset muscle soreness. *J. Athl. Train.* **1996**, *31*, 145.
93. Hasson, S.M.; Williams, J.; Signorile, J. Fatigue-induced changes in myoelectric signal characteristics and perceived exertion. *Can. J. Sport Sci.* **1989**, *14*, 99–102.
94. Vanderthommen, M.; Makrof, S.; Demoulin, C. Comparison of active and electrostimulated recovery strategies after fatiguing exercise. *J. Sports Sci. Med.* **2010**, *9*, 164–169.
95. Gupta, S.; Goswami, A.; Sadhukhan, A.K.; Mathur, D.N. Comparative study of lactate removal in short term massage of extremities, active recovery and a passive recovery period after supramaximal exercise sessions. *Int. J. Sports Med.* **1996**, *17*, 106–110. [CrossRef] [PubMed]
96. Bangsbo, J.; Graham, T.; Johansen, L.; Saltin, B. Muscle lactate metabolism in recovery from intense exhaustive exercise: Impact of light exercise. *J. Appl. Physiol. (1985)* **1994**, *77*, 1890–1895. [CrossRef] [PubMed]
97. Xie, Y.; Feng, B.; Chen, K.; Andersen, L.L.; Page, P.; Wang, Y. The Efficacy of Dynamic Contract-Relax Stretching on Delayed-Onset Muscle Soreness Among Healthy Individuals: A Randomized Clinical Trial. *Clin. J. Sport Med.* **2018**, *28*, 28–36. [CrossRef] [PubMed]
98. Torres, R.; Ribeiro, F.; Alberto Duarte, J.; Cabri, J.M. Evidence of the physiotherapeutic interventions used currently after exercise-induced muscle damage: Systematic review and meta-analysis. *Phys. Ther. Sport* **2012**, *13*, 101–114. [CrossRef]
99. Macdonald, G.Z.; Button, D.C.; Drinkwater, E.J.; Behm, D.G. Foam rolling as a recovery tool after an intense bout of physical activity. *Med. Sci. Sports Exerc.* **2014**, *46*, 131–142. [CrossRef] [PubMed]
100. Jay, K.; Sundstrup, E.; Sondergaard, S.D.; Behm, D.; Brandt, M.; Saervoll, C.A.; Jakobsen, M.D.; Andersen, L.L. Specific and cross over effects of massage for muscle soreness: Randomized controlled trial. *Int. J. Sports Phys. Ther.* **2014**, *9*, 82–91.
101. Fleckenstein, J.; Wilke, J.; Vogt, L.; Banzer, W. Preventive and Regenerative Foam Rolling are Equally Effective in Reducing Fatigue-Related Impairments of Muscle Function following Exercise. *J. Sports Sci. Med.* **2017**, *16*, 474–479. [PubMed]
102. Kalen, A.; Perez-Ferreiros, A.; Barcala-Furelos, R.; Fernandez-Mendez, M.; Padron-Cabo, A.; Prieto, J.A.; Rios-Ave, A.; Abelairas-Gomez, C. How can lifeguards recover better? A cross-over study comparing resting, running, and foam rolling. *Am. J. Emerg. Med.* **2017**, *35*, 1887–1891. [CrossRef] [PubMed]
103. Freiwald, J.; Baumgart, C.; Kühnemann, M.; Hoppe, M.W. Foam-Rolling in sport and therapy–Potential benefits and risks. *Sports Orthop. Traumatol.* **2016**, *32*, 258–266. [CrossRef]
104. Freiwald, J.; Baumgart, C.; Kühnemann, M.; Hoppe, M.W. Foam-Rolling in sport and therapy – Potential benefits and risks. *Sports Orthopaedics and Traumatology* **2016**, *32*, 267–275. [CrossRef]

105. Doering, T.M.; Reaburn, P.R.; Phillips, S.M.; Jenkins, D.G. Postexercise Dietary Protein Strategies to Maximize Skeletal Muscle Repair and Remodeling in Masters Endurance Athletes: A Review. *Int. J. Sport Nutr. Exerc. Metab.* **2016**, *26*, 168–178. [CrossRef] [PubMed]
106. Harper, A.E.; Miller, R.H.; Block, K.P. Branched-chain amino acid metabolism. *Annu. Rev. Nutr.* **1984**, *4*, 409–454. [CrossRef] [PubMed]
107. Foure, A.; Bendahan, D. Is Branched-Chain Amino Acids Supplementation an Efficient Nutritional Strategy to Alleviate Skeletal Muscle Damage? A Systematic Review. *Nutrients* **2017**, *9*, 1047. [CrossRef]
108. Salinas-Garcia, M.E.; Martinez-Sanz, J.M.; Urdampilleta, A.; Mielgo-Ayuso, J.; Norte Navarro, A.; Ortiz-Moncada, R. Effects of branched amino acids in endurance sports: A review. *Nutr. Hosp.* **2014**, *31*, 577–589. [CrossRef] [PubMed]
109. Hurley, C.F.; Hatfield, D.L.; Riebe, D.A. The effect of caffeine ingestion on delayed onset muscle soreness. *J. Strength Cond. Res.* **2013**, *27*, 3101–3109. [CrossRef]
110. Jouris, K.B.; McDaniel, J.L.; Weiss, E.P. The Effect of Omega-3 Fatty Acid Supplementation on the Inflammatory Response to eccentric strength exercise. *J. Sports Sci. Med.* **2011**, *10*, 432–438.
111. Su, Q.S.; Tian, Y.; Zhang, J.G.; Zhang, H. Effects of allicin supplementation on plasma markers of exercise-induced muscle damage, IL-6 and antioxidant capacity. *Eur. J. Appl. Physiol.* **2008**, *103*, 275–283. [CrossRef]

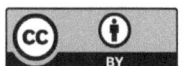

© 2019 by the authors. Licensee MDPI, Basel, Switzerland. This article is an open access article distributed under the terms and conditions of the Creative Commons Attribution (CC BY) license (http://creativecommons.org/licenses/by/4.0/).

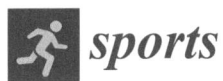

Review

Training and Competition Readiness in Triathlon

Naroa Etxebarria [1,*], Iñigo Mujika [2,3] and David Bruce Pyne [1]

1   Research Institute for Sport & Exercise, University of Canberra, Bruce ACT 2601, Australia; david.pyne@canberra.edu.au
2   Department of Physiology, Faculty of Medicine and Nursing, University of the Basque Country, Leioa 48940, Basque Country, Spain; inigo.mujika@inigomujika.com
3   Exercise Science Laboratory, School of Kinesiology, Faculty of Medicine, Universidad Finis Terrae, Santiago 7501015, Chile
*   Correspondence: naroa.etxebarria@canberra.edu.au; Tel.: +61-26201-6325

Received: 12 March 2019; Accepted: 25 April 2019; Published: 29 April 2019

Abstract: Triathlon is characterized by the multidisciplinary nature of the sport where swimming, cycling, and running are completed sequentially in different events, such as the sprint, Olympic, long-distance, and Ironman formats. The large number of training sessions and overall volume undertaken by triathletes to improve fitness and performance can also increase the risk of injury, illness, or excessive fatigue. Short- and medium-term individualized training plans, periodization strategies, and work/rest balance are necessary to minimize interruptions to training due to injury, illness, or maladaptation. Even in the absence of health and wellbeing concerns, it is unclear whether cellular signals triggered by multiple training stimuli that drive training adaptations each day interfere with each other. Distribution of training intensity within and between different sessions is an important aspect of training. Both internal (perceived stress) and external loads (objective metrics) should be considered when monitoring training load. Incorporating strength training to complement the large body of endurance work in triathlon can help avoid overuse injuries. We explore emerging trends and strategies from the latest literature and evidence-based knowledge for improving training readiness and performance during competition in triathlon.

Keywords: health; periodization; intensity; concurrent training; fatigue; quantification; monitoring; nutrition

1. Introduction

Triathlon is characterized by the multidisciplinary nature of the sport where swimming, cycling, and running are completed sequentially within the same event. The sport has a wide array of event formats, ranging from the mixed relay race (about 20 min), to the sprint distance race, lasting about 1 h, and the long-distance triathlon (Ironman), raced over an 8–9 h period at the elite level. In addition to the high training volumes typically undertaken for endurance sports, training for three different sporting disciplines simultaneously requires thoughtful planning of a large number of training sessions every week [1,2]. Large volumes of training can increase the incidence of illness and injuries, however, recent advances in knowledge in this area can minimize this risk while maximizing performance. This review examines the physiological (and biochemical) challenges of simultaneous multidisciplinary training and health risks associated with triathlon, individualized periodization and training strategies, and emerging trends in triathlon preparation.

The various formats and distances of triathlon racing all have their own discrete demands for different competition schemes. For example, in the main Olympic distance triathlon competition, a high level of sustained performance throughout the season is required, as the World Triathlon Series (eight events in 2019) reward the most consistent high-performing athlete with a World Champion title.

In contrast, the long-distance events, particularly the Ironman, demand a single stellar performance on the day, given the very small number of races a triathlete usually undertakes in a year and the grueling physical demands of the lengthy race. Finally, there is the newest addition to the Tokyo 2020 Olympics program, the mixed relay race where two male and two female athletes complete a super-sprint triathlon—300 m swim, 6.6 km bike, and 1 km run—before tagging off to a teammate. A rather short and intense performance display for a so-called endurance athlete. The intricacy of triathlon goes beyond the multidisciplinary nature of the sport, and expands to athlete physical and mental health, training monitoring, nutritional strategies, and many other aspects. Careful integration of existing and emerging factors contributing to performance outcomes (Table 1) should promote adaptation to training, reduce the risk of injury and illness, and optimize training and competition readiness.

Triathletes sustain high training loads with various combinations of intensity and volume of training, represented by power output measured in watts, during cycling, for example (external load), and the associated perceptual measures and physiological responses (internal load), such as rating of perceived exertion (RPE) and heart rate (HR), blood lactate, and oxygen consumption. The uncoupling of internal and external loads is used to assess the fatigue status of an athlete [3]. For example, using the cycling external load mentioned above, the power output may be maintained for the same duration; however, depending on the fatigue state of the athlete, this may be achieved with a high or low heart rate or a high or low perception of effort [3].

The dissociation between an HR response (internal load) to a known low exercise intensity, such as 150 W in cycling (external load), whereby the HR response is elevated in response to the relatively low absolute intensity (external load), might reveal a marked state of fatigue in an athlete. To achieve optimal training progression leading to best race performance, various training-load monitoring tools have been developed to assist athletes and coaches in evaluating the readiness to perform, risk of illness and/or injury, and readiness to return to play from injury [4,5]. These athlete/training monitoring tools can highlight apparent disparities between internal and external loads and help the coach identify any looming problems before they materialize or are substantially aggravated.

In triathlon, as is common in most other sports, experience, anecdotal reports, and scientific facts are integrated to make informed decisions on training prescription. However, translation of research outcomes into individual training plans can be challenging as each athlete is different and can respond to training stimuli in different ways [6]. Work-to-rest ratios, injury and illness episodes, and magnitude of adaptations to training stimuli will all influence the coach's decisions on individualized preparation for training and competition. Often, the best source for key information about optimizing training for athletes will come from the feedback provided by the athletes themselves [7]. Systematic athlete monitoring, anecdotal experience, and evidence-based knowledge will inform the coach to craft an integrated training plan individualized for each athlete.

1.1. Health First, Performance Follows

The primary aim of training is to prepare the triathlete for high-level competition. The journey to achieving this goal, however, will be different for most athletes. Individual requirements of frequency, volume, and intensity of training are different for each athlete, and an imbalance between training-induced fatigue and recovery can manifest in various ways. Some athletes suffer from excessive fatigue or overtraining, while others might succumb to injury or illness. During intensive training periods, carefully constructed individualized training plans should promote improvements in fitness capacities and performance, while avoiding setbacks. These setbacks are often caused by health-related issues (injuries) that follow sudden or abrupt increases or reductions in training loads [5]. Consistency in training is an important factor in optimizing the preparation process for competition, and an increased number of modified training weeks (due to illness or injury) can substantially reduce the chances of sporting success [8]. Adopting an integrated approach based on effective communication with a close relationship between the clinician (case manager) and the coach is a key for success [9].

Athlete training and athlete monitoring programs work in combination and typically incorporate training loads, health and well-being, physiological, dietary, and recovery strategies. A healthy immune system and a robust anatomical structure to avoid illness and injury are the foundations that support athletic training and competitive performance [8,10]. Most high-performing athletes will experience one or more significant health issues (or a sequence of them) that slow their progress in training at some point during a competitive season. The incidence of an injury per 1000 h of training has been reported as 0.7–1.4 during training and 9–19 during competition, most of which (50%) seems to derive from running, 43% from cycling, but only 7% with swimming [11]. Problems can take many forms from an acute injury, a more chronic condition that reaches breakpoint, or a temporary illness caused by sub-optimal nutritional intake, a long-haul travel-related episode, or the usual common cold. The long-distance triathlon requires a high intake of nutrients, especially carbohydrates, that can cause issues in the gastrointestinal tract [12,13]. Educating athletes and support staff for best practice in management of illness and preventative measures [14] is a major part of effective athlete health management (Table 1).

Table 1. General guidelines for illness prevention in athletes; adapted from Schwellnus et al. [14].

	Behavioral, Lifestyle, and Medical Strategies
Athletes are Advised to:	<ul><li>Minimize contact with infected people, young children, and animals;</li><li>Avoid crowds and minimize contact with people outside the team/support staff;</li><li>Keep at a distance to people who are coughing, sneezing, or have a "runny nose";</li><li>Wash hands regularly and effectively with soap and water, especially before meals;</li><li>Carry insect repellent, antimicrobial foam/cream, or alcohol-based hand washing gel;</li><li>Not share drinking bottles, cups, cutlery, towels, etc., with other people;</li><li>Choose beverages from sealed bottles, and avoid raw vegetables and undercooked meat;</li><li>Wear open footwear when using public showers and swimming pools;</li><li>Adopt strategies to facilitate good quality sleep at night and nap during the day.</li></ul>
Support Staff are Advised to:	<ul><li>Develop, implement, and monitor illness prevention guidelines for athletes and support staff; screening for airway inflammation disturbances (e.g., asthma, allergy);</li><li>Identify high-risk athletes to take precautions during training/competition;</li><li>Arrange for single-room accommodation during competition;</li><li>Update athletes' vaccines needed at home and for international travel.</li></ul>
	Training and Competition Load Management
Poor load management with ensuing maladaptation can be a risk factor for acute illness and overtraining. Changes in training load should be individualized in small increments <10%. General recommendations are:	<ul><li>Detailed training/competition plan, including post-event recovery strategies;</li><li>Training load monitoring, using measurements of external and internal load;</li><li>Adequate nutrition, hydration, sleep, relaxation strategies, and emotional support.</li></ul>
	Psychological Load Management
Psychological load (stressors) such as negative life event stress and daily hassles can increase the risk of illness in athletes. Clinical practical recommendations center on reducing state-level stressors and educating athletes, coaches, and support staff in proactive stress management:	<ul><li>Develop resilience strategies that help athletes manage negative life events, thoughts, emotions, and physiological states;</li><li>Education for stress management techniques, confidence building, and goal setting;</li><li>Reduce training/competition loads after negative life events to mitigate risk of illness;</li><li>Implement periodical stress assessments.</li></ul>

Table 1. *Cont.*

Measuring and Monitoring for Early Signs and Symptoms of Illness Over-Reaching and Overtraining	
An athlete's innate tendency is to continue to train and compete despite physical complaints or functional limitations. It is recommended that:	• Ongoing illness (and injury) surveillance systems should be implemented; • Athletes be monitored for subclinical signs of illness, such as non-specific symptoms; • Athletes be monitored for early symptoms and signs of over-reaching or overtraining.

1.2. Multidisciplinary Training—Interfering or Additive?

A challenge for many endurance sports including triathlon is understanding how the cellular level signaling responds to multiple modes of training. For example, skeletal muscle from endurance- and strength-trained individuals have diverse adaptive states, and simultaneous training for both endurance and strength results in a compromised adaptation, compared with training for either exercise modality alone [15], a phenomenon called the "interference effect" [16,17]. It is unclear how much interference occurs when simultaneously training for the three disciplines of swimming, cycling, and running. On the other hand, when multiple training stimuli are aligned in terms of timing, recovery, and balance between intensity and volume, the additive effects can yield central and certain peripheral physiological adaptations. This occurs when adaptations from different exercise modes are transferred a response, referred to as cross-training [18,19]. Despite limited evidence, a triathlete's running ability can improve from cycling-induced aerobic central adaptations and vice versa [20]. Maximizing the return from each training session by amplifying the biochemical pathways during training and recovery is a goal in any sport. This is especially the case in triathlon, where athletes deal with multiple disciplines that necessitate high to very high training loads. More research is required to fully understand the conjoined/simultaneous metabolic processes triggered by frequent training stimuli of varied duration, intensity, and exercising modes.

As sporting performances continue to improve, new strategies to maximize performance emerge, giving triathletes an edge in training and competition. In search of maximizing the training stimuli and consequent desired adaptations, the triathlete runs the risk of maladaptation. To avoid initiating metabolic pathways that might be detrimental to training progress, some basic understanding of metabolic signaling events is needed. Intra- and inter-individual variability in sports performance is largely due to metabolic flexibility and adaptation plasticity that underpin individual responses to training. Metabolic flexibility relies on the configuration of metabolic pathways that manage nutrient sensing, uptake, transport, storage, and utilization. This metabolic organization is mediated by synthesis, degradation, or activity regulation of key proteins or enzymes [21]. Metabolic flexibility underpins adaptation plasticity, accounting for substantial differences in the degree of adaptation or performance ability between individuals in response to the same training program. Adaptation plasticity is specific to the mode of exercise, timing, and individual responsiveness to different types of contractile activity [6]. However, peak induction for both metabolic and myogenic (muscle tissue) genes responsible for adaptation, generally occurs 4–8 h after an exercise bout. The mRNA (biologic messenger that translates exercise stimuli into anatomical, biochemical, and physiological adaptations) returns to pre-exercise levels within 24 h [22]. Triathletes undertake multiple training sessions a day, yielding a continuous overlay of molecular pathways in each 24 h window. Endurance training adaptations are dependent on the mode of exercise, the volume, intensity, and frequency of the contractile stimuli [23]. However, biological evidence to inform real world questions regarding volume, intensity, and timing of training stimuli for athletes is scarce. More understanding of these intracellular signaling cascades is needed to inform timing and sequence of training sessions for triathletes.

2. Training Periodization

The most important goal for coaches and triathletes is to maximize the competitiveness of the athletes, and design a well-controlled training program to ensure that peak performances are aligned with major triathlon competitions. Traditional training periodization, with its usual division of the training season into hierarchical preparatory, competitive, and transition periods, and structural components called macrocycles, mesocycles, and microcycles [24], provides coaches and athletes with basic guidelines for structuring and planning their training. In triathlon, top performances are often associated with periods of intensive training, followed by a taper, which involves a marked reduction in the training load for a few days before a major competition [25]. A taper intends to minimize a triathlete's habitual stressors, allowing physiological systems to undergo supercompensation [26]. An overload training period immediately preceding a taper may elicit larger subsequent performance gains in highly trained triathletes, but not in the presence of excessive fatigue, which increases the risk of training maladaptation and infection [27].

Although traditional periodization may be a perfectly valid strategy for long-distance triathletes targeting two or three major races in a season, a major limitation of this approach is its inability to elicit multiple peaks for repeated racing over the competitive season [28]. Elite triathletes competing in Olympic distance events have fewer opportunities to taper because repeated consistent top-level race performance is a key feature of the sport's competitive structure. Peaking strategies for multiple races will depend on the triathlete's level of fatigue after a race, or series of races, and the time frame between triathlons [25]. Block periodization, characterized by the sequencing of highly specialized accumulation, transmutation, and realization mesocycle blocks, could be a suitable alternative to traditional periodization for attaining multiple fitness and performance peaks throughout a competitive season [28]. The biological underpinnings of block-periodized endurance training have been reviewed recently [29].

Whatever the periodization approach, training prescription should be aligned with contemporary elite practice and evidence-based conceptual models, together with previous experiences, observations, and data, allowing contextualized decisions and effective management of the training process [30]. In this respect, multiple periodized approaches can be used at various points of an athlete's career or even within the same training season [31]. A flexible periodization strategy may also allow an Olympic distance triathlete to maintain high fitness throughout the season, which is often necessary to ensure high world and/or Olympic rankings. In this context, a world-class female triathlete was able to maintain a relatively high competitive level throughout an entire Olympic season (seventh place in the Triathlon World Ranking for 2012), and multiple fitness and performance peaks were achieved by means of planned training tapers in the lead-up to key international events [2].

A recent development in the topic of periodization is the concept of integrated periodization, which coordinates multiple training components best suited for a given training phase in an athlete's program. This concept could well represent a step towards best practice in triathlon training. The available evidence underpinning integrated periodization was recently reviewed, focusing on exercise training, recovery, nutrition, psychological skills, and skill acquisition as key factors by which athletic preparation can be optimized [32].

2.1. Training Intensity Distribution

The majority of competitive endurance events are performed at intensities close to an athlete's individual lactate threshold. However, observational studies on the training intensity distribution in various endurance sports, including swimming [33], cycling [34], running [35,36], and triathlon [2,31,37], show a strong focus on training at low-to-moderate intensities below the lactate threshold, with most of the remaining training time targeting high-intensity training at near-maximal and supramaximal intensities. This format of polarized training intensity distribution [38] is considered best practice to maximize adaptation at acceptable levels of physiological stress [39,40]. Well-trained endurance athletes show improvements in key variables related to endurance performance by manipulating training towards a polarized intensity distribution [41–44]. For example, a world-class female Olympic distance triathlete performed 74%, 88%, and 85% of her swim, bike, and run training, respectively, at intensities below her individual lactate threshold over an entire season [2]. Even higher percentages (82%, 91%, 88%) were reported in a world-champion long-distance paratriathlete [31]. In addition, faster Ironman performances are associated with longer training times at low-to-moderate intensities [37].

These somewhat paradoxical polarized training models may be explained by the greater effectiveness of both light and very intense exercise on aerobic phenotypic adaptations, linked to activation of intracellular signaling cascades. Upstream modulators of peroxisome proliferator-activated receptor-c coactivator (PGC) 1α expression influence mitochondrial biogenesis, oxidative phosphorylation, and other features of oxidative muscle fibers in skeletal muscle [45]. It has also been speculated that modern humans are physiologically better adapted to training modes similar to the exercise patterns that their hominid ancestors evolved on, which were mainly characterized by the prevalence of daily bouts of prolonged, low-intensity, aerobic-based activities, interspersed with periodic, short-duration, high-intensity bursts of activity [46].

2.2. Strength Training for Triathlon Performance

A well-planned and periodized strength training program should complement triathlon training throughout a season, allowing proper long-term athlete development, limiting the risk of injury, and eventually maximizing competition performance. Indeed, most elite triathletes nowadays combine their long, mostly aerobic swim, bike, and run training sessions with some form of strength training (i.e., concurrent training). Given the wide range in duration of the various triathlon events (e.g., ~approximately 20 min for an elite athlete racing in the mixed relay vs. approximately 8 to 9 h for elite male and female Ironman athletes, respectively), and the selective contribution to performance of upper- and lower-body muscle groups, both aerobic endurance and muscle strength are important to enhance competitive triathlon performance.

A recent meta-analysis highlighted the benefits and supported the implementation of strength training to complement the sport-specific aerobic training in middle- and long-distance events, irrespective of sport and level of athlete [47]. During the swim leg of a triathlon race, for instance, upper-body muscular strength and power should translate into increased ability to generate propulsive force in the water, improved stroke length and/or stroke rate, and increased free swimming speed [48]. Therefore, both dry-land and in-water strength training can be beneficial to performance during a triathlon swim [49]. Lower-body strength and power training can improve cycling ability and time trial performance [50,51] by reducing oxygen uptake, HR, blood lactate concentration, and RPE during prolonged cycling [52], and by eliciting an earlier peak torque during the pedal stroke [51]. Lower-body explosive strength training [53] and plyometric training [54] can also enhance running economy and performance. Well-trained triathletes performing a heavy weight training program in combination with their usual endurance training improved their maximal aerobic velocity, running economy, and hopping power [55], and delayed the onset of fatigue during prolonged submaximal cycling [56]. The beneficial effects of strength training on cycling and running economy and performance are confirmed by recent meta-analyses [47,57–59].

Greater effects on performance are yielded as a result of periodized heavy strength programs designed for maximal force development (e.g., 2–3 sets of 4 to 10 repetition maximum), involving sport-specific muscle groups and movements, focusing on performing the concentric phase of the lifts with maximal intended velocity, via two sessions per week for 12–24 weeks [47,60]. The improved endurance performance may relate to delayed activation of less efficient type II fibers, improved neuromuscular efficiency, conversion of fast-twitch type IIX fibers into more fatigue-resistant type IIA fibers, or improved musculo-tendinous stiffness [60], with no detrimental effects on maximal oxygen uptake and other markers of aerobic endurance [47,55]. In addition, strength training is considered the most effective exercise intervention to prevent overuse injuries in sport [61].

2.3. Quantification of Training and Competition Loads

Load is defined as the sport- and non-sport-related burden (single or multiple physiological, psychological, or mechanical stressors) as stimuli that are applied to a human biological system (including subcellular elements, a single cell, tissues, one or multiple organ systems, or the individual) [62]. Load can be applied to an athlete over varying time periods (seconds, minutes, and hours to days, weeks, months, and years) and magnitudes (i.e., duration, frequency, and intensity) [62]. Accurate and reliable quantification of the training load undertaken by an athlete is necessary to analyze and establish causal relationships between the training performed and the resultant physiological and performance adaptations [63–65]. Whatever the quantification methods used, they can be defined as quantifying either external or internal training load [3,66]. The external training load, which is measured independently of the internal workload [66], is an objective measure of the work that an athlete completes during either training or competition (e.g., hours of training, distance run, power output produced). However, other external factors, such as life events, daily hassles, or travel, may be equally meaningful [62].

In contrast the internal workload assesses the biological and psychological stress imposed by the training session, and is defined by disturbance(s) in homeostasis of the physiological and metabolic processes during the exercise training session [66]. Specific examples include measures such as HR (physiological/objective), RPE, or inventories for psychosocial stressors (psychological/subjective) [62] A recent study on the relationships between various training load measures in professional cycling showed that load measures based on RPE, HR, and power output are all reliable for quantifying training load in training and racing, and concluded that any method of training load quantification, which is consistently applied and discussed between coach and athlete may be equivalent in net value [67]. Several reports are available that summarize the most relevant workload quantification methods in long-duration cyclic sports [62,63,68]. Practical examples of their applications have been provided to adjust the training programs of elite athletes in accordance to their individualized stress/recovery balance [65]. It is noteworthy that a triathlon-specific load quantification method is available, which combines objective and subjective load coefficients and discipline-specific (i.e., swim, bike, run) weighting factors, but this method requires further scientific validation [69].

2.4. Monitoring Fatigue and Adaptation

Elite athletic preparation requires a fine balance between pushing the training and adaptation boundaries for performance, and avoiding negative outcomes, such as underperformance, injury, illness, or poor well-being [3,70]. Inappropriate loading may lead to excessive accumulated fatigue and maladaptive processes and increase injury risk by impairing factors, such as decision-making ability, coordination, and neuromuscular control. Excessive fatigue can contribute to increased risk of acute and overuse injuries [62]. The measurement and monitoring of fatigue and recovery in training and competition is a complex task requiring expertise in physiology, psychology, and sport science [71].

Elite triathletes' training loads can be extremely demanding, e.g., an average of 16 weekly sessions, with only 21 days of full rest over a 50-week Olympic season [2]. No single marker of an athlete's response to load consistently predicts maladaptation or injury [63], and a combination of external and internal load markers, subjective and objective measures is generally considered best practice. For instance, multiple biomarkers reflecting an athlete's positive adaptation or maladaptation to periods of intensive training demonstrate inconsistent findings, due in part to large inter-individual variability [72]. A systematic review of objective and subjective measures of athlete well-being to guide training and detect any progression toward negative health outcomes, and associated poor sports performance, indicated that athletes should report their subjective well-being on a regular basis (ideally daily), alongside other monitoring practices [68]. A multivariate approach, including physiological, biomechanical, cognitive, and perceptive monitoring, has been recommended to prevent maladaptation in highly trained triathletes [73]. Similarly, a recent study on the monitoring of professional road cyclists and elite swimmers during training camps provided further support for a multi-faceted approach to monitoring fatigue, recovery, and adaptation [70]. Furthermore, focusing on individual rather than group responses [72] and/or comparing individual to group day-to-day change in monitored variables may prove effective in flagging athletes potentially at risk of maladaptation [70].

3. Emerging Trends in Triathlete Preparation

Similar to other sports in the professional era, the competition structures, approaches to training, and support services in triathlon continue to evolve. While some national programs and professionally supported triathletes benefit from a well-resourced training and competition support program, most clubs and individual triathletes must take responsibility for managing their own preparations. While many evidence-based preparation strategies and practices are well established, new approaches continue to emerge as nations, programs, and individual coaches and athletes continually seek a competitive edge. Here, we highlight emerging trends in triathlon (and high-performance sports) that directly or indirectly influence training and competitive performance (see Table 2).

Table 2. Emerging new concepts in endurance training and triathlon to minimise fatigue, illness, and injury.

Factor	Traditional View	Emerging Trends
Psychological	• Acute events focus • Discipline seen as clinical • Minimal athlete education • No mental health priority	• Integrated model • Psychological skills training • Mental health
Training	• More is better philosophy • Rudimentary training monitoring	• Event formats dictating preparation • Load is not linear • Sophisticated training monitoring • Integrated periodization approach
Nutrition	• Macro- and micronutrient intake are important • Female Athlete Triad (low energy availability, menstrual dysfunction, and low bone mineral density)	• Timing on intake in relation to training and competition (i.e., periodized sports nutrition) • Relative energy deficiency (REDs) • New drink formulations and event-specific ingestion
Clinical/medical	• Healthcare provider-centered system • Treatment focus • Paper records	• Athlete-centered system • Prevention focus • Personalized medicine • Digital focus
Lifestyle factors, including hygiene, travel, sleep	• Competition focus • Training load focus • Treatment/management focus • Team responsibility	• Prevention or prophylactic focus • Self-responsibility • Travel management emphasized • Sleep management focus • More nuanced scheduling
Coordination	• Policy • Position statements • Guidelines	• Translation into practice • Implementation
Research	• Limited triathlon studies • Discipline-specific • Scientist-driven	• Triathlon-specific • Multi-disciplinary teams • Coach athlete involvement more clearly defined • Increasing technological involvement • More sophisticated data analyses

3.1. Psychological Factors

The traditional approach has in part focused on performance psychology to assist the athlete in their sporting pursuits. The psychologist has traditionally been more clinically oriented with only the occasional foray into the competition and training domains. Athletes often only sought assistance from a sports psychologist after some issue presented itself that caused problems at a personal or group level. In more recent times, psychology has broadened substantially to address a wide range of settings and issues. Mental toughness is often seen as an important factor and it appears that triathletes get stronger in this regard as they mature and obtain more race experience [74]. Another promising area is how athletes cope with mental fatigue arising from high level training and competition, and/or in combination with other lifestyle stresses [75]. Future work in mental fatigue will identify strategies for improving the ability of athletes to meet both the acute and chronic mental demands of high-volume training. Until recently, mental health issues were largely dealt with individually (in a private setting) and rarely in a team or public domain. Psychological skills training is increasingly undertaken proactively by athletes, while mental health issues are being dealt with in more confidence [76] and, in some high profile cases, chronicled in the public domain. It should be emphasized that sports and physical activity can be a positive factor in health-related quality of life in college-age individuals [77], so it is a matter of balancing the positive and negative factors of high level involvement in triathlon.

3.2. Training

Although the demands of training and competition are well understood, there are still coaches and athletes wedded to the more-is-better training philosophy. Progressions in training load should be periodized rather than strictly linear in nature, whatever the race distance. A range of external training load factors and baseline characteristics have been associated with an increased rate of injury and/or pain in endurance sports [78]. In contrast, more work is needed on effective markers of internal training loads. Somewhat contrary to common perception, the relationships between training volume and injury are more complex than a simple linear relationship between risk factors and occurrence of common injuries [79]. Work is now progressing on more uniform definitions and terms, better measures of internal and external training loads, and more sophisticated data analytics to improve the understanding of relationships between training and injury/illness risk. This information is needed to update current knowledge and prepare practical guidelines for the triathlon community.

3.3. Nutrition

Traditionally the focus of athlete nutrition has been on absolute and relative macro- and micro-nutrient intake. Triathlon has focused on carbohydrate intake, given its importance in fueling endurance training and competition formats, such as the Olympic distance and Ironman events. More recent work has highlighted the importance of timing of nutrient intake in relation to training and competition. New strategies are being promoted, such as "sleep low", which involves a sequential periodization of carbohydrate (CHO) availability and low glycogen recovery after "train high" glycogen-depleting interval training, followed by an overnight-fast and light intensity training ("train low") the following morning. [80]. In contrast, chronic ketogenic low-CHO high-fat diets might impair iron metabolism, aspects of immune function [81], performance, and well-being [82]. Further work is in progress to identify how diets can be individualized according to event demands, athlete background, training demands, and whether changes in body composition are required to improve performance.

During the 1990s and 2000s, the so-called female athlete triad was the predominant exercise model accounting for health issues in female athletes. The condition was characterized by athletes presenting with low energy availability, menstrual dysfunction, and low bone mineral density. In recent years, the relative energy deficiency (REDs) term has emerged, recognizing that low energy availability affects both female and male athletes, and a broader range of health and performance parameters, not just bone health and menstrual dysfunction [83]. Challenges around accurate clinical or laboratory measurement of energy availability, the perennial issue of body mass and composition management, and effective education strategies are currently being addressed. Further developments in this area will assist the goal of reducing the prevalence and incidence of injury and illness.

Heat stress and fluid replacement strategies are issues often faced during triathlon competition under hot and/or humid environmental conditions, particularly in the long-distance and Ironman formats. The benefits of carbohydrate content and fluid volume in sports drinks have been studied extensively and triathletes should pay particular attention to these matters [84]. However, greater reductions in body mass and higher post-competition core temperatures have been recorded in faster triathletes, indicating these competitors can push themselves harder and/or tolerate the effects of sweat loss and heat more effectively [85]. Investigators are continuing to develop innovative methods, such as ice slurry ingestion [86], new sports drink formulations, and manipulating drink content and timing before, during, and after training and competitive events, especially in the important hours after heavy exertion.

3.4. Clinical/Medical

Medical management is evolving from a healthcare and provider (medical doctor)-centered system, with a treatment focus and paper records that made consistency and retrieval of individual medical records difficult, to an athlete-centered system. New systems are evolving with an injury and illness prevention focus and personalized medicine, using the full suite of digital and technological solutions and systems. Improvements are also likely to come in the areas of improved biomedical testing (in immunological, oxidative stress-related fatigue and cardiovascular markers), improved clinician diagnoses, and field-based studies of race-related injuries and illnesses [87]. Personalized predictive medicine with a focus on genetics has arrived in clinical medicine, but will require additional metadata and biological validation to identify a comprehensive set of genes useful in sports [88]. Perception of injury and training risk factors among health professionals center primarily on training load and demographic characteristics. In one study, three common factors accounted for over 50% of the variance in injury risk in triathletes: The underlying training, health and medical monitoring, and preparation of the triathlete for competition [89]. This information points to the critical factors of training, monitoring, and competition preparations, all of which inform the upskilling of practitioners and training of the next generation of sports professionals.

3.5. Lifestyle Behaviours

Treatment and management priorities typically arise after an athlete has succumbed to fatigue, injury, or illness. In the future, however, increased attention will be given to prevention strategies, with athletes taking more self-responsibility for training, recovery, sleep, nutrition, and other factors. Sleep management or sleep hygiene is now a major focus of athlete preparation and research is driving new innovations and interventions to improve this important factor. Strategies for managing travel stress and jet lag should be implemented by triathletes embarking on long haul flights. Approaches for heat acclimation training and altitude training also continue to evolve. Hard-earned experience of athletes and coaches, and the results of research investigations, will generate more nuanced scheduling of heat and altitude training. Key themes for increasing the benefit of altitude and heat interventions include more effective preparatory training in the weeks before, implementation of more useful internal and external load measures, and nutritional strategies that maximize the adaptations needed to enhance performance at sea-level and altitude, and in temperate and hot environments [90].

3.6. Coordination

International federations, such as the International Triathlon Union (ITU), and national federations have traditionally managed competition and travel schedules; organized training, programs and tours; provided medical and scientific support both in domestic and international settings; and conducted coach–athlete education programs. This work requires substantial resourcing and policy development. The increasing professionalism, commercial funding, and sponsoring of programs, teams, and individuals has markedly changed the management and control of athlete programs and competition preparations. While this work in the organizational and management areas will continue, there is increasing need for clearer and more effective translation of expert knowledge (including coaches, triathletes, and support staff) and implementation of technology, research outcomes, and other improvements and innovations into national programs, clubs, competitions, and everyday training. Translation and innovation will require cooperation and communication between governing bodies, athlete and coaching groups, research entities, and across national borders.

3.7. Research

Despite the popularity of triathlon, the sport has received much less attention from industry and academic researchers than cycling, running, and swimming. Coaches and scientists in triathlon have to translate the outcomes from other sports to improve the management and performance of triathletes [91,92]. In the future, more triathlon-specific research will be conducted to promote best practice in the sport in junior, senior, and elite competitors. Triathletes and coaches will be more involved in research, rather than projects being driven largely by scientists and/or academic researchers. Like other sports, the focus of research is evolving from specific disciplines (for example, psychology, performance analysis, physiology, nutrition, medical and allied health) driven by scientists to multi-disciplinary research, fully integrating the coach and athlete. There will be more focus on technological innovation and sophisticated data analytics of training management and race performances.

Author Contributions: Conceptualization, N.E., I.M. and D.B.P.; methodology, N.E., I.M. and D.B.P.; investigation, N.E., I.M. and D.B.P.; resources, N.E., I.M. and D.B.P.; writing—original draft preparation, N.E., I.M. and D.B.P.; writing—review and editing, N.E., I.M. and D.B.P.; project administration, N.E.

Funding: This research received no external funding.

Acknowledgments: Iñigo Mujika was a recipient of a University of Canberra Distinguished International Visitor Award during the preparation of this manuscript.

Conflicts of Interest: The authors declare no conflict of interest.

References

1. Millet, G.P.; Vleck, V.E.; Bentley, D.J. Physiological requirements in triathlon. *J. Hum. Sport Exerc.* **2011**, *6*, 184–204. [CrossRef]
2. Mujika, I. Olympic preparation of a world-class female triathlete. *Int. J. Sports Physiol. Perform.* **2014**, *9*, 727–731. [CrossRef]
3. Halson, S.L. Monitoring training load to understand fatigue in athletes. *Sports Med.* **2014**, *44* (Suppl. 2), S139–S147. [CrossRef] [PubMed]
4. Gabbett, T.J.; Hulin, B.T.; Blanch, P.; Whiteley, R. High training workloads alone do not cause sports injuries: How you get there is the real issue. *Br. J. Sports Med.* **2016**, *50*, 444–445. [CrossRef] [PubMed]
5. Hulin, B.T.; Gabbett, T.J.; Lawson, D.W.; Caputi, P.; Sampson, J.A. The acute:chronic workload ratio predicts injury: High chronic workload may decrease injury risk in elite rugby league players. *Br. J. Sports Med.* **2016**, *50*, 231–236. [CrossRef]
6. Bouchard, C.; Rankinen, T.; Timmons, J.A. Genomics and genetics in the biology of adaptation to exercise. *Compr. Physiol.* **2011**, *1*, 1603–1648.
7. Coyne, J.O.C.; Gregory Haff, G.; Coutts, A.J.; Newton, R.U.; Nimphius, S. The current state of subjective training load monitoring-a practical perspective and call to action. *Sports Med. Open* **2018**, *4*, 58. [CrossRef]
8. Raysmith, B.P.; Drew, M.K. Performance success or failure is influenced by weeks lost to injury and illness in elite australian track and field athletes: A 5-year prospective study. *J. Sci. Med. Sport* **2016**, *19*, 778–783. [CrossRef]

9. Dijkstra, H.P.; Pollock, N.; Chakraverty, R.; Alonso, J.M. Managing the health of the elite athlete: A new integrated performance health management and coaching model. *Br. J. Sports Med.* **2014**, *48*, 523–531. [CrossRef] [PubMed]
10. Drew, M.K.; Raysmith, B.P.; Charlton, P.C. Injuries impair the chance of successful performance by sportspeople: A systematic review. *Br. J. Sports Med.* **2017**, *51*, 1209–1214. [CrossRef]
11. Zwingenberger, S.; Valladares, R.D.; Walther, A.; Beck, H.; Stiehler, M.; Kirschner, S.; Engelhardt, M.; Kasten, P. An epidemiological investigation of training and injury patterns in triathletes. *J. Sports Sci.* **2014**, *32*, 583–590. [CrossRef]
12. Jeukendrup, A.E.; Jentjens, R.L.; Moseley, L. Nutritional considerations in triathlon. *Sports Med.* **2005**, *35*, 163–181. [CrossRef]
13. Pfeiffer, B.; Stellingwerff, T.; Hodgson, A.B.; Randell, R.; Pottgen, K.; Jeukendrup, A.E. Nutritional intake and gastrointestinal problems during competitive endurance events. *Med. Sci. Sports Exerc.* **2012**, *44*, 344–351. [CrossRef] [PubMed]
14. Schwellnus, M.; Soligard, T.; Alonso, J.M.; Bahr, R.; Clarsen, B.; Dijkstra, H.P.; Gabbett, T.J.; Gleeson, M.; Hägglund, M.; Hutchinson, M.R.; et al. How much is too much? (part 2) international olympic committee consensus statement on load in sport and risk of illness. *Br. J. Sports Med.* **2016**, *50*, 1043–1052. [CrossRef]
15. Hickson, R.C. Interference of strength development by simultaneously training for strength and endurance. *Eur. J. Appl. Physiol. Occup. Physiol.* **1980**, *45*, 255–263. [CrossRef] [PubMed]
16. Fyfe, J.J.; Bishop, D.J.; Stepto, N.K. Interference between concurrent resistance and endurance exercise: Molecular bases and the role of individual training variables. *Sports Med.* **2014**, *44*, 743–762. [CrossRef] [PubMed]
17. Docherty, D.; Sporer, B. A proposed model for examining the interference phenomenon between concurrent aerobic and strength training. *Sports Med.* **2000**, *30*, 385–394. [CrossRef] [PubMed]
18. Tanaka, H. Effects of cross-training. Transfer of training effects on vo2max between cycling, running and swimming. *Sports Med.* **1994**, *18*, 330–339. [CrossRef]
19. Loy, S.F.; Hoffmann, J.J.; Holland, G.J. Benefits and practical use of cross-training in sports. *Sports Med.* **1995**, *19*, 1–8. [CrossRef]
20. Millet, G.P.; Candau, R.B.; Barbier, B.; Busso, T.; Rouillon, J.D.; Chatard, J.C. Modelling the transfers of training effects on performance in elite triathletes. *Int. J. Sports Med.* **2002**, *23*, 55–63. [CrossRef]
21. Vitkup, D.; Kharchenko, P.; Wagner, A. Influence of metabolic network structure and function on enzyme evolution. *Genome Biol.* **2006**, *7*, R39. [CrossRef]
22. Yang, Y.; Creer, A.; Jemiolo, B.; Trappe, S. Time course of myogenic and metabolic gene expression in response to acute exercise in human skeletal muscle. *J. Appl. Physiol. (1985)* **2005**, *98*, 1745–1752. [CrossRef] [PubMed]
23. Hawley, J.A. Adaptations of skeletal muscle to prolonged, intense endurance training. *Clin. Exp. Pharmacol. Physiol.* **2002**, *29*, 218–222. [CrossRef] [PubMed]
24. Matveyev, L.P. *Fundamentals of Sports Training*; Progress Publishers: Moscow, Russia, 1981.
25. Mujika, I. Tapering for triathlon competition. *J. Hum. Sport Exerc.* **2011**, *6*, 264–270. [CrossRef]
26. Mujika, I.; Le Meur, Y. The art and science of tapering. In *Complete Triathlon Guide*; Triathlon, U., Ed.; Human Kinetics: Champaign, IL, USA, 2012; Volume 255, pp. 131–144, 456.
27. Aubry, A.; Hausswirth, C.; Louis, J.; Coutts, A.J.; Le Meur, Y. Functional overreaching: The key to peak performance during the taper? *Med. Sci. Sports Exerc.* **2014**, *46*, 1769–1777. [CrossRef]
28. Issurin, V.B. New horizons for the methodology and physiology of training periodization. *Sports Med.* **2010**, *40*, 189–206. [CrossRef]
29. Issurin, V.B. Biological background of block periodized endurance training: A review. *Sports Med.* **2019**, *49*, 31–39. [CrossRef] [PubMed]
30. Kiely, J. Periodization paradigms in the 21st century: Evidence-led or tradition-driven? *Int. J. Sports Physiol. Perform.* **2012**, *7*, 242–250. [CrossRef] [PubMed]
31. Mujika, I.; Orbananos, J.; Salazar, H. Physiology and training of a world-champion paratriathlete. *Int. J. Sports Physiol. Perform.* **2015**, *10*, 927–930. [CrossRef] [PubMed]
32. Mujika, I.; Halson, S.; Burke, L.M.; Balague, G.; Farrow, D. An integrated, multifactorial approach to periodization for optimal performance in individual and team sports. *Int. J. Sports Physiol. Perform.* **2018**, *13*, 538–561. [CrossRef]

33. Mujika, I.; Chatard, J.C.; Busso, T.; Geyssant, A.; Barale, F.; Lacoste, L. Effects of training on performance in competitive swimming. *Can. J. Appl. Physiol.* **1995**, *20*, 395–406. [CrossRef] [PubMed]
34. Sanders, D.; Myers, T.; Akubat, I. Training-intensity distribution in road cyclists: Objective versus subjective measures. *Int. J. Sports Physiol. Perform.* **2017**, *12*, 1232–1237. [CrossRef]
35. Esteve-Lanao, J.; San Juan, A.F.; Earnest, C.P.; Foster, C.; Lucia, A. How do endurance runners actually train? Relationship with competition performance. *Med. Sci. Sports Exerc.* **2005**, *37*, 496–504. [CrossRef]
36. Stellingwerf, T. Case study: Nutrition and training periodization in three elite marathon runners. *Int. J. Sport Nutr. Exerc. Metab.* **2012**, *22*, 392–400. [CrossRef]
37. Muñoz, I.; Cejuela, R.; Seiler, S.; Larumbe, E.; Esteve-Lanao, J. Training-intensity distribution during an ironman season: Relationship with competition performance. *Int. J. Sports Physiol. Perform.* **2014**, *9*, 332–339. [CrossRef] [PubMed]
38. Seiler, K.S.; Kjerland, G.O. Quantifying training intensity distribution in elite endurance athletes: Is there evidence for an "optimal" distribution? *Scand. J. Med. Sci. Sports* **2006**, *16*, 49–56. [CrossRef]
39. Seiler, S. What is best practice for training intensity and duration distribution in endurance athletes? *Int. J. Sports Physiol. Perform.* **2010**, *5*, 276–291. [CrossRef]
40. Hydren, J.R.; Cohen, B.S. Current scientific evidence for a polarized cardiovascular endurance training model. *J. Strength Cond. Res.* **2015**, *29*, 3523–3530. [CrossRef] [PubMed]
41. Esteve-Lanao, J.; Foster, C.; Seiler, S.; Lucia, A. Impact of training intensity distribution on performance in endurance athletes. *J. Strength Cond. Res.* **2007**, *21*, 943–949. [PubMed]
42. Ingham, S.A.; Fudge, B.W.; Pringle, J.S. Training distribution, physiological profile, and performance for a male international 1500-m runner. *Int. J. Sports Physiol. Perform.* **2012**, *7*, 193–195. [CrossRef]
43. Neal, C.M.; Hunter, A.M.; Brennan, L.; O'Sullivan, A.; Hamilton, D.L.; DeVito, G.; Galloway, S.D. Six weeks of a polarized training-intensity distribution leads to greater physiological and performance adaptations than a threshold model in trained cyclists. *J. Appl. Physiol. (1985)* **2013**, *114*, 461–471. [CrossRef]
44. Stoggl, T.; Sperlich, B. Polarized training has greater impact on key endurance variables than threshold, high intensity, or high volume training. *Front. Physiol.* **2014**, *5*, 33. [CrossRef] [PubMed]
45. Laursen, P.B. Training for intense exercise performance: High-intensity or high-volume training? *Scand. J. Med. Sci. Sports* **2010**, *20* (Suppl. 2), 1–10. [CrossRef] [PubMed]
46. Boullosa, D.A.; Abreu, L.; Varela-Sanz, A.; Mujika, I. Do olympic athletes train as in the paleolithic era? *Sports Med.* **2013**, *43*, 909–917. [CrossRef] [PubMed]
47. Berryman, N.; Mujika, I.; Arvisais, D.; Roubeix, M.; Binet, C.; Bosquet, L. Strength training for middle- and long-distance performance: A meta-analysis. *Int. J. Sports Physiol. Perform.* **2018**, *13*, 57–63. [CrossRef]
48. Mujika, I.; Crowley, E. Strength training for swimmers. In *Concurrent Aerobic and Strength Training*; Schumann, M., Rønnestad, B.R., Eds.; Springer: Cham, Switzerland, 2019; pp. 369–396.
49. Crowley, E.; Harrison, A.J.; Lyons, M. The impact of resistance training on swimming performance: A systematic review. *Sports Med.* **2017**, *47*, 2285–2307. [CrossRef]
50. Aagaard, P.; Andersen, J.L.; Bennekou, M.; Larsson, B.; Olesen, J.L.; Crameri, R.; Magnusson, S.P.; Kjaer, M. Effects of resistance training on endurance capacity and muscle fiber composition in young top-level cyclists. *Scand. J. Med. Sci. Sports* **2011**, *21*, e298–e307. [CrossRef]
51. Rønnestad, B.R.; Hansen, J.; Hollan, I.; Ellefsen, S. Strength training improves performance and pedaling characteristics in elite cyclists. *Scand. J. Med. Sci. Sports* **2015**, *25*, e89–e98. [CrossRef] [PubMed]
52. Rønnestad, B.R.; Hansen, E.A.; Raastad, T. Strength training improves 5-min all-out performance following 185 min of cycling. *Scand. J. Med. Sci. Sports* **2011**, *21*, 250–259. [CrossRef]
53. Paavolainen, L.; Hakkinen, K.; Hamalainen, I.; Nummela, A.; Rusko, H. Explosive-strength training improves 5-km running time by improving running economy and muscle power. *J. Appl. Physiol. (1985)* **1999**, *86*, 1527–1533. [CrossRef]
54. Saunders, P.U.; Telford, R.D.; Pyne, D.B.; Peltola, E.M.; Cunningham, R.B.; Gore, C.J.; Hawley, J.A. Short-term plyometric training improves running economy in highly trained middle and long distance runners. *J. Strength Cond. Res.* **2006**, *20*, 947–954.
55. Millet, G.P.; Jaouen, B.; Borrani, F.; Candau, R. Effects of concurrent endurance and strength training on running economy and vo2 kinetics. *Med. Sci. Sports Exerc.* **2002**, *34*, 1351–1359. [CrossRef]

56. Hausswirth, C.; Argentin, S.; Bieuzen, F.; Le Meur, Y.; Couturier, A.; Brisswalter, J. Endurance and strength training effects on physiological and muscular parameters during prolonged cycling. *J. Electromyogr. Kinesiol.* **2010**, *20*, 330–339. [CrossRef] [PubMed]
57. Barnes, K.R.; Kilding, A.E. Strategies to improve running economy. *Sports Med.* **2015**, *45*, 37–56. [CrossRef] [PubMed]
58. Denadai, B.S.; de Aguiar, R.A.; de Lima, L.C.; Greco, C.C.; Caputo, F. Explosive training and heavy weight training are effective for improving running economy in endurance athletes: A systematic review and meta-analysis. *Sports Med.* **2017**, *47*, 545–554. [CrossRef] [PubMed]
59. Balsalobre-Fernandez, C.; Santos-Concejero, J.; Grivas, G.V. Effects of strength training on running economy in highly trained runners: A systematic review with meta-analysis of controlled trials. *J. Strength Cond. Res.* **2016**, *30*, 2361–2368. [CrossRef]
60. Rønnestad, B.R.; Mujika, I. Optimizing strength training for running and cycling endurance performance: A review. *Scand. J. Med. Sci. Sports* **2014**, *24*, 603–612. [CrossRef] [PubMed]
61. Lauersen, J.B.; Bertelsen, D.M.; Andersen, L.B. The effectiveness of exercise interventions to prevent sports injuries: A systematic review and meta-analysis of randomised controlled trials. *Br. J. Sports Med.* **2014**, *48*, 871–877. [CrossRef] [PubMed]
62. Soligard, T.; Schwellnus, M.; Alonso, J.M.; Bahr, R.; Clarsen, B.; Dijkstra, H.P.; Gabbett, T.; Gleeson, M.; Hägglund, M.; Hutchinson, M.R.; et al. How much is too much? (part 1) international olympic committee consensus statement on load in sport and risk of injury. *Br. J. Sports Med.* **2016**, *50*, 1030–1041. [CrossRef] [PubMed]
63. Borresen, J.; Lambert, M.I. The quantification of training load, the training response and the effect on performance. *Sports Med.* **2009**, *39*, 779–795. [CrossRef] [PubMed]
64. Mujika, I. The alphabet of sport science research starts with q. *Int. J. Sports Physiol. Perform.* **2013**, *8*, 465–466. [CrossRef]
65. Mujika, I. Quantification of training and competition loads in endurance sports: Methods and applications. *Int. J. Sports Physiol. Perform.* **2017**, *12* (Suppl. 2), S2-9–S2-17. [CrossRef]
66. Lambert, M.I. Quantification of endurance training and competition loads. In *Endurance Training: Science and Practice*; Mujika, I., Ed.; Iñigo Mujika S.L.U.: Vitoria-Gasteiz, Basque Country, 2012; pp. 21–28.
67. van Erp, T.; Foster, C.; de Koning, J.J. Relationship between various training load measures in elite cyclists during training, road races and time trials. *Int. J. Sports Physiol. Perform.* **2019**, *14*, 493–500. [CrossRef] [PubMed]
68. Saw, A.E.; Main, L.C.; Gastin, P.B. Monitoring the athlete training response: Subjective self-reported measures trump commonly used objective measures: A systematic review. *Br. J. Sports Med.* **2016**, *50*, 281–291. [CrossRef] [PubMed]
69. Cejuela Anta, R.; Esteve-Lanao, J. Training load quantification in triathlon. *J. Hum. Sport Exerc.* **2011**, *6*, 218–232. [CrossRef]
70. Saw, A.E.; Halson, S.L.; Mujika, I. Monitoring athletes during training camps: Observations and translatable strategies from elite road cyclists and swimmers. *Sports* **2018**, *6*, 63. [CrossRef] [PubMed]
71. Kellmann, M.; Bertollo, M.; Bosquet, L.; Brink, M.; Coutts, A.J.; Duffield, R.; Erlacher, D.; Halson, S.L.; Hecksteden, A.; Heidari, J.; et al. Recovery and performance in sport: Consensus statement. *Int. J. Sports Physiol. Perform.* **2018**, *13*, 240–245. [CrossRef]
72. Greenham, G.; Buckley, J.D.; Garrett, J.; Eston, R.; Norton, K. Biomarkers of physiological responses to periods of intensified, non-resistance-based exercise training in well-trained male athletes: A systematic review and meta-analysis. *Sports Med.* **2018**, *48*, 2517–2548. [CrossRef] [PubMed]
73. Le Meur, Y.; Hausswirth, C.; Natta, F.; Couturier, A.; Bignet, F.; Vidal, P.P. A multidisciplinary approach to overreaching detection in endurance trained athletes. *J. Appl. Physiol. (1985)* **2013**, *114*, 411–420. [CrossRef]
74. Jones, M.I.; Parker, J.K. An analysis of the size and direction of the association between mental toughness and olympic distance personal best triathlon times. *J. Sport Health Sci.* **2019**, *8*, 71–76. [CrossRef] [PubMed]
75. Russell, S.; Jenkins, D.; Smith, M.; Halson, S.; Kelly, V. The application of mental fatigue research to elite team sport performance: New perspectives. *J. Sci. Med. Sport* **2018**. [CrossRef]
76. Souter, G.; Lewis, R.; Serrant, L. Men, mental health and elite sport: A narrative review. *Sports Med. Open* **2018**, *4*, 57. [CrossRef]

77. Snedden, T.R.; Scerpella, J.; Kliethermes, S.A.; Norman, R.S.; Blyholder, L.; Sanfilippo, J.; McGuine, T.A.; Heiderscheit, B. Sport and physical activity level impacts health-related quality of life among collegiate students. *Am. J. Health Promot.* **2018**. [CrossRef]
78. Johnston, R.; Cahalan, R.; O'Keeffe, M.; O'Sullivan, K.; Comyns, T. The associations between training load and baseline characteristics on musculoskeletal injury and pain in endurance sport populations: A systematic review. *J. Sci. Med. Sport* **2018**, *21*, 910–918. [CrossRef]
79. Kienstra, C.M.; Asken, T.R.; Garcia, J.D.; Lara, V.; Best, T.M. Triathlon injuries: Transitioning from prevalence to prediction and prevention. *Curr. Sports Med. Rep.* **2017**, *16*, 397–403. [CrossRef] [PubMed]
80. Marquet, L.A.; Hausswirth, C.; Molle, O.; Hawley, J.; Burke, L.; Tiollier, E.; Brisswalter, J. Periodization of carbohydrate intake: Short-term effect on performance. *Nutrients* **2016**, *8*, 755. [CrossRef] [PubMed]
81. McKay, A.K.; Peeling, P.; Pyne, D.B.; Welvaert, M.; Tee, N.; Leckey, J.J.; Sharma, A.P.; Ross, M.L.; Garvican-Lewis, L.A.; Swinkels, D.W.; et al. Chronic adherence to a ketogenic diet modifies iron metabolism in elite athletes. *Med. Sci. Sports Exerc.* **2019**, *51*, 548–555. [CrossRef]
82. Mujika, I. Case study: Long-term low-carbohydrate, high-fat diet impairs performance and subjective well-being in a world-class vegetarian long-distance triathlete. *Int. J. Sport Nutr. Exerc. Metab.* **2018**, *13*, 1–6. [CrossRef]
83. Mountjoy, M.L.; Burke, L.M.; Stellingwerff, T.; Sundgot-Borgen, J. Relative energy deficiency in sport: The tip of an iceberg. *Int. J. Sport Nutr. Exerc. Metab.* **2018**, *28*, 313–315. [CrossRef] [PubMed]
84. Burke, L.M.; Mujika, I. Nutrition for recovery in aquatic sports. *Int. J. Sport Nutr. Exerc. Metab.* **2014**, *24*, 425–436. [CrossRef]
85. Del Coso, J.; González, C.; Abian-Vicen, J.; Salinero Martín, J.J.; Soriano, L.; Areces, F.; Ruiz, D.; Gallo, C.; Lara, B.; Calleja-González, J. Relationship between physiological parameters and performance during a half-ironman triathlon in the heat. *J. Sports Sci.* **2014**, *32*, 1680–1687. [CrossRef]
86. Stevens, C.J.; Dascombe, B.; Boyko, A.; Sculley, D.; Callister, R. Ice slurry ingestion during cycling improves olympic distance triathlon performance in the heat. *J. Sports Sci.* **2013**, *31*, 1271–1279. [CrossRef]
87. Vleck, V.; Millet, G.P.; Alves, F.B. The impact of triathlon training and racing on athletes' general health. *Sports Med.* **2014**, *44*, 1659–1692. [CrossRef] [PubMed]
88. Mattsson, C.M.; Wheeler, M.T.; Waggott, D.; Caleshu, C.; Ashley, E.A. Sports genetics moving forward: Lessons learned from medical research. *Physiol. Genom.* **2016**, *48*, 175–182. [CrossRef] [PubMed]
89. Gosling, C.M.; Forbes, A.B.; Gabbe, B.J. Health professionals' perceptions of musculoskeletal injury and injury risk factors in australian triathletes: A factor analysis. *Phys. Ther. Sport* **2013**, *14*, 207–212. [CrossRef] [PubMed]
90. Saunders, P.U.; Garvican-Lewis, L.A.; Chapman, R.F.; Periard, J.D. Special environments: Altitude and heat. *Int. J. Sport Nutr. Exerc. Metab.* **2019**, 1–27. [CrossRef]
91. Pyne, D.B.; Etxebarria, N. Lost in translation: Getting your research message across. In *Sport Science: Current and Future Trends for Performance Optimization*; Morouço, P., Takagi, H., Fernandes, R.J., Eds.; ESECS/Instituto Politécnico de Leiria: Leiria, Portugal, 2018; pp. 10–23.
92. Millet, G.P.; Bentley, D.J.; Vleck, V.E. The relationships between science and sport: Application in triathlon. *Int. J. Sports Physiol. Perform.* **2007**, *2*, 315–322. [CrossRef] [PubMed]

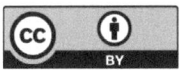

© 2019 by the authors. Licensee MDPI, Basel, Switzerland. This article is an open access article distributed under the terms and conditions of the Creative Commons Attribution (CC BY) license (http://creativecommons.org/licenses/by/4.0/).

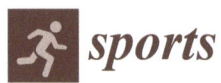

Case Report

Late-Presenting Swimming-Induced Pulmonary Edema: A Case Report Series from the Norseman Xtreme Triathlon

Jørgen Melau [1,2,3,*], Martin Bonnevie-Svendsen [2], Maria Mathiassen [4], Janne Mykland Hilde [5], Lars Oma [6] and Jonny Hisdal [1,2,7]

1. Institute of Clinical Medicine, University of Oslo, 0316 Oslo, Norway; jonny.hisdal@medisin.uio.no
2. Department of Vascular Surgery, Oslo University Hospital, 0424 Oslo, Norway; martin.bonnevie@gmail.com
3. Prehospital Division, Vestfold Hospital Trust, 3103 Toensberg, Norway
4. Department of Cardiology, Telemark Hospital Trust, 3710 Skien, Norway; maria.mathiassen@gmail.com
5. Department of Cardiology, Akershus University Hospital, 1478 Loerenskog, Norway; janne.mykland.hilde@ahus.no
6. Baerum Hospital, Vestre Viken Hospital Trust, 3004 Drammen, Norway; lars.oma@mac.com
7. Institute for Surgical Research, Oslo University Hospital, 0424 Oslo, Norway
* Correspondence: jorgen@melau.no

Received: 16 April 2019; Accepted: 31 May 2019; Published: 3 June 2019

Abstract: Swimming-induced pulmonary edema (SIPE) may develop during strenuous physical exertion in water. This case series reports on three cases of suspected late-presenting SIPE during the Norseman Xtreme Triathlon. A 30-year-old male professional (PRO) triathlete, a 40-year-old female AGE GROUP triathlete and a 34-year-old male AGE GROUP triathlete presented with shortness of breath, chest tightness and coughing up pink sputum during the last part of the bike phase. All three athletes reported an improvement in breathing during the first major uphill of the bike phase and increasing symptoms during the downhill. The PRO athlete had a thoracic computed tomography, and the scan showed bilateral ground glass opacity in the peripheral lungs. The male AGE GROUP athlete had a normal chest x-ray. Both athletes were admitted for further observation and discharged from hospital the following day, with complete regression of symptoms. The female athlete recovered quickly following pre-hospital oxygen treatment. Non-cardiogenic pulmonary edema associated with endurance sports is rare but potentially very dangerous. Knowledge and awareness of possible risk factors and symptoms are essential, and the results presented in this report emphasize the importance of being aware of the possible delayed development of symptoms. To determine the presence of pulmonary edema elicited by strenuous exercise, equipment for measuring oxygen saturation should be available for the medical staff on site.

Keywords: SIPE; endurance; triathlon; open water; swimming

1. Introduction

Swimming-induced pulmonary edema (SIPE) is a potentially dangerous complication during strenuous exercise with the possibility of accompanying misdiagnosis. Cough, dyspnea, hemoptysis and hypoxemia may develop after surface swimming or diving, often in young, healthy individuals. The condition is relatively rare, but an increasing number of cases of SIPE is being reported in triathletes [1]. Episodes are more likely to occur in highly fit individuals undertaking strenuous or competitive swims. A study of American triathletes reported an association between SIPE and hypertension [1]. Other potential risk factors included diabetes, fish oil use, long course triathlons, wearing a wetsuit and female sex [1]. SIPE usually resolves spontaneously within 24 hours, or with beta2 adrenergic agonist or diuretic therapy, but can be fatal if not treated [2,3]. Individuals who develop SIPE often have recurrences under the same conditions [4,5]. Increased awareness among health professionals and organizers, in addition to early detection of symptoms of SIPE, are therefore warranted to avoid life-threatening episodes during future extreme triathlon competitions.

Previous case reports have described cases with sudden onset of shortness of breath during swimming, and shortly after the swimming phase of a triathlon resulting in withdrawal from the race [6–9]. There are also reports of athletes completing entire triathlon events with symptoms of SIPE during the bike and run legs [10]. In this case series, we report three cases of slowly progressing pulmonary edema with resultant race withdrawal, one after 122 km and two cases after 180 km, respectively, during the Norseman Extreme Triathlon in 2016, 2017 and 2018. All three cases were diagnosed with swimming-induced pulmonary edema (SIPE) and displayed an undulating symptom behaviour not previously described in the literature. Two athletes were admitted to hospital for further examination, and one athlete did not need hospitalization.

2. Case Report

A 30-year-old male PRO triathlete, a 40-year-old female AGE GROUP athlete and a 34-year-old AGE GROUP athlete, all with no history of medical illness, who regularly competed at long distance triathlons presented with shortness of breath, chest tightness and coughing up pink sputum during the last part of the bike phase of a full distance triathlon race. Ambient air temperature varied between 6 and 8 °C and the water temperature was around 14.2 to 14.4 °C during the races in 2016 and 2017 and somewhat higher in 2018 with an air temperature of 10 °C and water temperature at 17.5 °C. The PRO male athlete had completed the same competition the previous 3 years without any medical complications. The female and the male AGE GROUP athletes entered their first Extreme triathlon, but they had both previously completed several full Ironman competitions without symptoms of SIPE. As part of another study during the same competition, normal spirometry was performed the day before the race for both the PRO athlete and the female athlete. Written informed consent for publication was obtained from all athletes.

During the swim, all athletes wore a well-fitted wetsuit and neoprene swim cap. They later reported that they felt increasingly breathless and were struggling to keep the usual pace in the water just minutes after the start. None of them reported that they had aspirated during the swim.

The bike leg during the Norseman Extreme Triathlon starts with approximately 40 km uphill, from sea level to 1245 m above sea level (Figure 1).

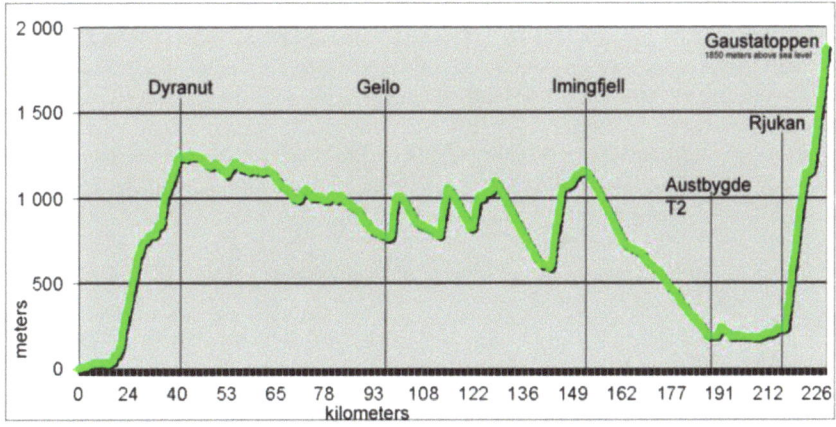

Figure 1. The elevation profile for the Norseman Extreme Triathlon.

All athletes reported an improvement in breathing during the first major uphill (1245 m elevation over 40 km) of the bike phase and reported increasing symptoms during the downhill. The female athlete contacted the medical crew due to shortness of breath and coughing pink sputum after about 122 km. During the clinical examination, she presented mild facial edema, jugular vein distention and lip cyanosis. Peripheral capillary oxygen saturation (SpO_2) was measured to 88%, and she was coughing up pink sputum. No signs of airway obstruction were found, and she denied any previous history of allergies. The athlete was taken out of the competition by one of the race doctors. She was transferred to the nearest local medical center for further treatment but recovered quickly after being treated with oxygen and hospitalization was not indicated. The male athletes managed to complete the 180 km long bike phase, but due to coughing and increased shortness of breath, they were both forced to withdraw from the race just a few meters into the run phase.

The PRO athlete was examined by one of the race doctors immediately after withdrawal. The medic reported end-expiratory crackles bilaterally and a productive cough with pink sputum. He had facial edema but no cyanosis. He was transferred to the nearest hospital, approximately 1 h away for further examination.

On arrival, his blood pressure was 105/62 mmHg, respiratory rate 20 breaths/min, heart rate 84 beats/min and oxygen saturation was 96% on room air. A laboratory examination showed a serum sodium level of 142 mEq/L, B-natriuretic peptide (BNP) level of 26 pmol/L (normal range < 10 pmol/L), troponin T 76 ng/L (normal range < 10 ng/L), C-reactive protein 23 mg/L (normal range < 5 mg/L), hemoglobin 12.1 g/dL and D-dimer 0.7 mg/L (normal range < 0.5 mg/L). An electrocardiogram (ECG) showed sinus rhythm with incomplete right bundle branch block (RBBB). He had normal findings on clinical examination.

Arterial blood gas results were; pH 7.48, pCO_2 4.84 kPa, pO_2 9.39 kPa, bicarbonate 26.2 mmol/L, base excess 3.4 mmol/L and lactate 2.7 mmol/L.

An echocardiogram was performed at arrival at the emergency department that showed a well-contracting, normal-sized left ventricle and mildly dilated right ventricle. The end-diastolic impression of the intraventricular septum led to suspected high pulmonary artery pressure.

At the hospital, he was initially diagnosed with suspected pulmonary embolism and transferred to a larger regional hospital for a thoracic computed tomography (CT) scan. The findings included bilateral ground glass opacity in the peripheral lungs but no pulmonary embolism. Due to the complete regression of symptoms, no treatment other than rehydration and oxygen was given during hospitalization. He was discharged from hospital the following day.

At a 1-month follow-up-examination, the athlete had fully recovered with complete regression of CT findings and echocardiogram changes. He was diagnosed with swimming-induced pulmonary edema.

The male AGE GROUP athlete called the emergency number directly and was not examined by a race doctor. After completing the bike phase (180 km), he experienced increased shortness of breath and coughing with pink sputum. When examined by the paramedics he presented with heavy coughing. SpO_2 was measured to 90%. He was transferred to the nearest hospital for further examinations, which was the same hospital as the PRO athlete was transferred to two years earlier. On arrival, his blood pressure was 123/70 mmHg, respiratory rate 16 breaths/min, heart rate 70 beats/min and oxygen saturation was 93% on room air. A laboratory examination showed a serum sodium level of 142 mEq/L, troponin T 101 ng/L (normal range < 10 ng/L), C-reactive protein 8 mg/L (normal range < 5 mg/L), hemoglobin 13 g/dL and D-dimer 0.4 mg/L (normal range < 0.5 mg/L). An ECG showed sinus rhythm with pathological R-progression in V1 to V6. Clinical examination reported end-expiratory crackles bilaterally but otherwise normal findings.

Arterial blood gas results were; pH 7.46, pCO_2 5.01 kPa, pO_2 8.20 kPa, bicarbonate 25.9 mmol/L, base excess 2.6 mmol/L and lactate 2.2 mmol/L.

No echocardiogram was performed. He was given diuretics and was discharged from the hospital with complete regression of symptoms the following day.

3. Discussion

All three athletes presented in this report experienced a debut of shortness of breath during the swim phase of an extreme triathlon competition with symptomatic progression throughout the following bike phase. Upon presentation for medical personnel, all athletes displayed decreased levels of oxygen saturation, of which two were measured pre-hospital. Pulmonary edema would negatively impact ventilation and thereby, oxygen saturation. In the presented cases, the use of on-site pulse oxiometry served to strengthen the suspicion of potential SIPE.

During hospital examination, the PRO athlete had several blood biomarkers outside of the normal range. In our experience, results of not yet published data suggest this is a common and potentially normal finding in asymptomatic participants of extreme triathlons. His RBBB was considered a normal variant as often seen in young, well-trained athletes. Following an echocardiogram ruling out cardiac failure, and CT scan revealing no signs of emboli but the presence of ground glass opacity, the clinical picture best fits that of SIPE.

The ECG of the AGE GROUP athlete displayed pathological R-progression in V1 to V6, which was also considered a normal variant in well-trained endurance athletes. Due to his elevated troponin levels, ischemic cardiac disease cannot be ruled out entirely as a potential etiology. However, this athlete had no known risk factors for ischemic heart disease, and this differential diagnosis would not account for symptomatic improvement during uphill cycling. As such, the overall clinical presentation is arguably more suggestive of SIPE.

To the best of our knowledge, the female athlete did not undergo diagnostic blood tests or radiographic examinations. Therefore, the possibility of other differential diagnoses, such as angio-oedema or asthma attack, cannot be ruled out entirely. Nevertheless, we would argue that the absence of obstructive symptoms, no prior history of allergies, and quick symptom regression following oxygen treatment suggests SIPE is the more likely diagnosis.

Despite the early presentation of symptoms, the athletes were able to bike several hours before getting attention by the medical crew. They further reported symptom relief during uphill and aggravation of symptoms during downhill biking. To our knowledge, this undulating symptom behavior has yet to be described in the literature and may provide insight into contributing mechanisms to SIPE.

Although SIPE is commonly referred to as a rare condition, there are frequent reports of incidences during triathlon races. We have identified at least 16 reported cases published in the period 2010 to 2019 [6–10]. Symptoms appear to debut with sudden onset of shortness of breath during swimming. This may be severe enough to prompt immediate withdrawal from the race, or may gradually worsen, including hemoptysis, throughout the bike and run phase of a race. When examining 31 asymptomatic Ironmen participants with chest sonography pre- and post-race, Pingitore and colleagues observed subclinical signs of increased pulmonary water content in 23 athletes (74%) [11]. They also found a significant correlation between increased water content and cardiac-related variables and NH_2-terminal pro-brain natriuretic peptide (NT-proBNP). A study on autopsies following triathlon deaths found a greater proportion of left ventricular hypertrophy (LVH) among deceased triathletes compared to what was expected in the triathlon population [12]. With LVH being a proposed risk factor for SIPE, the authors hypothesize that SIPE may well be a significant contributor to swimming-related deaths in triathlon.

Further contributors to the development of SIPE have been described to include whole-body immersion including face immersion, cold water, use of wet suit and/or swim cap, sudden physical exertion, and any situation that could raise central blood pressure on the race morning, such as excessive hydration or anxiety. Previous studies have hypothesized that SIPE-prone individuals develop hypertension and elevated left ventricular (LV) end-diastolic pressure when exposed to cold, increased oxygen intake and exercise, although more recent studies show that cold exposure is not a prerequisite for developing SIPE [3,13]. Furthermore, elevated levels of cardiac troponin T and abnormal left ventricular function following Ironman races have been suggested as a possible link to pulmonary edema [14].

A unique factor related to immersion in both swimming and diving is the well-documented fluid shift that occurs due to pressure effects on venous blood pooling. Studies have demonstrated a 600 to 700 mL shift of blood from the venous system into the central circulation when immersed to the neck, which in turn increases lung vascular volume and likely contributes to the development of pulmonary edema [15]. This fluid shift may lead to right and LV stroke volume mismatch potentially similar to that seen in other forms of acute heart failure [16]. The Frank-Starling mechanism that normally will counteract the stroke volume imbalance is likely to have reached its physiological limit during a triathlon. This results in the accumulation of fluid in the lungs. Systemic venous constriction and redistribution of blood from the peripheral circulation will maintain the right ventricular filling pressures, and the ongoing stroke volume difference will result in pulmonary edema.

Triathletes typically aim to minimize hydrodynamic drag and to this end wear tightly fitted wetsuits. The potential role of wetsuit use in the development of SIPE is not clearly understood. However, it has been suggested that tight-fitting wetsuits may increase cardiac preload, and thereby, contribute to the development of SIPE [1]. The authors are aware of several SIPE cases where athletes have avoided reoccurrence when replacing tight wetsuits with more loosely fitted suits. Although more research is needed, it may be that the fitting and use of wetsuits is a modifiable risk factor for SIPE.

Once the alveolar–capillary membrane has been disrupted, any elevation in capillary pressure would be expected to facilitate a fluid shift to the alveoli. During exercise, pulmonary vascular pressure remains high [17]. If pulmonary edema is already established, cycling and running may, therefore, maintain or worsen an existing pulmonary edema. Interestingly, all three athletes presented in this report reported symptom relief during uphill cycling and aggravation during downhills. The Norseman Xtreme Triathlon cycling course is characterized by hills of long durations, altitudes of up to 1245 m above sea level and shifting weather conditions. Rain and air temperatures as low as 6 to 10 °C are not uncommon in the more exposed parts of the course. Preliminary results from yet unpublished temperature recordings of the Norseman Xtreme Triathlon participants suggests considerable terrain-associated changes in core temperature during the cycling leg. One could hypothesize that the combination of cold air, high speeds and resulting core temperature drop during downhills result in peripheral vasoconstriction that facilitates increased pulmonary artery pressure. whereas the higher heart rates and increased thermogenic heat produced during uphills might lead to a decrease in peripheral vascular resistance. Along with lower speeds and a more upright riding position, this may reverse a fluid shift to the pulmonary circulation and lung tissue and potentially explain the reported symptom improvement during uphill cycling.

Triathletes are often adept at experiencing discomfort and continuing racing despite fatigue and dyspnea, and a pulmonary edema in development may, therefore, go unrecognized. However, racing in the absence of SIPE usually involves higher exertion in uphills than downhills. The presence of symptom improvement going uphill and worsening dyspnea and cough during downhill cycling may help athletes distinguish SIPE in development from the respiratory stress of physiological exertion.

The presented results underscore that race medics should be familiar with the potential for slow progression and late presentation of SIPE. Biking and running may sustain and worsen an ongoing SIPE, and symptoms, such as facial swelling and coughing, may present very late in the race, especially if the race is hilly. Symptoms might be relieved when going uphill and worsen during downhill sections of the bike ride, and cold weather may aggravate the condition. A focus on symptoms and devices to measure SpO_2 in the field may facilitate early detection of symptoms of this potentially fatal complication. Symptoms of SIPE usually resolve after normalization of the physiologic environment and by supportive treatment, such as oxygen therapy and occasionally β2-agonists [18]. Furthermore, the athlete should be aware of the increased possibility of recurrent episodes [19].

Summary of take-home messages:

- Athletes and race crews should recognize the common symptoms of SIPE;

- These include shortness of breath, cough and blood-stained sputum;
- Triathletes with SIPE may present for medical examination very late in the race;
- Symptoms may improve during uphill and worsen during downhill cycling;
- Pulse oximeters may assist race medics in identifying potential cases of SIPE;
- SIPE is usually self-limiting upon cessation of exertion, but hospitalization, oxygen therapy or beta2/diuretic therapy may be warranted.

Author Contributions: Investigation J.M.; M.M.; J.M.H.; L.O.; M.B.-S., and J.H. Writing—original draft preparation M.M.; J.M.; Writing—reviewing and editing J.M.; M.B.-S.; J.H. Supervision J.H.

Funding: This research received no external funding.

Acknowledgments: The authors would like to thank the Norseman Xtreme Triathlon organization, crew, and race director. The results of this study are presented clearly, honestly, and without fabrication, falsification, or inappropriate data manipulation.

Conflicts of Interest: The authors declare no conflict of interest.

References

1. Miller, C.C., III; Calder-Becker, K.; Modave, F. Swimming-induced pulmonary edema in triathletes. *Am. J. Emerg. Med.* **2010**, *28*, 941–946. [CrossRef] [PubMed]
2. Cochard, G.; Arvieux, J.; Lacour, J.M.; Madouas, G.; Mongredien, H.; Arvieux, C.C. Pulmonary edema in scuba divers: Recurrence and fatal outcome. *Undersea Hyperb. Med.* **2005**, *32*, 39–44. [PubMed]
3. Slade, J.B., Jr.; Hattori, T.; Ray, C.S.; Bove, A.A.; Cianci, P. Pulmonary edema associated with scuba diving: Case reports and review. *Chest* **2001**, *120*, 1686–1694. [CrossRef] [PubMed]
4. Adir, Y.; Shupak, A.; Gil, A.; Peled, N.; Keynan, Y.; Domachevsky, L.; Weiler-Eavell, D. Swimming-induced pulmonary edema: Clinical presentation and serial lung function. *Chest* **2004**, *126*, 394–399. [CrossRef] [PubMed]
5. Koehle, M.S.; Lepawsky, M.; McKenzie, D.C. Pulmonary oedema of immersion. *Sports Med.* **2005**, *35*, 183–190. [CrossRef] [PubMed]
6. Smith, R.; Brooke, D.; Kipps, C.; Skaria, B.; Subramaniam, V. A case of recurrent swimming-induced pulmonary edema in a triathlete: The need for awareness. *Scand. J. Med. Sci. Sports* **2017**, *27*, 1130–1135. [CrossRef] [PubMed]
7. Yamanashi, H.; Koyamatsu, J.; Nobuyoshi, M.; Murase, K.; Maeda, T. Exercise-Induced Pulmonary Edema in a Triathlon. *Case Rep. Med.* **2015**. [CrossRef] [PubMed]
8. Casey, H.; Dastidar, A.G.; MacIver, D. Swimming-induced pulmonary oedema in two triathletes: A novel pathophysiological explanation. *J. R. Soc. Med.* **2014**, *107*, 450–452. [CrossRef] [PubMed]
9. Ma, J.L.; Dutch, M.J. Extreme sports: Extreme physiology. Exercise-induced pulmonary oedema. *Emerg. Med. Australas.* **2013**, *25*, 368–371. [CrossRef] [PubMed]
10. Beale, A.; Gong, F.F.; La Gerche, A. Exercise-induced pulmonary edema in endurance triathletes. *Int. J. Cardiol.* **2016**, *203*, 980–981. [CrossRef] [PubMed]
11. Pingitore, A.; Garbella, E.; Piaggi, P.; Menicucci, D.; Frassi, F.; Lionetti, V.; Piarulli, A.; Catapano, G.; Lubrano, V.; Passera, M.; et al. Early subclinical increase in pulmonary water content in athletes performing sustained heavy exercise at sea level: Ultrasound lung comet-tail evidence. *Am. J. Physiol. Heart Circ. Physiol.* **2011**, *301*, H2161–H2167. [CrossRef] [PubMed]
12. Moon, R.E.; Martina, S.D.; Peacher, D.F.; Kraus, W.E. Deaths in triathletes: Immersion pulmonary oedema as a possible cause. *BMJ Open Exerc. Med.* **2016**, *2*, e000146. [CrossRef] [PubMed]
13. Hampson, N.B.; Dunford, R.G. Pulmonary edema of scuba divers. *Undersea Hyperb. Med.* **1997**, *24*, 29–33. [PubMed]
14. Vleck, V.E.; Millet, G.P.; Alves, F.B. The impact of triathlon training and racing on athletes' general health. *Sports Med.* **2014**, *44*, 1659–1692. [CrossRef] [PubMed]
15. Hong, S.K.; Cerretelli, P.; Cruz, J.C.; Rahn, H. Mechanics of respiration during submersion in water. *J. Appl. Physiol.* **1969**, *27*, 535–538. [CrossRef] [PubMed]

16. MacIver, D.H.; Townsend, M. A novel mechanism of heart failure with normal ejection fraction. *Heart* **2008**, 446–449. [CrossRef] [PubMed]
17. Naeije, R.; Chesler, N. Pulmonary circulation at exercise. *Compr. Physiol.* **2012**, *2*, 711–741. [PubMed]
18. Gründig, H.; Nikolaidis, P.T.; Moon, R.E.; Knechtle, B. Diagnosis of Swimming Induced Pulmonary Edema—A Review. *Front Physiol.* **2017**, *8*, 652. [CrossRef] [PubMed]
19. Hull, J.H.; Wilson, M.G. The breathless swimmer: Could this be swimming-induced pulmonary edema? *Sports Med.–Open* **2018**, *4*, 51. [CrossRef] [PubMed]

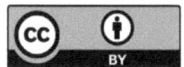

© 2019 by the authors. Licensee MDPI, Basel, Switzerland. This article is an open access article distributed under the terms and conditions of the Creative Commons Attribution (CC BY) license (http://creativecommons.org/licenses/by/4.0/).

MDPI AG
Grosspeteranlage 5
4052 Basel
Switzerland
Tel.: +41 61 683 77 34

Sports Editorial Office
E-mail: sports@mdpi.com
www.mdpi.com/journal/sports

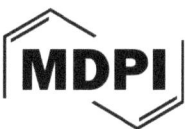

Disclaimer/Publisher's Note: The title and front matter of this reprint are at the discretion of the Guest Editors. The publisher is not responsible for their content or any associated concerns. The statements, opinions and data contained in all individual articles are solely those of the individual Editors and contributors and not of MDPI. MDPI disclaims responsibility for any injury to people or property resulting from any ideas, methods, instructions or products referred to in the content.

www.ingramcontent.com/pod-product-compliance
Lightning Source LLC
LaVergne TN
LVHW072323090526
838202LV00019B/2338